Neurosurgical Treatment of Movement Disorders

AANS Publications Committee
Isabelle M. Germano, MD, Editor

Neurosurgical Topics

The American Association of Neurological Surgeons

Library of Congress Catalog
ISBN: 1-879284-58-8

Neurosurgical Topics ISBN: 0-9624246-6-8

Printed in U.S.A.

The American Association of Neurological Surgeons
22 South Washington Street
Park Ridge, Illinois 60068

This publication is published under the auspices of the Publications Committee of the American Association of Neurological Surgeons (AANS). However, this should not be construed as indicating endorsement or approval of the views presented by the AANS, or by its committees, commissions, affiliates, or staff.

Warren R. Selman, MD, Chairman
AANS Publications Committee

Joanne B. Needham, AANS Staff Editor

AANS1.75M898

Neurosurgical Topics SERIES

FORTHCOMING BOOKS

1998

Calvarial and Dural Reconstruction
Edited by Setti S. Rengachary, MD, and Edward C. Benzel, MD

Intracranial Endoscopic Neurosurgery
Edited by David F. Jimenez, MD

Geriatric Neurosurgery
Edited by Warren R. Selman, MD, and Edward C. Benzel, MD

1999

Craniocerebral Missile Wounds, Volumes 1 and 2
Edited by Bizhan Aarabi, MD, and Howard H. Kaufman, MD

Neural Tube Defects, Volumes 1 and 2
Edited by J. Gordon McComb, MD, and Joan L. Venes, MD

Dedication

To my parents, Francesco and Lucetttta,

in acknowledgment of their understanding and support.

Contents

LIST OF CONTRIBUTORS

Ron L. Alterman, MD
Assistant Professor of Neurosurgery
New York University Center for the Study and Treatment of Movement Disorders
New York, New York

Roy A. E. Bakay, MD
Professor of Neurosurgery
Emory University
Atlanta, Georgia

Alim Louis Benabid, MD, PhD
Department of Clinical and Biological Neurosciences
Joseph Fourier University of Grenoble
Hôpital A. Michallon
Grenoble, France

Reina Benabou, MD, PhD
Assistant Neurologist
Division of Functional Neurosurgery
Hospital das Clinicas
University of Sao Paulo Medical School
Sao Paulo, Brazil

Claude M. Bertrand, CC, MD, FRCS(C)
Emeritus Professor, Surgery
Université de Montreal
Emeritus Chief, Division of Neurosurgery
Notre-Dame Hospital
Montreal, Quebec, Canada

Cesar V. Borlongan, PhD
Assistant Professor
Division of Neurosurgery
University of South Florida
Tampa, Florida

Mitchell F. Brin, MD
Associate Professor of Neurology
Director, Movement Disorders
The Mount Sinai Medical Center
New York, New York

Giovanni Broggi, MD
Professor and Chairman
Department of Neurosurgery
Istituto Nazionale Neurologico "C. Besta"
Milan, Italy

Kim J. Burchiel, MD, FACS
John Raaf Professor and Chairman
Department of Neurological Surgery
Oregon Health Sciences University
Portland, Oregon

Dominique Caparros-Lefebvre, MD, PhD
Department of Neurology
CHU Pointe à Pitre
French West Indies

Mahlon R. DeLong, MD
Chairman and Professor
Department of Neurology
Emory University School of Medicine
Atlanta, Georgia

David Eidelberg, MD
Director, Movement Disorders Center and Functional Brain Imaging Laboratory
Professor of Neurology
Department of Neurology
North Shore University Hospital
Manhasset, New York

Thomas B. Freeman, MD
Associate Professor
Director, Neural Reconstruction Program
Division of Neurosurgery
Department of Pharmacology and Experimental Therapeutics
University of South Florida
Tampa, Florida

Isabelle M. Germano, MD
Associate Professor of Neurosurgery and Neurology
The Mount Sinai School of Medicine
Director of Stereotaxy and Functional Neurosurgery
The Mount Sinai Medical Center
New York, New York

Robert A. Hauser, MD
Associate Professor
Director, The Movement Disorders Center
Department of Neurology
University of South Florida
Tampa, Florida

M. Peter Heilbrun, MD
Professor and Chairman
Department of Neurosurgery
University of Utah School of Medicine
Salt Lake City, Utah

Douglas A. Holt, MD
Assistant Professor
Division of Infectious Diseases
University of South Florida
Tampa, Florida

William D. Hutchison, PhD
Assistant Professor
Division of Neurosurgery
University of Toronto
The Toronto Hospital, Western Division
Toronto, Ontario, Canada

Joseph Jankovic, MD
Professor of Neurology
Director, Parkinson's Disease Center and Movement Disorders Clinic
Baylor College of Medicine
Houston, Texas

Peter J. Jannetta, MD
Walter E. Dandy Professor and Chairman
Department of Neurosurgery
University of Pittsburgh School of Medicine
Presbyterian University Hospital
Pittsburgh, Pennsylvania

Ken Kazumata, MD
Research Fellow
Functional Brain Imaging Laboratory
North Shore University Hospital
Manhasset, New York

Patrick Kelly, MD
Professor and Chairman
New York University Center for the Study and Treatment of Movement Disorders
New York, New York

Jeffrey H. Kordower, PhD
Professor
Department of Neurological Sciences
Rush-Presbyterian-St. Lukes Medical Center
Chicago, Illinois

Anthony E. Lang, MD
Professor of Neurology
Division of Neurology
Toronto Western Hospital
Toronto, Ontario, Canada

Andres Lozano, MD, PhD, FRCS(C)
Associate Professor
Division of Neurosurgery
University of Toronto
The Toronto Hospital, Western Division
Toronto, Ontario, Canada

Mark R. McLaughlin, MD
Department of Neurosurgery
University of Pittsburgh School of Medicine
Presbyterian University Hospital
Pittsburgh, Pennsylvania

Lauren V. Moran, BA
Research Assistant
Functional Brain Imaging Laboratory
North Shore University Hospital
Manhasset, New York

C. Warren Olanow, MD, FRCP(C)
Professor and Chairman
Department of Neurology
The Mount Sinai Medical Center
New York, New York

Richard K. Osenbach, MD
Assistant Professor
Department of Neurosurgery
Medical University of South Carolina
Charleston, South Carolina

Daniel P. Perl, MD
Director, Neuropathology Division
The Mount Sinai Medical Center
New York, New York

Pierre Pollak, MD
Department of Clinical and Biological Neurosciences
Joseph Fourier University of Grenoble
Hôpital A. Michallon
Grenoble, France

Paul R. Sanberg, PhD
Professor
Director, The Neuroscience Program
Division of Neurosurgery
Department of Pharmacology and Experimental Therapeutics
University of South Florida
Tampa, Florida

Philip A. Starr, MD, PhD
Assistant Professor of Neurosurgery
University of California
San Francisco, California

Ronald R. Tasker, MD, FRCS(C)
Professor
Department of Surgery
University of Toronto
Division of Neurosurgery
The Toronto Hospital, Western Division
Toronto, Ontario, Canada

Jerrold L. Vitek, MD, PhD
Associate Professor of Neurology
Emory University
Atlanta, Georgia

Donald J. Weisz, PhD
Associate Professor
Departments of Neurosurgery, Neurology, and Otolaryngology
The Mount Sinai School of Medicine
New York, New York

Thomas Wichmann, MD
Assistant Professor
Department of Neurology
Emory University School of Medicine
Atlanta, Georgia

Bo-Yi Yang, PhD
Research Assistant Professor
Departments of Neurosurgery, Neurology, and Otolaryngology
The Mount Sinai School of Medicine
New York, New York

AANS Publications Committee

Home Study Examination Information

Neurosurgical Treatment of Movement Disorders
Isabelle M. Germano, MD, Editor
Released August 1, 1998
CME Credits Expiration: August 1, 2001

The American Association of Neurological Surgeons (AANS) is accredited by the Accreditation Council for Continuing Medical Education (ACCME) to sponsor Continuing Medical Education (CME) for physicians. *Neurosurgical Topics* Series Home Study Examinations were planned and produced in accordance with the ACCME Essentials.

The AANS designates this CME activity for a maximum of 15 hours in category 1 credit toward the AMA Physician's Recognition Award. Each physician should claim only the number of hours that he or she actually spent studying the CME enduring material.

Participants have 3 years from the date of publication shown on this enduring material to complete the Home Study Examination Questions, submit the evaluation form, and request category 1 credit. For a copy of the Home Study Examination Questions, please refer to the enclosed card or contact the AANS at 847-692-9500.

The Home Study Examination is available in printed or electronic format. The test is to be self-scored. A CME certificate will be mailed upon submission of the evaluation form along with a $30 processing fee.

After reading this book, a physician should be able to:

- describe the classification, pathophysiology, pathology, and clinical presentation of movement disorders
- review the current medical treatment of movement disorders
- define the current indications for surgical intervention of movement disorders
- appraise the technical aspects of surgical procedures used in the treatment of movement disorders
- identify the limitations and advantages of these techniques
- develop a multidisciplinary approach to the treatment of movement disorders

Preface

Parkinson's disease is the second most frequent cause of neurological disability in the United States. Since the original description as *paralysis agitans* at the turn of the 20th century, knowledge of its pathogenesis has advanced dramatically. Now, Parkinson's and other neurological disorders characterized by excessive or insufficient movements are well recognized and known as movement disorders. As our knowledge of these diseases continues to expand, medical treatments to ameliorate the symptoms are better understood, widely employed, and highly successful. However, the beneficial therapeutic effects are often of limited duration. Modern microsurgical computer-guided techniques, combined with advances in electrophysiology and anesthesia, have led to a resurgence of interest in neurosurgical treatment for movement disorders.

Intended as a comprehensive yet practical guide for neurosurgeons and neurologists, this volume reviews the mechanisms, pathophysiology, and medical management of movement disorders and describes the indications, techniques, and outcomes of neurosurgical procedures used to treat these common and disabling conditions. The technical details on surgical procedures for movement disorders provided in this book make it unique and valuable for a team approach to neurosurgical treatment of movement disorders.

Isabelle M. Germano, MD
New York, New York
1998

PART A

Overview

CHAPTER 1

Classification of Movement Disorders

Joseph Jankovic, MD, and Anthony E. Lang, MD

This introductory chapter is intended to provide an overview of phenomenological and etiological classifications of movement disorders. Movement disorders are a group of neurological symptoms, signs, or diseases manifested by either slowness and poverty of movement, so-called "hypokinesias," or excessive, abnormal involuntary movements, so-called "hyperkinesias." Parkinson's disease is the best example of a hypokinetic movement disorder. Hyperkinetic movement disorders include tremor, dystonia, chorea, tics, myoclonus, stereotypies, and a variety of miscellaneous movement disorders. Most, but not all, movement disorders are thought to be caused by a dysfunction in the basal ganglia. The important role of the basal ganglia in motor control, muscle tone, posture, and some cognitive processes is becoming increasingly recognized. Extraordinary progress has been achieved in the understanding of neurochemical and physiological abnormalities underlying various basal ganglia diseases. These advances have contributed to the development of new pharmacological and surgical approaches.

The analysis of patients with movement disorders requires observations that are not usually included in the standard neurological examination. Prior to deciding where in the nervous system the disease process is located and then what that process is, the clinician must first observe and examine the patient to define the phenomenology and to classify the movement disorder. Abnormal movements must be considered a clinical sign for which there are many causes. Most types of movement disorders can be seen in pure form with no known or established cause. These primary ("essential" or "idiopathic") disorders must be distinguished from the secondary ("symptomatic") disorders.

The International Classification of Diseases, Tenth Revision: Neurological Adaptation (ICD-10 NA) has been recently completed as a result of collaboration between the World Health Organization and the Movement Disorder Society (Table 1). The primary purpose of this classification is to facilitate an organized approach to differential diagnosis, epidemiological studies, international communication, education, and clinical research. Although the need to maintain strict compatibility between ICD-10 NA and

TABLE 1

The International Classification of Diseases, Tenth Revision: Neurological Adaptation (ICD-10 NA)*

Extrapyramidal and Movement Disorders

Parkinson's disease

Includes idiopathic parkinsonism, paralysis agitans; excludes Guamanian-type parkinsonism-dementia complex, diffuse Lewy body disease

- Classical type
- Akinetic type
- Tremor type
- Postural instability/gait difficulty type
- Hemiparkinsonism
  - Sporadic
  - Familial

Secondary parkinsonism

Excludes parkinsonism in diseases classified elsewhere

Malignant neuroleptic syndrome

Drug-induced secondary parkinsonism (e.g., dopamine receptor blockers, antiemetic drugs, dopamine depleters, lithium, flunarizine, cinnarizine, diltiazem)
- Active drug reaction
- Tardive drug reaction

Secondary parkinsonism due to other external agents (e.g., manganese poisoning, carbon monoxide, cyanide, methanol, carbon disulfide, 1-methyl-4-phenyl-1,2,3,6-tetrahydropyridine [MPTP])

Postencephalitic parkinsonism
- Postencephalitic parkinsonism, encephalitis lethargica
- Other postinfectious parkinsonism
  - Excludes parkinsonism in infectious diseases classified elsewhere, slow virus or prior infection of central nervous system

Other secondary parkinsonism (e.g., head injury, sequelae of intracranial injury)
- Excludes psychogenic parkinsonism

Secondary parkinsonism, unspecified

Parkinsonism in diseases classified elsewhere

Parkinsonism in sporadic degenerative diseases classified elsewhere (parkinsonism plus syndromes); e.g., parkinsonism in:
- Alzheimer's disease
- corticobasal ganglionic degeneration
- dentato-rubral-pallido-luysian atrophy
- diffuse Lewy body disease
- Guamanian-type parkinsonism-dementia complex
- Hallervorden-Spatz disease
- olivopontocerebellar degeneration
- pallido-pyramidal-dentato-luysian degeneration
- progressive supranuclear ophthalmoparesis (Steele-Richardson-Olszewski)
- Shy-Drager syndrome
- striatonigral degeneration
- multisystem degeneration with dysautonomia (multiple system atrophy)

Parkinsonism in familial degenerative and metabolic diseases classified elsewhere; e.g., parkinsonism in:
- Huntington's disease
- dopa-responsive dystonia
- subacute necrotizing encephalopathy (Leigh's disease)
- Wilson's disease (hepatocerebral degeneration)

Parkinsonism in infectious diseases classified elsewhere; e.g., parkinsonism in:
- acquired immunodeficiency syndrome (AIDS)
- Creutzfeldt-Jakob disease
- Gerstmann-Straussier-Scheinker disease
- subacute sclerosing panencephalitis
- syphilis

Parkinsonism in other diseases classified elsewhere; e.g.,
- brain tumor
- cerebrovascular disease
- noncommunicating (obstructive) hydrocephalus
- normal pressure hydrocephalus
- paraneoplastic disease
- psychogenic disease
- syringomesencephalia

Other degenerative diseases of the basal ganglia

Hallervorden-Spatz disease
- Pigmentary pallidal degeneration
- Other specified pallidal degeneration

TABLE 1 (cont'd)

THE INTERNATIONAL CLASSIFICATION OF DISEASES, TENTH REVISION: NEUROLOGICAL ADAPTATION (ICD-10 NA)*

Progressive supranuclear ophthalmoplegia (ophthalmoparesis)
  Idiopathic (Steele-Richardson-Olszewski)
  Vascular (multi-infarct)

Striatonigral degeneration

Other specified degenerative diseases of basal ganglia
    Excludes multisystem degeneration with dysautonomia (multiple system atrophy), olivopontocerebellar degeneration, Wilson's disease (hepatolenticular degeneration)
  Hemiparkinson-hemiatrophy syndrome
  Corticobasal ganglionic degeneration (cortico-dentato-nigral degeneration with neuronal achromasia)
  Pallido-pyramidal-dentato-luysian degeneration
  Dentato-rubral-pallido-luysian atrophy
  Guamanian-type parkinsonism, parkinsonism-dementia-amyotrophic lateral sclerosis complex of Guam
    Excludes Western Pacific-type motor neuron disease
  Parkinsonism associated with calcification of the basal ganglia
    Idiopathic sporadic (Fahr's disease)
    With hypoparathyroidism
    With pseudohypoparathyroidism
    Familial basal ganglia calcifications

Degenerative disease of the basal ganglia, unspecified

Dystonia

  Excludes athetoid cerebral palsy, dystonia (dyskinesia) in diseases classified elsewhere

Drug-induced dystonia (e.g., manganese, carbon disulfide, cyanide)
  Acute drug-induced dystonia
  Acute drug-induced dyskinesia
  Tardive dystonia
  Tardive dyskinesia
  Other specified drug-induced dystonia (e.g., drug-induced oculogyric crises)

Idiopathic familial dystonia
  Autosomal dominant familial dystonia (with DYT I gene on 9q34)
  Nonclassic dystonia
  Atypical dystonia
  Dopa-responsive dystonia, idiopathic diurnal dystonia, Segawa variant, hereditary progressive dystonia, guanosine triphosphate cyclohydrolase I 14q22.1-q22.2 gene defect
  Myoclonic dystonia
  Rapid-onset dystonia
  X-linked recessive dystonia-parkinsonism complex (Lubag)
  Hereditary juvenile parkinsonism-dystonia complex
  Familial dystonia with other specified inheritance
    Generalized dystonia, familial
    Hemidystonia, familial
    Axial dystonia, familial
    Cranial dystonia, familial
      Ocular dystonia, familial
      Orofacial dystonia, familial
    Laryngeal dystonia, familial
    Cervical dystonia, familial
    Limb dystonia, familial
      Arm/hand dystonia, familial (writer's/musician's/other occupational cramps)
      Leg/foot dystonia, familial
    Multiple or combined types of idiopathic familial dystonia

Idiopathic nonfamilial dystonia
  Generalized dystonia, nonfamilial
  Hemidystonia, nonfamilial
  Axial dystonia, nonfamilial
  Other cranial dystonia, nonfamilial
      Excludes blepharospasm, idiopathic orofacial dystonia
    Ocular dystonia, nonfamilial (idiopathic oculogyric crises)
      Excludes drug-induced dystonia
  Laryngeal dystonia, nonfamilial (isolated spasmodic dysphonia)
  Limb dystonia, nonfamilial
    Arm/hand dystonia, nonfamilial (writer's/musician/other occupational cramps)
      Excludes writer's and occupational cramps of psychogenic origin
    Leg/foot dystonia, nonfamilial
  Multiple or combined types of idiopathic nonfamilial dystonia
  Other types of idiopathic nonfamilial dystonia

TABLE 1 (cont'd)

The International Classification of Diseases, Tenth Revision: Neurological Adaptation (ICD-10 NA)*

Spasmodic torticollis (idiopathic cervical dystonia)
- Excludes torticollis NOS, familial cervical dystonia
- Spasmodic torticollis
- Spasmodic retrocollis
- Spasmodic anterocollis
- Spasmodic laterocollis
- Other specified cervical dystonia

Idiopathic orofacial dystonia
- Excludes familial orofacial dystonia
- Orofacial dyskinesia
- Edentulous orofacial dyskinesia
- Isolated oromandibular dystonia

Blepharospasm (idiopathic cranial dystonia, Meige's syndrome)

Other dystonia
- Excludes atlantoaxial subluxation, congenital muscular contractions, dystonia in diseases classified elsewhere, seizure-induced twisting postures
- Paroxysmal dystonias
  - Sporadic kinesigenic dystonia
  - Familial kinesigenic dystonia
  - Sporadic nonkinesigenic dystonia
  - Familial nonkinesigenic dystonia
  - Tonic spasm of multiple sclerosis
  - Paroxysmal nocturnal dystonia
- Sandifer syndrome (pseudodystonia with anteroflexion associated with gastrointestinal reflux in young chidren)
- Secondary dystonia NOS
- Pseudodystonia NOS

Dystonia, unspecified

Other extrapyramidal and movement disorders

Essential tremor
- Excludes tremor NOS, isolated rest tremor
- Isolated head tremor
- Isolated facial tremor
- Isolated vocal tremor
- Isolated hand tremor
- Shuddering attacks of childhood
- Multiple-site tremor
  - Sporadic
  - Familial

Drug-induced tremor

Other specified forms of tremor
- Excludes tremor in diseases classified elsewhere
- Kinetic (intention) tremor
- Physiological tremor
- Dystonic tremor
- Orthostatic tremor
- Task-specific (e.g., handwriting) tremor
- Midbrain type tremor
- Isolated rest tremor

Myoclonus
- Excludes ataxia with myoclonus (Ramsay Hunt syndrome), epilepsia partialis continua, facial myokymia, hemifacial spasm, myoclonic epilepsy, myoclonus in diseases classified elsewhere
- Cortical type diffuse myoclonus
- Focal or multifocal cortical type myoclonus
- Essential myoclonus (Friedreich's paramyoclonus multiplex)
- Oculopalatal myoclonus
- Segmental spinal myoclonus
- Propriospinal myoclonus
- Peripheral myoclonus
- Sleep (hypnic) myoclonus
- Postanoxic action myoclonus (Lance-Adams)
- Other specified myoclonic disorders

Drug-induced chorea (e.g., dopamine receptor blockers, antiemetic drugs, dopaminergic drugs, psychostimulants, toxins)

Other chorea, chorea NOS
- Excludes chorea in diseases classified elsewhere, chorea NOS with heart involvement, Huntington's disease (Huntington's chorea), Huntington's disease–juvenile onset (<20 years), Huntington's disease–late onset (>50 years), rheumatic chorea, Sydenham's chorea
- Chorea gravidarum
- Chorea associated with hormone therapy
- Hemichorea
- Neuroacanthocytosis (choreoacanthocytosis)
- Benign hereditary chorea
- Kinesigenic choreoathetosis

Drug-induced tics and other tics of organic origin
- Excludes Gilles de la Tourette's syn-

TABLE 1 (cont'd)

THE INTERNATIONAL CLASSIFICATION OF DISEASES, TENTH REVISION: NEUROLOGICAL ADAPTATION (ICD-10 NA)*

drome, tics NOS, tics in diseases classified elsewhere

Drug-induced tics

Tics of organic origin not related to drug, secondary tic NOS

Other specified extrapyramidal and movement disorders

Paroxysmal nocturnal limb movement disorder

Painful legs (or arms) moving toes (or fingers) syndrome

Sporadic restless legs syndrome (Ekbom)

Familial restless legs syndrome with or without periodic movements

Stiff-person syndrome (stiff-man syndrome)

Ballismus/hemiballismus

Opsoclonus-myoclonus syndrome (dancing eyes, dancing feet syndrome)

Stereotypies

Excludes edentulous orofacial dyskinesia, epileptic automatisms, Gilles de la Tourette's syndrome, orofacial dyskinesia, psychogenic stereotypies, restless legs syndrome, stereotyped movement disorder, stereotypies in:

- autism
- diseases classified elsewhere
- mental retardation
- Rett's syndrome
- schizophrenia
- tardive dyskinesia

Akathisia not related to drugs

Excludes drug-induced akathisia

Extrapyramidal and movement disorder, unspecified

Extrapyramidal and movement disorders in diseases classified elsewhere

Dystonia, hemidystonia, and dyskinesia in diseases classified elsewhere; e.g., dystonia in:

- ataxia telangiectasia
- corticobasal ganglionic degeneration
- Hallervorden-Spatz disease
- hereditary spastic paraplegia
- Huntington's disease
- Joseph's disease
- juvenile neuronal ceroid lipofuscinosis
- Lesch-Nyhan syndrome
- multiple sclerosis
- neuroacanthocytosis
- Nieman-Pick disease type C
- pallidal degeneration
- Parkinson's disease
- progressive supranuclear ophthalmoparesis (Steele-Richardson-Olszewski)
- reflex sympathetic dystrophy
- Rett's syndrome
- multisystem degeneration with dysautonomia (multiple system atrophy)
- subacute necrotizing encephalopathy (Leigh's disease)
- Wilson's disease (hepatolenticular degeneration)

Chorea and hemichorea in diseases classified elsewhere; e.g., chorea in:

- hyperthyroidism
- neuroacanthocytosis
- systemic lupus erythematosus

Excludes chorea gravidarum, chorea NOS with heart involvement, Huntington's disease, rheumatic chorea, Sydenham's chorea

Tremor in diseases classified elsewhere; e.g., tremor in:

- brain tumor
- cerebrovascular disease
- head injury

Myoclonus in diseases classified elsewhere; e.g., myoclonus in:

- Alzheimer's disease
- brain tumor
- Creutzfeldt-Jakob disease
- cerebrovascular disease
- head injury
- metabolic encephalopathy
- olivopontocerebellar atrophy
- progressive myoclonic ataxia (Ramsay Hunt syndrome)

Tics in diseases classified elsewhere

Stereotypies in diseases classified elsewhere; e.g., stereotypies in:

- autism
- mental retardation
- Rett's syndrome
- schizophrenia

*Modified from Jankovic.[3] NOS = not otherwise specified.

TABLE 2

PARKINSONISM PLUS SYNDROMES: DIFFERENTIAL DIAGNOSIS*

	PD	PSP	SDS	SND	OPCA	CBGD	DLBD	PDACG
Bradykinesia	+	+	+	+	±	+	±	+
Rigidity	+	+	+	+	+	+	±	+
Gait disturbance	+	+	+	+	+	+	±	+
Tremor	+	–	–	–	±	±	–	+
Ataxia	–	–	±	–	+	–	–	+
Dysautonomia	±	±	+	±	±	–	±	±
Dementia	±	+	±	–	–	±	+	+
Dysarthria/dysphagia	±	+	±	+	+	+	±	+
Dystonia	±	±	–	±	–	+	–	–
Eyelid apraxia	–	+	±	±	–	±	–	±
Limb apraxia	–	–	–	–	–	+	±	–
Motor neuron disease	–	–	±	±	–	–	–	+
Myoclonus	±	–	–	±	±	+	±	–
Neuropathy	–	–	±	–	±	–	–	–
Oculomotor deficit	–	+	±	–	+	+	±	±
Sleep impairment	±	±	+	±	±	–	±	–
Asymmetric findings	+	–	–	±	–	+	–	–
Levodopa response	+	±	±	±	±	–	–	–
Levodopa dyskinesia	+	–	–	±	–	–	–	–
Family history	±	–	–	–	–	–	–	–
Putaminal T-2 hypointensity	–	±	+	+	+	–	–	–
Lewy bodies	+	–	±	±	±	±	+	–

* PD = Parkinson's disease; PSP = progressive supranuclear palsy; SDS = Shy-Drager syndrome; SND = striatonigral degeneration; OPCA = olivopontocerebellar atrophy (the familial forms of OPCA are included among the genetic forms of spinocerebellar atrophies); CBGD = corticobasal ganglionic degeneration; DLBD = diffuse Lewy body disease; PDACG = parkinsonism-dementia-amyotrophic lateral sclerosis complex of Guam; + = present; – = not present; ± = may or may not be present. Reproduced from Jankovic [7] with permission.

the original ICD-10 has sometimes resulted in awkward and seemingly illogical placement or sequencing of certain categories, the ICD-10 NA represents an important advancement in the attempt to develop a universally accepted categorization of neurological diseases.

BRADYKINESIA

Bradykinesia is the clinical hallmark of hypokinetic (parkinsonian) disorders (Table 2). Other features that typically accompany bradykinesia include rigidity, tremor, and gait and balance difficulties. Bradykinesia may be clinically manifested by slowness of limb and body movements, reduced blinking and lack of facial expression, monotonous speech, and slowness in activities of daily living. "Freezing" or "motor blocks" are viewed by some as extreme forms of bradykinesia. About 75% of patients exhibiting the cardinal signs of parkinsonism have primary or idiopathic parkinsonism, known as Parkinson's disease. The others have secondary or heredodegenerative forms of parkinsonism (Table 3). It is beyond the scope of this chapter to review the clinical, pharmacological, and imaging features that help to differentiate Parkinson's disease from the atypical forms of parkinsonism (see Table 2). Features that support a diagnosis of Parkinson's disease include the asymmetric presence of a resting tremor and a good (and usually

TABLE 3

CLASSIFICATION OF PARKINSONISM

Primary (idiopathic) parkinsonism

- Parkinson's disease
- Juvenile parkinsonism

Multisystem degeneration ("parkinsonism plus")

- Progressive supranuclear palsy (PSP)
- Multiple system atrophy (MSA)
- Striatonigral degeneration (SND or MSA-P)
- Olivopontocerebellar atrophy (OPCA or MSA-C)
- Shy-Drager syndrome (SDS)
- Lytico-Bodig or parkinsonism-dementia-amyotrophic lateral sclerosis complex of Guam (PDACG)
- Corticobasal ganglionic degeneration (CBGD)
- Progressive pallidal atrophy
- Parkinsonism-dementia complex
- Pallidopyramidal disease

Heredodegenerative Parkinsonism

- Hereditary juvenile dystonia-parkinsonism
- Autosomal dominant Lewy body disease
- Huntington's disease
- Wilson's disease
- Hereditary ceruloplasmin deficiency
- Hallervorden-Spatz disease
- Olivopontocerebellar and spinocerebellar degeneration
- Machado-Joseph disease
- Familial amyotrophy-dementia-parkinsonism
- Disinhibition-dementia-parkinsonism-amyotrophy complex
- Gerstmann-Strausler-Scheinker disease
- Familial progressive subcortical gliosis
- Lubag (X-linked dystonia-parkinsonism)
- Familial basal ganglia calcification
- Mitochondrial cytopathies with striatal necrosis
- Ceroid lipofuscinosis
- Familial parkinsonism with peripheral neuropathy
- Parkinsonian-pyramidal syndrome
- Neuroacanthocytosis
- Hereditary hemochromatosis

Secondary (acquired, symptomatic) parkinsonism

- Infectious: postencephalitic, AIDS, subacute sclerosing panencephalitis, Creutzfeldt-Jakob disease, prion diseases
- Drugs: dopamine receptor blocking drugs (antipsychotic, antiemetic drugs), reserpine, tetrabenazine, alpha-methyl-dopa, lithium, flunarizine, cinnarizine
- Toxins: MPTP, carbon monoxide, manganese, mercury, carbon disulfide, cyanide, methanol, ethanol
- Vascular: multi-infarct, Binswanger's disease
- Trauma: pugilistic encephalopathy
- Other: parathyroid abnormalities, hypothyroidism, hepatocerebral degeneration, brain tumor, paraneoplastic disease, normal pressure hydrocephalus, noncommunicating hydrocephalus, syringomesencephalia, hemiatrophy-hemiparkinsonism, peripherally induced tremor and parkinsonism, and psychogenic disease

* Modified from Jankovic.[7]

sustained) response to levodopa. Early falls, significant oculomotor disturbance, and early prominent dysautonomia, in addition to other clinical features atypical for Parkinson's disease, are important clues to an alternative diagnosis.

TREMOR

Tremor can be defined as a rhythmical oscillation of a body part. Tremors usually have a relatively fixed periodicity, although on clinical inspection the rate may appear irregular. Tremor is usually further subdivided on the basis of the position, posture, or motor activity necessary to bring it about (Table 4). A resting tremor is seen when the body part is in complete repose. Maintenance of a posture, such as extending the arms parallel to the floor, reveals a postural tremor, whereas moving the body part to and from a target brings out kinetic or intention tremor. Occasionally, a tremor is seen only with certain actions or limb positions. "Primary writing tremor" is possibly the most common example of such task-specific tremors. Orthostatic tremor, an example of a position-specific tremor, is an uncommon and frequently unrecognized high-frequency tremor involving the

TABLE 4

Classification and Differential Diagnosis of Tremors*

Rest tremors

- Parkinson's disease
- Other parkinsonian syndromes (less commonly)
- Midbrain ("rubral") tremor: rest < postural < kinetic
- Wilson's disease (also acquired hepatocerebral degeneration)
- Essential tremor—only if severe: rest < < postural and action

Postural and action ("terminal") tremor

- Physiological tremor
- Exaggerated physiological tremor (these factors can also aggravate other forms of tremor)
  - Stress, fatigue, anxiety, emotion
  - Endocrine: hypoglycemia, thyrotoxicosis, pheochromocytoma, adrenocorticosteroids
  - Drugs and toxins: beta agonists, dopamine agonists, amphetamines, lithium, tricyclic antidepressants, neuroleptics, theophylline, caffeine, valproic acid, alcohol withdrawal, mercury ("hatter's shakes"), lead, arsenic, others
- Essential tremor (familial or sporadic) ? subtypes
- Primary writing tremor
- With other CNS disorders:
  - Parkinson's disease
  - Other akinetic-rigid syndromes
  - Idiopathic dystonia, including focal dystonias
  - With peripheral neuropathy
  - Charcot-Marie-Tooth syndrome (controversial as to whether to call this the Roussy-Levy syndrome)
  - Variety of other peripheral neuropathies (especially dysgammaglobulinemia)
  - Cerebellar tremor

Kinetic (intention) tremor

- Disease of cerebellar "outflow" (dentate nucleus and superior cerebellar peduncle): multiple sclerosis, trauma, tumor, vascular disease, Wilson's syndrome, acquired hepatocerebral degeneration, drugs, toxins (e.g., mercury), others

Miscellaneous rhythmical movement disorders

- Psychogenic tremor
- Orthostatic tremor
- Rhythmical movements in dystonia (dystonic tremor)
- Rhythmical myoclonus (segmental myoclonus; e.g., palatal or branchial myoclonus, spinal myoclonus, limb myorhythmia)
- Oscillatory myoclonus
- Asterixis
- Clonus
- Epilepsia partialis continua
- Hereditary chin quivering
- Spasmus nutans
- Head bobbing with third ventricular cysts
- Nystagmus

* CNS = central nervous system. Modified from Weiner and Lang.[11]

proximal lower limbs and trunk when the patient stands for any period of time. Table 4 lists a variety of other rhythmical movements that can sometimes be confused with tremor.

Chorea

Chorea consists of irregular, unpredictable, brief, jerky, continuous movements that progress randomly from one part of the body to another (Table 5). The movements are brisk and abrupt in some cases (e.g., Sydenham's chorea), whereas in others, they are slower and more flowing (e.g., Huntington's disease). The term "choreoathetosis" has been used in this latter situation, in which chorea may be combined with features of dystonia and athetosis.

TABLE 5

ETIOLOGICAL CLASSIFICATION OF CHOREA*

Developmental/aging choreas Physiological chorea of infancy Cerebral palsy—anoxic, kernicteric Minimal cerebral dysfunction Buccal-oral-lingual dyskinesia and edentulous orodyskinesia in the elderly Senile chorea (probably several causes) *Hereditary choreas* Huntington's disease Benign hereditary chorea Neuroacanthocytosis Other CNS "degenerations": olivopontocerebellar atrophy, Azorean disease, ataxia telangiectasia, tuberous sclerosis, Hallervorden-Spatz disease, dentato-rubral-pallido-luysian atrophy, familial calcification of basal ganglia, others Neurometabolic disorders: Wilson's disease, Lesch Nyhan, lysosomal storage disorders, amino acid disorders, Leigh's disease, porphyria *Drug-induced choreas* Neuroleptics (tardive dyskinesia) Antiparkinsonian drugs Amphetamines Tricyclic antidepressants Oral contraceptives Anticonvulsants Anticholinergics Others *Toxin-induced choreas* Alcohol intoxication and withdrawal Anoxia Carbon monoxide Manganese Mercury Thallium Toluene	*Metabolic* Hyperthyroidism Hypoparathyroidism (various types) Pregnancy (chorea gravidarum) Hyper- and hyponatremia, hypomagnesemia, hypocalcemia Hypo- and hyperglycemia (latter may cause hemichorea, hemiballismus) Acquired hepatocerebral degeneration Nutritional—e.g., beriberi, pellagra, vitamin B12 deficiency in infants *Infectious* Sydenham's chorea Encephalitis lethargica Various other infections and postinfectious encephalitides, including Creutzfeldt-Jakob disease *Immunological* Systemic lupus erythematosus (including antinuclear factor-negative cases with lupus anticoagulant) Henoch-Schonlein Others rarely—sarcoidosis, multiple sclerosis, Behcet's syndrome, polyarteritis nodosa, myeloproliferative disorder *Vascular* (often hemichorea) Infarction Hemorrhage Arteriovenous malformation Polycythemia rubra vera Migraine *Tumors* *Trauma*, including subdural and epidural hematoma *Miscellaneous*, including paroxysmal choreoathetosis

*Modified from Shoulson.[10]

BALLISMUS

Ballismus comprises wide-amplitude flinging movements, usually involving the proximal limbs, most often on only one side of the body (hemiballismus). Occasionally bilateral movements occur (biballismus or paraballismus). Ballismus is believed to be at one end of the chorea spectrum, because many patients demonstrate additional distal choreic movements and, as recovery occurs, hemiballismus often transforms into a milder hemichoreic state.

TABLE 6

Etiological Classification of Dystonia*

Primary dystonia
- Sporadic
- Inherited
  - Classic autosomal dominant (Oppenheim's) dystonia (DYTI gene, 9q34)
  - Adult-onset cranial-cervical dystonia (DYT6 gene, 8p21)
  - Adult-onset cervical dystonia (18p)

Secondary dystonia
- Dystonia plus syndromes
  - Sporadic
  - Inherited
    - Myoclonic dystonia (18)
    - Dopa-responsive dystonia (guanosine triphosphate cyclohydrolase I, 14q22.1)
    - Rapid-onset dystonia-parkinsonism
    - X-linked dystonia-parkinsonism (Lubag, DYT3 gene, Xq13)
- Associated with neurodegenerative disorders
  - Sporadic
    - Parkinson's disease
    - Progressive supranuclear palsy
    - Multiple system atrophy
    - Corticobasal ganglionic degeneration
    - Multiple sclerosis
    - Central pontine myelinolysis
  - Inherited
    - Wilson's disease
    - Huntington's disease
    - Juvenile parkinsonism-dystonia
    - Progressive pallidal degeneration
    - Hallervorden-Spatz disease
    - Hypoprebetalipoproteinemia (HARP syndrome), acanthocytosis, retinitis pigmentosa, and pallidal degeneration
    - Joseph's disease
    - Ataxia telangiectasia
    - Neuroacanthocytosis
    - Rett's syndrome
    - Intraneuronal inclusion disease
    - Infantile bilateral striatal necrosis
    - Familial basal ganglia calcifications
    - Spinocerebellar degeneration
    - Olivopontocerebellar atrophy
    - Hereditary spastic paraplegia with dystonia
    - X-linked dystonia parkinsonism or Lubag (pericentromeric)
    - Deletion of 18q
- Associated with metabolic disorders
  - Amino acid disorders
    - Glutaric acidemia
    - Methylmalonic acidemia
    - Homocystinuria
    - Hartnup's disease
    - Tyrosinosis
  - Lipid disorders
    - Metachromatic leukodystrophy
    - Ceroid lipofuscinosis
    - Dystonic lipidosis ("sea blue" histiocytosis)
    - Gangliosidoses, GM1 and GM2 variants
    - Hexosaminidase A and B deficiency
  - Miscellaneous metabolic disorders
    - Wilson's disease
    - Mitochondrial encephalopathies: Leigh's disease, Leber's disease
    - Lesch-Nyhan syndrome
    - Triosephosphate isomerase deficiency
    - Vitamin E deficiency
    - Biopterin deficiency
    - Aromatic L-amino acid decarboxylase deficiency
- Due to a known, specific cause
  - Perinatal cerebral injury and kernicterus: athetoid cerebral palsy, delayed onset dystonia
  - Infection: viral encephalitis, encephalitis lethargica, Reye's syndrome; subacute sclerosing panencephalitis, Creutzfeldt-Jakob disease, AIDS
  - Other: tuberculosis, syphilis, acute infectious torticollis
  - Paraneoplastic brain stem encephalitis
  - Cerebral vascular or ischemic injury
  - Brain tumor
  - Arteriovenous malformation
  - Head trauma and brain surgery
  - Peripheral trauma
  - Toxins: manganese, carbon monoxide, carbon disulfide, methanol, disulfiram, wasp sting
  - Drugs: levodopa, bromocriptine, antipsychotics, metoclopramide, fenfluramine, flecainide, anticonvulsants, certain calcium channel blockers, ergots

TABLE 6 (cont'd)

ETIOLOGICAL CLASSIFICATION OF DYSTONIA*

Other hyperkinetic syndromes associated with dystonia	Syringomyelia
Tic disorders with dystonic tics	Arnold-Chiari malformation
Paroxysmal dyskinesias	Trochlear nerve palsy
Paroxysmal kinesigenic dyskinesia	Vestibular torticollis
Paroxysmal nonkinesigenic dyskinesia	Posterior fossa mass
Paroxysmal exertion-induced dyskinesia	Soft tissue neck mass
Paroxysmal hypnogenic dyskinesia	Congenital postural torticollis
Hypnogenic dystonia (probably a seizure disorder)	Congenital Klippel-Feil syndrome
Psychogenic	Isaac's syndrome
Pseudodystonia	Sandiffer's syndrome
Atlantoaxial subluxation	Satoyoshi syndrome
	Stiff-person syndrome
	Ventral hernia

*Modified from Jankovic and Fahn.[8]

DYSTONIA

Dystonia can be defined as a disorder dominated by sustained muscle contractions that frequently cause twisting and repetitive movements or abnormal postures (Table 6). Dystonic movements may be slow and twisting. Prolonged dystonic spasms result in characteristic posturing of various body parts. In addition, dystonic movements may be quite rapid, resembling the shock-like jerks of myoclonus. Dystonia may also be manifested by rhythmical movements, present especially when the patient actively attempts to resist the involuntary dystonic movement. This dystonic tremor can be abolished if the patient is asked to relax and allow the body part to move in the direction of the dystonic pull. The wide range of abnormal movement types that occur in dystonic syndromes is often a source of misdiagnosis. Patients with dystonia may also demonstrate a postural and action tremor of the limbs similar to essential tremor.

The term "action dystonia" refers to dystonic movements and postures that are specific to selected actions or positions. Many patients use a variety of peculiar tricks to lessen the severity of their abnormal movements. These features have frequently encouraged a misdiagnosis of hysteria. The adult-onset, idiopathic focal and segmental dystonias are the most common dystonic disorders seen in neurological practice. These include cranial dystonia (blepharospasm, oromandibular/lingual dystonia), laryngeal dystonia (spasmodic dysphonia), cervical dystonia (spasmodic torticollis) and other axial dystonias, and dystonic writer's cramp and other "occupational spasms."

TICS

Tics are the most varied of all movement disorders (Table 7). Tics are usually abrupt, transient, stereotypical, coordinated movements that vary in intensity and are repeated at irregular intervals. The movements are most often brief and jerky (clonic); however, slower, more prolonged movements (tonic or dystonic) may also occur. Patients typically demonstrate a wide array of simple and complex motor or vocal tics as well as a number of associated symptoms, including hyperactivity, attention deficit disorder, and obsessive-compulsive disorder. Several other features are helpful in distinguishing this movement disorder from other dyskinesias. Patients usually experience an inner urge to make

TABLE 7

CLASSIFICATION OF TICS

Physiological tics

- Mannerisms

Pathological tics

- Primary
  - Sporadic
    - Transient motor or phonic tics (<1 year)
    - Chronic motor or phonic tics (>1 year)
    - Adult-onset (recurrent) tics
    - Tourette's syndrome
  - Inherited
    - Tourette's syndrome
    - Huntington's disease
    - Primary dystonia
    - Neuroacanthocytosis
- Secondary ("Tourettism")
  - Infections: encephalitis, Creutzfeldt-Jakob disease, Sydenham's chorea
  - Drugs: stimulants, levodopa, carbamazepine, phenytoin, phenobarbital, antipsychotics (tardive tics)
  - Toxins: carbon monoxide
  - Developmental: static encephalopathy, mental retardation syndromes, chromosomal abnormalities
  - Other: head trauma, stroke, neurocutaneous syndromes, chromosomal abnormalities, schizophrenia, neuroacanthocytosis degenerative disorders

Related disorders

- Stereotypies
- Self-injurious behaviors
- Hyperactivity syndrome
- Compulsions
- Excessive startle
- Jumping Frenchmen of Maine, latah, myriachit

*Modified from Jankovic.[4]

the movement themselves, and this premonitory urge is temporarily relieved by the execution of the tic. Tics are voluntarily suppressible for variable periods of time, but this usually occurs at the expense of mounting inner tension and the need to perform the tic. Voluntary suppression, however, is not specific for tics and several other types of abnormal movements also may be suppressed for short periods of time.

MYOCLONUS

Myoclonus can be defined as sudden, brief, shock-like involuntary movement that may be caused by both active muscle contraction (positive myoclonus) or inhibition of ongoing muscle activity (negative myoclonus) (Table 8). Asterixis is the most common example of negative myoclonus. The differential diagnosis of myoclonus is quite broad, and there is a wide range of clinical patterns of myoclonus. Frequency, amplitude, distribution, rhythmicity, and response to stimuli vary greatly from patient to patient. The frequency varies from single, rare jerks to constant, repetitive contractions. The amplitude may range from a small contraction that fails to move a joint to a very large jerk that moves the entire body. The distribution ranges from focal involvement of one body part, to segmental (involving two or more contiguous regions), to multifocal, to generalized. When the jerks occur bilaterally, they may be symmetrical or asymmetrical. When they occur in more than one region, they may be synchronous in two body parts (within milliseconds) or asynchronous. Myoclonus is usually arrhythmic and irregular, but in some patients it is very regular (rhythmical) and in others there may be jerky oscillations that last for a few seconds and then fade away (oscillatory). Myoclonic jerks may occur spontaneously, without a clear precipitant, or as a response to a wide variety of stimuli. This stimulus sensitivity may occur in response to sudden noise, light, visual threat, pinprick or touch, or muscle stretch. Attempted movements (or even the intention to move) may initiate the muscle jerks (action or intention myoclonus).

TABLE 8

Eiological Classification of Myoclonus*

Physiological myoclonus (normal subjects)
- Sleep jerks (hypnic jerks)
- Anxiety-induced
- Exercise-induced
- Hiccup (singuitus)
- Benign infantile myoclonus with feeding

Essential myoclonus (no known cause and no other gross neurological deficit)
- Hereditary
- Sporadic

Epileptic myoclonus (seizures dominate; no encephalopathy, at least initially)
- Fragments of epilepsy, isolated epileptic myoclonic jerks, epilepsia partialis continua, idiopathic stimulus-sensitive myoclonus, photosensitive myoclonus, myoclonic absences in petit mal epilepsy
- Childhood myoclonic epilepsies, infantile spasms, myoclonic astatic epilepsy (Lennox-Gastaut syndrome), cryptogenic myoclonus epilepsy (Aicardi's syndrome), awakening myoclonus epilepsy of Janz
- Benign familial myoclonic epilepsy (Rabot)
- Progressive myoclonic epilepsy: Baltic myoclonus (Unverricht-Lundborg disease)

Symptomatic myoclonus (progressive or static encephalopathy dominates)
- Storage disease: Lafora body disease, lipidoses (e.g., GM2 gangliosidosis, Tay-Sachs disease), Krabbe's disease, ceroid-lipofuscinosis [Batten/Kufs disease], sialidosis ("cherry-red spot")
- Spinocerebellar degeneration: Ramsay Hunt syndrome (several etiologies), Friedreich's ataxia, ataxia telangiectasia
- Basal ganglia degenerations: Wilson's disease, torsion dystonia, Hallervorden-Spatz disease, corticobasal ganglionic degeneration, progressive supranuclear palsy, Huntington's disease, Parkinson's disease, multiple system atrophy, dentato-rubro-luysian atrophy
- Mitochondrial encephalopathies
- Dementias: Creutzfeldt-Jakob disease, Alzheimer's disease
- Viral encephalopathies: subacute sclerosing panencephalitis, encephalitis lethargica, arbor virus encephalitis, herpes simplex encephalitis, postinfectious encephalitis
- Metabolic: hepatic failure, renal failure, dialysis syndrome, hyponatremia, hypoglycemia, infantile myoclonic encephalopathy (polymyoclonus) (± neuroblastoma), nonketotic hyperglycemia, multiple carboxylase deficiency
- Toxic encephalopathies: bismuth, heavy-metal poisoning, methyl bromide, DDT, drugs including levodopa, tricyclic antidepressants, others
- Physical encephalopathies: post-hypoxia (Lance-Adams), posttraumatic, heat stroke, electric shock, decompression injury
- Focal CNS damage: post-stroke, post-thalamotomy, tumor, trauma, olivodentate lesions (palatal myoclonus), spinal cord lesions (segmental/spinal myoclonus)
- Rarely, nerve root, plexus, or peripheral nerve disorders

*Modified from Fahn et al.[2]

Stereotypy

Stereotypy is an involuntary, patterned, repetitive, continuous, coordinated, purposeless or ritualistic movement, posture, or utterance. Stereotypy may be simple, as exemplified by a repetitive tongue protrusion or body-rocking movements, or complex, such as self-caressing, crossing and uncrossing of legs, marching in place, and pacing (Table 9). This movement disorder is typically present in patients with tardive dyskinesia. Other causes of stereotypy include mental retardation, autism, Rett's syndrome, schizophrenia, and other developmental and psychiatric disorders.

TABLE 9

STEREOTYPIES*

Physiological
Mannerisms
Pathological
Mental retardation
Autism (Kanner's infantile autism, Asperger's syndrome)
Rett's syndrome
Williams syndrome
Tardive dyskinesia
Akathisia
Neuroacanthocytosis
Schizophrenia
Catatonia
Obsessive-compulsive disorder
Tourette's syndrome
Restless legs syndrome
Epileptic automatism
Psychogenic

*Modified from Jankovic.[5]

TABLE 10

CLASSIFICATION OF PAROXYSMAL DYSKINESIAS*

Paroxysmal kinesigenic dyskinesia
Paroxysmal non-kinesigenic dyskinesia
Paroxysmal exertion-induced dyskinesia
Paroxysmal nocturnal dyskinesia
Paroxysmal psychogenic dyskinesia
Each category includes:
Short-lasting (<5 minutes)
Idiopathic: familial/sporadic
Secondary
Long-lasting (>5 minutes)
Idiopathic: familial/sporadic
Secondary

*Modified from Demirkiran and Jankovic.[1]

OTHER MANIFESTATIONS

Certain types of dyskinesias occur intermittently rather than in a persistent fashion. This is typical of tics and some forms of myoclonus. Rarely, patients with chorea and/or dystonia have bouts of sudden-onset, short-lived involuntary movements known as paroxysmal dyskinesias (Table 10). Action dystonia could be confused with a paroxysmal dyskinesia; however, in the former, the abnormal movement consistently occurs in response to the specific action, rather than occurring in a periodic or unpredictable manner.

Abnormal or excessive startle occurs in a number of disorders. In some patients, the only problem is an exaggerated response to startle that habituates poorly after repeated stimuli. In others, there is an abnormal response to the stimuli that normally evoke a startle response. Hyperekplexia, or "startle disease," is the best known example of pathological startle, now known to be associated with a mutation in the gene for a subunit of the glycine receptor. A variety of other unusual disorders, first described in the 19th century together with Tourette's syndrome, manifest as excessive startle, including the jumping Frenchmen of Maine, latah, and myriachit. These latter disorders also demonstrate sudden striking out, echo phenomena, automatic obedience, and several other, less common features.

The term "akathisia" refers to a sense of restlessness and the feeling of a need to move. This disorder may be accompanied by a variety of "akathitic," stereotypic movements, including repetitive rubbing, crossing and uncrossing the arms, stroking the head and face with the hands, repeatedly picking at clothing, abduction and adduction of limbs or digits, crossing and uncrossing the legs, swinging or up-and-down pumping of the legs, shifting weight, rocking, marching in place while sitting or standing, or pacing. Patients may even have vocalizations such as moans, grunts, and shouts. Whether true akathitic movements can occur in the absence of the subjective sense of needing to move remains controversial. Akathisia is usually a complication of therapy with dopamine receptor blockers.

Restless legs syndrome is another disorder in which most movements occur secondary to the subjective need to move. The patient typically complains of sensory disturbances in the legs

TABLE 11

NEUROLEPTIC-INDUCED MOVEMENT DISORDERS

Acute, Transient	*Chronic, Persistent*
Dystonic reaction	Tardive stereotypy
Parkinsonism	Tardive chorea
Akathisia	Tardive dystonia
Neuroleptic malignant syndrome	Tardive akathisia
	Tardive tics
	Tardive myoclonus
	Tardive tremor
	Persistent parkinsonism
	Tardive sensory syndrome

*Modified from Jankovic.[6]

(less often in the arms), including pins and needles, creeping or crawling, aching, itching, stabbing, heaviness, tension, burning, or coldness. These complaints are usually experienced when lying down or when elevating the legs in the evening. This condition is commonly associated with insomnia and another movement disorder known as periodic movements of sleep (sometimes inappropriately termed "nocturnal myoclonus"). These periodic, slow, sustained (1-2 seconds) movements range from synchronous to asynchronous dorsiflexion of the big toes and feet to triple flexion of one or both legs. More rapid myoclonic movements or slower, prolonged dystonic-like movements of the feet and legs also may be present in these patients while awake.

Painful legs and moving toes is an unusual but well-defined movement disorder most often involving the lower limbs. Rarely, a similar disorder can be seen in the upper limbs. The movements are not usually the main source of disability or concern. On the other hand, most of these patients complain bitterly of the accompanying deep pulling or searing pain in the lower limb and foot. These patients demonstrate continuous, rhythmical wriggling or writhing of the toes, with the ankle and proximal muscles of the legs being involved less often. In some cases, there is a history of nerve insult or injury and the examination may demonstrate evidence of peripheral nerve dysfunction.

Hemifacial spasm is the best recognized "peripheral movement disorder." Here the movement consists of irregular tonic and clonic contractions involving the muscles innervated by the ipsilateral seventh cranial nerve. Eyelid twitching usually is the first symptom, followed at variable intervals by lower facial muscle involvement. In rare cases of bilateral involvement, the spasms are asynchronous on the two sides, in contrast to dystonic blepharospasm. In addition to hemifacial spasm, there are other peripheral movement disorders such as fasciculations and myokymia, and some movement disorders, particularly dystonia and tremor, can occur after peripheral trauma.

The nature and extent of the investigation of the patient presenting with a movement disorder will vary depending on the clinical circumstances. When the historical and clinical features are characteristic of certain conditions (e.g., familial essential tremor, Tourette's syndrome), further investigations may be unnecessary. This also applies to certain well-recognized drug-induced movement disorders (Table 11). Table 12 provides an approach to the investigation of movement disorders. The importance of excluding Wilson's disease cannot be overemphasized in view of its treatability and universally fatal outcome if left undiagnosed.

REFERENCES

1. Demirkiran M, Jankovic J: Paroxysmal dyskinesias: clinical features and classification. **Ann Neurol 38:** 571-579, 1995
2. Fahn S, Marsden CD, Van Woert MH: Definition and classification of myoclonus. **Adv Neurol 43:**1-5, 1986
3. Jankovic J: International Classification of Diseases, Tenth Revision: Neurological Adaptation (ICD-10 NA): Extrapyramidal and movement disorders. **Mov Disord 10:**533-540, 1995
4. Jankovic J: Phenomenology and classification of tics, in Jankovic J (ed): **Tourette Syndrome, Neurologic Clinics.** Philadelphia, Pa: WB Saunders, 1997, Vol 15, pp 267-275
5. Jankovic J: Stereotypies, in Marsden CD, Fahn S (eds): **Movement Disorders - 3.** London: Butterworth-Heinemann, 1994, pp 503-517
6. Jankovic J: Tardive syndromes and other drug-induced movement disorders. **Clin Neuropharmacol 18:**197-214, 1995
7. Jankovic J: Treatment of parkinsonian syndromes, in Kurlan R (ed): **Treatment of Movement Disorders.** Philadelphia, Pa: JB Lippincott, 1995, pp 95-114

TABLE 12

INVESTIGATION OF MOVEMENT DISORDERS*

Investigation	Movement Disorder					
	A	C	HB	D	T	M
Routine hematology (including sedimentation rate)	+	+	+	+	–	+
Routine biochemistry (including Ca^{++}, uric acid, liver function tests)	+	+	+	+	±	+
Serum Cu, ceruloplasmin (with or without 24-hour urine Cu, liver biopsy, radiolabeled Cu studies)	++	++	–	++	±	+
Slit-lamp examination	++	++	–	++	±	+
Thyroid function	±	++	–	+	–	+
Antistreptolysin O test, Anti-DNAse B, antihyaluronidase	–	+	–	±	±	–
Antinuclear factor, lupus erythematosis cells, other immunological studies, anticardiolipin antibodies, VDRL test	±	++	+	+	–	+
Blood acanthocytes	+	+	–	+	+	±
Lysosomal enzymes	+	+	–	+	±	+
Urine organic and amino acids	±	+	–	+	-	+
Urine oligosaccharides and mucopolysaccharides	±	+	–	+	-	+
Serum lactate and pyruvate	±	+	–	+	-	+
DNA tests for gene mutations	±	±	–	±	-	±
Bone marrow for storage cells, including EM	±	+	–	+	-	+
EM of leukocytes; biopsy of liver/skin/conjunctiva	±	+	–	+	-	+
Nerve/muscle biopsy	±	+	–	+	-	+
Oligoclonal bands	±	+	+	+	-	±
Computed tomography, magnetic resonance imaging	++	++	++	++	±	++
Electroencephalography	+	+	–	+	+	++
Electromyography and nerve conduction studies	+	+	–	+	+	+
Evoked potentials	+	+	–	+	–	++
Electroretinogram	±	+	–	+	–	+
Neuropsychological testing	±	±	–	–	±	–

*Modified from Lang.[9] The extent of investigation will depend on factors such as age at onset, nature of progression, and presence of historical or clinical atypical features suggesting a secondary cause of the movement disorder in question. A = akinetic rigid syndrome; C = chorea; HB = hemiballism; D = dystonia; T = tics; M = myoclonus; VDRL = Venereal Disease Research Laboratory; EM = electron microscopy; ++ = very important or frequently useful; + = sometimes helpful; ± = questionably helpful; – = rarely, if ever, helpful.

8. Jankovic J, Fahn S: Dystonic disorders, in Jankovic J, Tolosa E (eds): **Parkinson's Disease and Movement Disorders.** 3rd ed. Baltimore, Md: Williams & Wilkins, 1998 (In press)
9. Lang AE: Movement disorder symptomatology, in Bradley WG, Daroff RB, Fenichel GM, et al (eds): **Neurology in Clinical Practice.** London: Butterworth-Heinemann, 1996, pp 299-320
10. Shoulson I: On chorea. **Clin Neuropharmacol 9** (Suppl 2):S85-S99, 1986
11. Weiner WJ, Lang AE: **Movement Disorders: A Comprehensive Survey.** Mount Kisco, NY: Futura, 1989

CHAPTER 2

HISTORY OF SURGERY FOR MOVEMENT DISORDERS

ALIM LOUIS BENABID, MD, PHD, DOMINIQUE CAPARROS-LEFEBVRE, MD, PHD, AND PIERRE POLLAK, MD

In every stage of neurosurgical history, the methods used were the result of a compromise between necessity (to cure the symptoms of a disease, namely, movement disorders) and available techniques and concepts of the era (pathophysiological understanding of movement disorder mechanisms, particularly for Parkinson's disease). Modern improvements in methodology and stereotactic localization, particularly in European centers, has provided greater accuracy for lesion placement and improved results.[93]

Before levodopa received widespread acceptance for the treatment of Parkinson's disease, stereotactic surgery was the most successful treatment for tremor and rigidity. The major criticism of this neurosurgical contribution was the often superficial and unblinded clinical assessment of the results (the early reports would probably be rejected by referees today), and the lack of correlation between the actual (and not the claimed) target and clinical symptoms. To give credit where it is due, in this early period the mortality rate was low: Bertrand et al[25] reported no postoperative deaths in more than 500 consecutive cases. We must at least acknowledge neurosurgeons' good will, as they consistently tried and reported new methods to improve the accuracy of target localization. They used increasingly precise morphological methods, from ventriculography to magnetic resonance imaging (MRI), and functional electrophysiological recording, from as early as 1940[113] to the major contribution of the French groups.[6-8,56-59,73-76,152,153]

Whether the very first surgical procedures trying to improve tremor and other movement disorders were designed on the basis of clear neurophysiological data is perhaps an anachronic question. Indeed, when surgeons began using ablative therapy for movement disorders, the localization theories for parkinsonism and related diseases lacked their current precision and implicated mainly the pallidum, excluding other structures such as the networks that have been studied in the last 30 years. The role of the substantia nigra in the occurrence of parkinsonian signs had never been suggested until it was demonstrated by Trétiakoff[157] in his thesis of 1919; it remained under discussion until 1970. Meanwhile, neurosurgeons did not wait for the conclusion of these long-lasting anatomical and pathological debates. They continued to assess various targets empirically to discover optimum sites for effective lesioning. Better understanding of basal ganglia function has induced, and in turn benefited from, brainstorming sessions among neuroscientists. Therefore, designation of the best targets, according to a precise risk-to-benefit ratio and with worldwide consensus, could be a reality in the near future. This statement requires per se a detailed and reproducible evaluation of clinical status before, during, and after surgery; this was unfortunately often missing in the earlier history of ablative surgery, and thus did not allow precise comparisons of the various techniques. However, the history of the understanding of the basal ganglia is intimately linked, and should be analyzed in parallel, to the history of movement disorder surgery. Ideas evolved in parallel processes for methods, targets, and indications, but will have to be described separately.

As neurosurgery is at the end of a convergent stream of clinical needs, of physiological and pathological data, and of methods, its history pertains also to evolution. This chapter uses as sources previously well-documented reviews on pallidotomy,[77] the basal ganglia,[128, 131,133] and neurosurgery for movement disorders.[137] The epistemological process that can be outlined through the history of movement disorder surgery is emphasized. This may lead to some redundancy, which in some ways mirrors the nonlinear approach neurosurgeons have used during nearly half a century.

The Impact of Levodopa

The major event that affected the treatment of Parkinson's disease was the discovery of levodopa (L-DOPA). Thus, the surgical approaches to Parkinson's disease can be divided into three eras: the pre-levodopa, levodopa, and post-levodopa periods.

The Pre-Levodopa Era

The epoch prior to the discovery of L-DOPA was characterized by the search for cures for the symptom triad of tremor, rigidity, and akinesia. During this era, the input of neurosurgeons was paramount, although poor clinical assessment of patients and questionable assessment of lesion sites do not allow us to take full advantage of the early results in trying to understand the basal ganglia system.

Pallidotomy

Interest was centered on the pallidum at this time because of the emerging physiopathological concepts of Hassler[78-80] and the incidental observation made by Cooper[47] that vascular lesions of the anterior choroidal artery induced ischemic damage in the pallidum that was responsible for the clinical improvement of patients. Leksell's careful practice allowed 75% of his patients to resume work, with neither mortality nor visual deficit and very rare motor deficit; part of his large series was left unpublished and became public, thanks to Laitinen et al, in 1992.[95]

The effects of pallidotomy were mild for akinesia and rigidity, but significant for tremor, and results could be spectacular when they were not plagued by complications or side effects. Most neurologists had one or more patients with disappointing results, mainly side effects such as motor neglect or hemiparesis. Although the results of pallidotomy were poor for tremor and mild for akinesia and rigidity, and despite the fact that a large German series showed that immediate good results still would leave only 50% of patients usefully improved over the long term, this surgery was, along with thalamotomy, the only available treatment for Parkinson's disease in the pre-levodopa era. The need for a large number of operations to avoid long waiting lists pushed neurosurgeons to develop quicker, freehand procedures.[24,26] Such practices as using leukotomes as probes, with neither stereotaxy nor electrophysiological delineation, but only pneumoencephalography, probably helped accelerate the decline of the method and its prompt disappearance when L-DOPA was discovered.

Thalamotomy

The need to optimize the effect of ablative surgery on tremor led researchers to the thalamus and its subnuclei, mainly the ventral intermediate (VIM) nucleus, which can be considered the most satisfactory target for tremor control but is disappointing for akinesia and rigidity. For this reason, Gillingham[70] in 1960 tried to associate pallidotomy with thalamotomy, performing the second procedure later if needed.

The Levodopa Era

Growing interest in biochemical research led to the discovery of the role of dopamine in Parkinson's disease, the use of L-DOPA, and the abandonment of thalamotomy (and of all surgical methods). The discovery of dopamine was credited to Guggenheim in 1913, but the depletion of striatal dopamine in Parkinson's disease was not demonstrated until almost 50 years later; treatment with L-DOPA started in the period 1961-1965. When the drug was available worldwide, Parkinson's disease began to be viewed as a medical, rather than a surgical, disorder. Patients were referred to neurologists, who usually rejected the surgical alternative because of its bad reputation. The number of stereotactic procedures dramatically decreased.

The therapeutic effect of L-DOPA and other dopaminergic agonists was so spectacular that the number of thalamotomies per year strikingly diminished and almost disappeared. Neurosurgical therapy for movement disorders was thought to be dead, especially because the remaining indications, such as dystonias, tremors of multiple sclerosis, and posttraumatic and post-stroke movement disorders, were poorly improved by thalamotomy. Even essential tremor, which was the best indication for thalamotomy, suffered from this new medical therapy, although it was totally inefficient for essential tremor. Neurologists had come to consider the risks of surgery as unacceptable in view of the apparently safe and presumably reversible effects of dopaminergic treatment.

However, after less than 10 years of L-DOPA treatment, the first unexpected side effects of the drug were observed. Neurologists and their patients faced the dramatic and disabling abnormal involuntary movements that now not only limited the use of the "miracle" drug but also added a new chapter to the history of the movement disorders they had been used to treat. The development of other classes of drugs brought their own complications, some of them in the psychiatric range.[111] The heyday of L-DOPA treatment thus abated.

The Post-Levodopa Era

From a neurosurgical point of view, the post-levodopa period has been characterized by the rebirth of neurosurgical methods. The reintroduction of pallidotomy[95] provided a cure for the disabling side effects of L-DOPA and allowed patients to enjoy the benefits of their medical treatment. Also, the development of deep brain stimulation immediately fascinated, or at least attracted, neurologists due to its reversibility, low complication rate, and good results. A new era of functional surgery was born.

The rejection of postoperative deficits, previously acceptable because of the lack of choice, motivated the search for less aggressive methods. Grafting appeared as a suitable solution for the replacement of defective neurotransmitters, and ablative methods were replaced by inhibitory techniques that would even be applied to the abnormal involuntary movements that were side effects of the medical treatment.

Historical Evolution of Surgical Approaches for Parkinson's Disease

Open Surgical Approach

Surgery for disabling movement disorders was first used at the end of the 19th century. Because phrenology was prominent at the time, a further aim was to localize functions of cortical and subcortical areas. It began with corticectomy in the premotor area to cure choreoathetosis.[85] A smaller corticectomy, limited to Broadman's areas 4 and 6, also induced a motor deficit and delayed seizures.[40] Despite its severe side effects in dystonia or chorea, as well as a 10%-30% mortality rate,[94,162] this procedure was later applied to parkinsonian tremor but met with little success.[41,134] In 1940, Meyers,[113] preserving the pyramidal tract through a transventricular approach, resected two thirds of the caudate nucleus with good results, which were retrospectively attributed to the section of pallidofugal fibers. Browder,[36] on the contrary, in 1948 used an approach through the caudate and deliberately sectioned the anterior limb of the internal capsule, resulting in a high rate of mortality after bilateral surgery. These approaches had some effect on tremor and rigidity through the postoperative deficit they often induced, but they were often devastating to patients. Consequently, any improvement of the surgical approach to the basal ganglia, such as subfrontal, transfrontal, and transtemporal approaches for ansotomy[56-59] or for internal pallidotomy,[73] reduced the mortality rate, with an improvement of 40%-80% in rigidity and tremor. During the same period, section of fiber bundles took aim at motor efferent pathways. Such procedures included pyramidotomy,[123] pedunculotomy,[160] cordotomy or tractotomy at the cervical level, including anterolateral extrapyramidal cordotomy,[135,136] and mesencephalic tractotomy.[77] Afferent pathways were also sectioned via rhizotomy.[62] These procedures induced less motor deficit, but were also less effective.[136]

Operative complications not only meant drawbacks but sometimes led to significant progress in concepts and methods. This is what happened with Cooper,[47] who, in 1953, while performing a pedunculotomy in a postencephalitic patient, had lesioned the anterior choroidal artery and had to ligate it. This was followed by an improvement in the patient's symptoms and opened the way to a series of interventions using deliberate ligation of the choroidal artery. The effects were presumed to be due to an ischemic lesion of the pallidum, but there was another consequence as well, that of infarction of the internal capsule, which was responsible for an unacceptable mortality rate of about 13%. To avoid this, Cooper directly targeted the pallidum, into which, through a lateral transtemporal approach guided by pneumoencephalography, he inserted a catheter to inject alcohol.[48,52,53] Despite attempts to check the localization of the catheter, the lesion sites were not always where expected, which led once more to progress when it was discovered that the thalamus could be an even better target. These open surgical procedures had in common that the intended target could not be precisely localized and there was no way to prove they had been reached. This eventually led to the performance of more accurate and precisely positioned lesions and prepared the way for stereotaxy.

Stereotactic Approach

As early as 1897, a frame fixed on the skull of a patient was used to remove bullets, which had been previously localized with two perpendicular x-rays taken from Crooks tubes hung on the frame; this was casually presented in a Parisian newspaper (Remy and Contremoulins: Le chercheur de projectiles, L'illustration, 27 November 1897). Much later, Spiegel and Wycis[146,147,149] performed the first acknowledged stereotactic procedure, in 1947, on a psychiatric patient. They also performed stereotactic pallidotomy in patients with movement disorders.[149]

Various stereotactic frames were developed to ensure motionless head position in patients and thus a precise trajectory, allowing neurosurgeons to avoid errors of lesion placement and to reach the target with a precision of 0.5-1 mm. However, early attempts to attain a near-perfect procedure were sometimes disappointing, for various reasons. The poor quality of some stereotactic frames was responsible for the lack of precision of the final target area. These early attempts at localization contributed to the development of neurophysiology, which began in 1962 with Guiot et al[75] and others.[7,8,69,152,153] The localization of lesions progressed according to several types of information: anatomical landmarks, electrophysiological activity of various nuclei, and, later, stimulation effects may have led to more accurate targets.

Evolution of Ideas About Targets

The anatomical distinction between cortex, white matter, and the basal ganglia had been described as early as the 17th century by Willis, and in greater detail in the 18th century by Vicq d'Azyr, who first described a segregated thalamus.[128,131,133] The search for relationships between anatomical sites or structures and physiological functions was dominated by such luminaries as Charcot and Pitres (1877),[46] Broca (1861),[35] Bastian (1909),[17] and others, who proved through now-famous patient observations that cerebral functions could be impaired by focal lesions. The basal ganglia became a center of interest with the results of clinicopathological studies on disorders such as Huntington's disease, lethargic encephalitis, and of course the observation of degeneration of the substantia nigra.[157,160] Later, observations of putamenal necrosis following carbon dioxide intoxication provided additional data. The functions of the basal ganglia were for a long time based upon the use of such crude tools as lesions and stimulation. The results were disappointing, because lesions often did not produce visible deficits and stimulation could not reproduce specific behaviors or functions. This was due to the insufficient or erroneous concepts of the organization of the basal ganglia and thalamus; however, it contributed to the evolution of knowledge and led to the concepts of functional loops or networks, which we are just starting to understand.[128,131,133] The major breakthrough was made many years later, with the discovery of striatal dopamine depletion and the logically expected improvement in parkinsonian symptoms by L-DOPA.[27] Further understanding of the regulation of movement and of movement disorders will require considerable integration of data from various sources: anatomical, connective, chemical, and electrophysiological (in terms of patterns, not only excitatory or inhibitory inputs), as well as data from pathology and from surgery.

Guridi and Lozano[77] (1997) stressed that Spatz's demonstration in 1927,[145] of the concept of an extrapyramidal system (including the striatum, pallidum, subthalamic nucleus, substantia nigra, red nucleus, and dentate nucleus) was a major step in the evolution of neurosurgical concepts of movement disorders. Percheron et al[128] in 1994 carefully described the long, sometimes erratic, often misleading, and still incomplete evolution of ideas on the basal ganglia system. Whatever the level of understanding of this system was, it provided a more rational and functional substrate for what must be recognized as an experimental approach in human patients with movement disorders. In an early series of 16 patients (1942, 1959), Meyers,[115,117] in an attempt to alleviate the hyperkinetic and hypertonic features of parkinsonism and similar disorders—chorea, athetosis, and dystonia—severed or extirpated structures such as the caudate head (his first target, which he resected intentionally on the basis of the emerging concept of the extrapyramidal system), the ansa lenticularis, the anterior limb of the internal capsule, and the oral third of the globus pallidus and of the putamen. Encouraging results were observed mainly in parkinsonian patients, in whom tremor could be abolished and rigidity significantly improved but never cured. His continuing investigations showed that the most effective lesion sites were the ansa lenticularis (ansotomy of the pallidofugal fibers) and the anterior limb of the internal capsule. These areas could be lesioned without inducing signs of pyramidal dysfunction, which were customary following previously used surgical procedures such as cervical chordotomy, motor and premotor cortical extirpation, and the later-developed lateral midbrain crusotomy. These surgical methods were not directed at the pathophysiological changes of the disorders for they were not known until recently, but at the motor symptoms, which were expected to be reduced by alteration of the cerebral motor function areas.

The Striatum

Resection of the caudate nucleus, whether or not associated with the putamen and anterior limb of the internal capsule was carried out by Meyers[113-117] in the 1940s and 1950s, using a transventricular approach as others were doing. The published results varied from 45% to 62% for good outcome for tremor, but the mortality rate also varied from 12% to 41%. Striatal targets are no longer used for lesioning and have not yet been used for stimulation; however, they have triggered a specific interest in neural graft surgery. The striatum appears to be the main, if not the only, site of projection from the dopamine cells of the pars compacta of the substantia nigra, which connect with D_1 and D_2 receptor-bearing striatal cells. These striatal cells, according to the parallel process model,[10] project through two different pathways onto the pallidal (and pars reticulata of the substantia nigra [SNr]) neurons, either directly or indirectly (through a relay in the external segment of the globus pallidus [GPe], which exerts a gamma-aminobutyric acid [GABA]ergic action on the cells of the subthalamic nucleus, which in turn produce glutamatergic outputs) onto the GABAergic targets in the SNr and the internal segment of the globus pallidus (GPi).[129] Then, a meaningful strategy would be to reinnervate the deafferented striatum by grafting dopamine cells into it, which could deliver the missing dopamine locally to the D_1 and D_2 dopamine-sensitive neurons. The large size of the striatum and its good stereotactic accessibility are additional factors that make it an ideal target.

The GPi and Related Targets

Although its function is not completely determined yet (is it purely motor? involved in motivation? in learning skills? in cognition? are its connections cortical? limbic? hippocampal? thalamic?), the pallidum is a target that neurosurgeons appreciate because of its size and consequent visibility. On MRI it appears with high accuracy and spatial resolution. However, this large nucleus has a spatially and somatotopically complex organization; accurate localization of the site of a lesion or of electrode implantation is difficult and requires a local functional assessment. This is made even more difficult because of its shape; the pallidum is wider in its anterior part than in its posterior tail, which continuously narrows.

Despite these facts, the pallidum is periodically subject to renewed interest,[71,72] as is the case currently. Initially targeted following the serendipitous observations of Cooper[47] in 1953, its role as an ablative target was rationalized by a series of experimental works and by the introduction of stereotactic methods. Despite an extensive and often rigorous practice,[151] it was abandoned after poor results for akinesia and rigidity and better results of the thalamic targets for tremor in the pre-levodopa era. Cooper also extensively studied the clinical effectiveness and the surgical complications of targeting different parts of the pallidum. Spiegel and Wycis[148] and later Gillingham[70] targeted the pallidum or the ansa as the efferent gateway of the basal ganglia. Narabayashi and colleagues[118,119] did the same, on the basis that parkinsonism was believed to result from an imbalance between the pallidum and the striatum. The size of the pallidum and the fact that its complex organization was not yet totally understood prevented precise localization of the target for a lesion. Leksell, in a systematic approach to this problem, investigated the different parts of this nucleus and found that the posteromedial part of the GPi was the most efficient target. The heterogeneity of the GPi is due to its afferent as well as its efferent connections. The sensorimotor area of the pallidum is mostly ventroposterior and medial,[54,84,91,124,125] while the pallidotomies of the pre-levodopa era mostly involved the anterodorsal part of the GPi, and sometimes even the GPe.

During the post-levodopa era, a new disorder of iatrogenic origin appeared, which rapidly led to abnormal involuntary movements. No medical treatment was available for it and it did not consistently respond to thalamotomy. Laitinen and colleagues[95] have recently resuscitated the GPi as a target through the posterolateral ventral pallidectomy. They explained this revival by a slight modification to the original Leksell technique. Success was essentially due to the remarkable effects on abnormal involuntary movements, although outcome for akinesia, rigidity, and tremor is reported as variable. The clinical improvement, as compared to Leksell's reported results, remains to be demonstrated.

One must not be indifferent to the variability of the results reported in different series, which could be related to an underlying substrate rather than purely to variability between the skills of various teams. Even though early neurosurgical reports often lacked careful clinical assessment and precise localization of the lesion or the electrodes, the variability in results could be related to the inherent variability of localization in a large structure that encompasses heterogeneous anatomical elements, such as aggregates of neuronal bodies defining subnuclear segregation of the pallidum, or bundles of efferent fibers in the ansa lenticularis and fasciculus lenticularis. The considerable amount of experimental data provided in 1971 by DeLong and his group[54] and others[61] neither improved these results nor alleviated the complications reported after bilateral procedures. The recent introduction of chronic electrical stimulation/inhibition of the GPi[130,134] will allow for a more precise dissection of physiological effects related to localization.

The Thalamus and Its Subnuclei

Interest has centered on the thalamus as a result of both fortuitous observation and deliberate anatomical investigation. In the 1950s, studies by Cooper[48,52,53] of postmortem controls of surgical lesions aimed at the pallidum showed that parts of the thalamus (ventral lateral nucleus) were sometimes destroyed and still were consistent with a good functional effect on tremor. In the early 1960s, because of the disappointing results of pallidal surgery in German investigations, Hassler et al[78,79] studied pallidal projections in pallidotomy autopsy cases and showed that pallidofugal fibers, originating from the GPi, projected to the anterior lateral nuclei of the thalamus. It was then confirmed that thalamotomy could replace pallidotomy[32,78,79] for the relief of tremor. Consequently, an empirical effort was made to delineate the smallest site where lesions could achieve the best results with minimal side effects. This culminated in the identification of a low and lateral nucleus of the thalamus, which clearly appeared to be the VIM nucleus identified by Hassler's group and others.[78,79,122,164]

The VIM nucleus is composed of large, darkly stained neurons, located between the ventral lateral nucleus and the ventral caudal or ventral posterior nuclei in higher primates. Its function is difficult to understand, as it is anatomically defined by cerebellar and vestibular afferents[130,132] and physiologically defined by its kinesthetic afferents. A short-latency field potential is produced by electrical stimulation of large afferent fibers in the contralateral limb,[122,164] and some neurons may respond to passive activation of joints and muscles and exhibit neuronal activity synchronous with tremor in patients during surgical procedures.[7,8,19-21,99,100,122,164] This is a matter of debate, as no proprioceptive afferent from the spinal cord has been observed and as experimental sectioning of sensory afferents has not suppressed tremor in animal studies.[6,96] However, recent intraoperative observations, including those by the authors, support the kinesthetic afferent hypothesis: postoperative stimulation of the VIM nucleus in parkinsonian patients stops tremor without including any cerebellar symptoms, which would appear, however, if the intensity of stimulation current was increased far above the tremor suppression threshold, corresponding to an increased and unassessable current spread. This fits in with the observation that thalamotomy induces fewer cerebellar symptoms (8.6%) than subthalamotomy (40.8%), which comes closer to the cerebellothalamic projections.[164] However, these concepts are not mutually exclusive, as the observation of anatomical connections does not impose their participation in every function related to a given structure. This also has obviously important implications in the understanding of tremor mechanisms.

If the VIM nucleus has replaced the ventral lateral nucleus in the search for the best target for tremor suppression, with the help of microrecordings, centrum medianum-parafascicularis, which has been proposed for chronic stimulation by Andy,[11] is still under evaluation. Its cholinergic afferents suggest it could have a prominent role in the control of tremor.

Similarly, the ventral oral posterior and ventral oral anterior nuclei are periodically claimed to be better targets than the VIM nucleus for rigidity, dystonia, or abnormal movements. However, this will remain an academic discussion until good anatomical and clinical correlation with indisputable localization data has been provided.

The pulvinar now seems to be an obsolete target for tremor or pain control. Moreover, its role in cognitive processes and language suggests that lesioning it would induce many adverse effects.[51]

The Subthalamic Nucleus

Subthalamic lesions are known to produce ballismus and hypotonia. Historically, many surgical lesions have been localized in a region called "the subthalamic area." In fact, these were probably in the cerebellar afferents of the thalamus, namely, the fields of Forel.[12,78,79] This is different from the subthalamic nucleus (STN), or corpus luysi, which is a structure well defined anatomically (almond-shaped and located above the lateral border of the substantia nigra), chemically (filled with a dense population of glutamatergic neurons), and functionally (receiving GABAergic afferents from the GPe and sending its glutamatergic efferents to the GPi and the SNr). It has been demonstrated that the neuronal firing rate in the STN is exacerbated in Parkinson's disease (patients and animal models) and that its destruction or inhibition[3,13,22,23] suppresses parkinsonian symptoms. Due to the reversibility and the low morbidity of chronic electrical neuroinhibition of the STN, this procedure has been commonly used in parkinsonian patients since 1993.[101] If current results are confirmed by further clinical evaluation, the STN could be one of the best targets for functional neurosurgery to treat Parkinson's disease.

The Cerebral Cortex

History has not shown that cortical lesions can suppress tremor, even if positron emission tomography (PET) studies have revealed overactivity of motor and premotor areas in the presence of tremor. However, neurophysiological recordings have demonstrated the presence of rhythmic discharges synchronous with tremor. The hypothesis that the cerebral cortex could be a target is supported, however, by the intraoperative observation that stimulation of the premotor cortex suppresses rest tremor in parkinsonian patients[163] (Tsubokawa T, Yamamoto T, Katayama Y: Chronic thalamic stimulation for relief of ballistic involuntary movement. XIIth Meeting of the World Society for Stereotactic and Functional Neurosurgery. Ixtapa, Mexico, October 11-15, 1993) and by the recent observation of improvement in posttraumatic tremor following chronic cortical motor area stimulation.[121] However, the use of the cortex as a target is impeded by the risk of stimulation-induced seizures, which cannot be easily predicted or prevented by careful evaluation of current intensity.

Other Potential Targets

Lesions of the cerebellar nuclei were tested in the treatment of parkinsonism, with poor results.[156] The dentate nucleus was removed during open procedures, with a high mortality rate, and stereotactic dentatectomy was proposed in the treatment of spasticity and dystonia, with a relative improvement in pyramidal spasticity.[81,165]

Ablative Surgical Techniques For Parkinson's Disease

Several ablative techniques to interrupt, destroy, or inactivate the functional target have been used over the years. Mechanical probes (blades and leukotomes) were the first tools used in these surgical procedures. Ligation of the anterior choroidal artery, as defined by Cooper[47] in 1953 from the serendipitous process following pedunculotomy, was used for a period of time but remains the only example of such a technique.

Chemical lesions were used in freehand targeting of the pallidum and also in other stereotactic procedures, such as frontobasal leukotomy. Alcohol was the earliest neurotoxic agent and has now been replaced, at least in experimental situations, by specific agents such as kainic acid or ibotenic acid. Cooper, when carrying out chemopallidectomy,[48,53] found it difficult to know whether the alcohol was restricted to the pallidum or extended to thalamopallidal connections. He then designed a method using catheters equipped with balloons, which allowed an initial injection of etopalin to prevent the reflux of alcohol that was later injected into the cavity made by the balloon. With much experience using this method, he was able to report high levels of success, with up to 90% of rigidity alleviated and 85% of tremor, and a mortality rate that decreased to 2.5%.[52] Narabayashi[118] used procaine hydrochloride to simulate lesions and then created permanent lesions by mixing procaine oil with wax.

Ultrasonography was used a few years later in an attempt to more accurately control the size of the lesions.[117] Temperature extremes of either hot or cold were, and sometimes still are, used to make lesions in various parts of the brain.[50,98] With thermal lesions, it is easier to control the size, and this procedure also allows reversible simulation by small changes in temperature before permanent lesioning.

In order to create reliable and reproducible lesions in size, beta-emitters such as yttrium-90 pellets were used by Talairach et al[153] and others[31] in stereotactic thalamotomy and pallidotomy. This allowed precise intraoperative assessment of the site of the lesion (unmistakably shown by the yttrium pellet) and of its size (known to be reliable from animal studies). The drawback was that the effect usually took time to be established and thus did not allow intraoperative control of the efficiency of the procedure.

Radiofrequency lesions have been the most

frequently employed method, allowing initial stimulation and even recording of neural activity through the electrodes. The lesion can be progressively increased in size to obtain an intraoperatively controllable effect. Radiofrequency, which acts by liberating heat through the mechanism of energy loss by Eddy-Foucault currents, induces a local coagulation of cellular proteins without the creation of vapor bubbles, microexplosions, or rupture of vessels that can be observed during electrical coagulation. A large amount of literature has been devoted to the correlation between the size of the lesion and the parameters of electrocoagulation.

Augmentative Surgical Techniques for Parkinson's Disease

Electrical Stimulation

Therapeutic applications of electrical stimulation of the brain go back to the early history of biology, when Scribonius Largus discovered that the sensory shocks experienced by human beings in contact with torpedo fish could cure or heal rheumatic diseases, as is depicted in some Pompeiian mosaics. These sensory effects, which were later related to electricity through the pioneering work of Volta,[45] demonstrate that biological cells can both produce and be sensitive to electricity. It is striking that bioelectricity as well as various attempts to use it therapeutically were intensively investigated and saw tremendous popularity during previous centuries, from Aldini's experiments on humans in Italy to Mesmer's social entertainment in Paris, in the late 18th century.

For various reasons, no doubt mainly technological because it was not easy to produce electricity, these techniques fell into oblivion. The rebirth of bioelectricity came with the discovery of the electrical nature of nerve impulses, in the electrophysiological work of Lapique and others on electrical excitability and conduction properties of nerves, and finally, in 1952, with the breakthrough of the elucidation of the membrane potential by Hodgkin and Huxley,[83] who with Katz won a Nobel prize. Since that time, electrical stimulation has been associated with excitation of neural structures. The negative electrode being the most effective, it has by extrapolation been considered the "active" electrode.

Transposition of these fundamental discoveries to in vivo practice in the 19th century was done essentially in experimental procedures investigating the response of neural structures to excitation, first in animals (Aldini in Italy following his uncle Volta)[45] and then in humans (Hitzig and Fritsch[82] following Aldini). The electrical activity of living tissues also was recorded, which led to the development of electrocardiography and electroencephalography. The demonstration of a relationship between epilepsy and abnormal electrical activity of the brain was probably the major event to promote the study of bioelectricity among the medical community, and specifically the neurological and neurosurgical fields.

The parallel development of the concept of noninvasive therapy led to neurostimulation methods, considered to be "neuroaugmentive," as opposed to ablative or destructive, procedures. Therefore, a wide spectrum of neurostimulation procedures was investigated, including transcutaneous nerve stimulation, epidural spinal cord stimulation, cortical cerebellar stimulation, and deep brain stimulation targeting the opioid neural structures of the periaqueductal gray matter and the somatosensory nuclei of the thalamus. This period of investigation has extended from the early 1950s up to the present and has been essentially aimed at the treatment of pain, but also of rigidity, epilepsy, and movement disorders. The effect of chronic stimulation on movement disorders was observed and reported long ago but did not lead to a firm conclusion. Along with its effect on pain, this was brought to the therapeutic level by Bechtchereva et al[18] in 1972.

Neurostimulation has been directed at various structures, including the somatosensory thalamus[112,142] the centrum medianum-parafascicularis,[11] the cerebellum and the dentate nucleus,[50,51] and the VIM nucleus.[8,30,43,154] Various frequencies have also been used, such as 30 Hz in the ventral posterolateral (VPL) nucleus of the thalamus,[112,142] 75-150 Hz in the medial thalamus,[33] and 300 Hz in the ventral caudal and VPL nuclei.[154] The movement disorders treated have included cerebellar tremor of multiple sclerosis,[33] dyskinesias from sensory deafferentation,[112,142] or spasticity, Huntington's chorea, dystonia, torticollis, and others.

It was during the practice of neurostimulation, mainly during intraoperative electrophysiological investigations, that a clear relationship was established between the electrical frequency and the clinical effects,[19-21] which led to a new concept of high-frequency electrical neuroinhibition. The safety, reversibility, and adaptability of electrical neuroinhibition opened new clinical investigations of various targets, ranging from previous targets of destructive stereotaxy (such as the thalamus and pallidum) to structures previously considered untouchable (such as the STN).

Neurostimulation has been applied since the 19th century. In the beginning it was done with crude electrical instruments, resulting in disappointing effects such as diffuse motor contractions.[60] Horsley and Beevor[86] reported the cortical stimulation experiments done by Ferrier. Many years later, electrical stimulation of the septum,[80] the periventricular gray matter and brain stem,[15] the internal capsule,[2] the striatum,[55] and the VPL nucleus[87] was proposed for pain relief, using stereotactic procedures. This long-lasting experience with brain stimulation showed, as expected, that chronic low-voltage stimulation was well tolerated by neuronal and glial cells. Precise subcortical electrical discharges were applied to assess the efficacy of the chosen targets intraoperatively.[24,161] This technique was then applied by many neurosurgeons, because suppression of tremor by transient electrical inhibition was at least an improvement before making an irreversible lesion. Some investigators left stimulating electrodes implanted for hours or days and observed that tremor relief continued, without the development of tolerance.[11,23] Chronic cerebellar stimulation was also tried for spasticity due to cerebral palsy and for intractable epilepsy.[159] Benabid et al[21] in 1987 permanently implanted electrodes in patients who had undergone previous contralateral thalamotomy (to prevent the possible adverse effects of bilateral lesions), and later extended the technique to unilateral or bilateral stimulation. This procedure was further developed by other teams.[9,31,143,144] The lack of neuronal lesions after long-term stimulation[44] encouraged the investigation of new targets, the GPi[143,144] and the STN.[101]

Electrical Inhibition

In 1967, Guiot et al[74] wrote: "Sterotactic surgery has won its title of nobility: it is called 'functional surgery.' However, its goal is to destroy cellular centers or to interrupt neural pathways. It is therefore purely suppressive." This is no longer true, because we now have the means to achieve the same end, with reversible neural inhibition (of cells or fibers). Similarly, in 1961, Talairach et al[153] wrote that "this new orientation of a truly functional surgery of Parkinson's disease principally concerns afferents . . . aiming at the modification of the functional status of complex neuronal networks, involved in control and regulation of motor activity and tone, rather than destroying hypothetical subcortical centers. . . ." This replaced "procedures more directly anatomically aimed at the [motor] effector at various levels . . . at the cost of variably reversible motor deficits." This tendency toward a more functional stereotaxy has created the need for less destructive methods.

Effects of Thalamic Electrical Stimulation on Movement Disorders and Tremor

Cerebral and, later, thalamic electrical discharges were first applied in experimental conditions, when electrical devices were reliable enough to avoid large cerebral lesions due to uncontrollable current intensity. The reason for these early experiments was to assess what happened when a current was applied to neurons.

The first long-lasting electrical stimulations were done at the origin of rather heroic and important studies,[34,112] beginning in the 1960s. These researchers implanted electrodes on the surface of the visual cortex of a blind nurse[34] or in the thalamus of patients suffering from chronic intractable pain.[112] The results of these experiments had several interesting effects. First, the "cranial taboo," which held that devices cannot be placed into a human brain without the certainty of a direct benefit, had been broken and this did not provoke the serious social and intellectual repercussions that many had feared.[64] Second, these studies demonstrated that chronic electrical impulses applied to neurons and glial cells with an implanted foreign device were well tolerated in humans. This question could have taken years to resolve using only animal experiments.

Discovery of the Relationship Between High Frequency and Inhibitory Effects

The effects of electrical stimulation on movement disorders was observed as soon as it was used, which was initially as an intraoperative investigational method. The resulting data did not produce a clear-cut conclusion, as these papers did not have as the primary aim the systematic demonstration of the relationship between stimulation parameters and induced effects. Stimulation was reported as sometimes improving and sometimes worsening tremor. Stimulation frequencies varied from 30 to 300 Hz.[120] The fact that it could be used as therapy was enough to lead some neurosurgeons[11,33,112,142,154] to try it as a chronic method. However, these attempts did not provide convincing, long-lasting effects, in part because strict frequency conditions were not observed, and therefore were discontinued.

During the authors' practice of thalamotomy, the systematic use of stimulation at 30 and 100 Hz intraoperatively showed clearly that tremor was not controlled or was worsened at 30 Hz (it could be precisely driven even at frequencies of <10 Hz) and was consistently and totally suppressed at 100 Hz, in a fully reversible manner. This led the authors to propose this method to patients who had undergone a previous unilateral thalamotomy.[21] The results were so striking that the method was immediately used as a first intention technique and performing deep brain lesions has not stopped since that time.

Replacement of Thalamotomy by High-Frequency Stimulation or Neuroinhibition and Extension to Other Targets

Chronic implanted devices had been used in experimental pain treatment since 1970. At that time, there was no ethical opposition to the application of the same technique to movement disorders. The good results of the technique led to the worldwide development of deep brain stimulation to treat movement disorders and to the suggestion that other targets than the VIM nucleus be tried.

Basic research had proved that the STN was a key structure in the organization of the basal ganglia and that its destruction suppressed parkinsonian symptoms in monkeys exposed to 1-methyl-4-phenyl-1,2,3,6-tetrahydropyridine (MPTP).[13,23,97] As lesioning of the STN could not be performed in humans, it was then proved that electrical neuroinhibition could achieve the same effects as lesioning in the same monkey model,[22] which made the first human application possible.[101] Following the same logic, the GPi, already validated by pallidotomy, became another target for electrical neuroinhibition.[144]

Grafting Neural Tissue

In the treatment of Parkinson's disease, grafting cells competent in the production of the missing neurotransmitter opens a new chapter aimed at treating the cause of the disease rather than suppressing its consequences. This field of research has expanded tremendously during the last decade. There is no doubt that a new chapter remains to be written, concerning applications of gene therapy to restoring cells to their lost primary functions. The necessity of performing local transfection will mandate these methods being registered in the field of neurosurgery.

Today an experimental procedure, neural tissue grafting, will undoubtedly be a major component of the therapeutic armamentarium in the future. Grafting neural tissue into the brain is one of the dreams that would, in theory, be able to change human destiny. This is probably why these methods have overcome the enormous ethical, biological, and technical difficulties they have encountered, although they still have poor therapeutic efficacy. First performed a century ago,[155] they became a subject of scientific interest and intense investigation in the 1970s.

The experimental period started with the successful grafting of monoamine neurons,[150] fetal dopaminergic neurons,[28,29,66] and adrenal gland[67] in rat models of Parkinson's disease (such as the denervated striatum in rodents that had previously undergone unilateral injections of 6-hydroxydopamine, producing extensive lesions of the substantia nigra).[28,29] Since then, it has been convincingly demonstrated that functional recovery depends on graft survival and dopaminergic fiber ingrowth into the denervated striatum, forming abundant synaptic contacts with the striatal neurons.[68] The graft also receives fibers from the host brain[110] and is metabolically and physiologically active.[138,141] Moreover, human fetal dopaminergic neurons are able to survive transplantation into the denervated striatum of immunosuppressed or athymic rats.[37,88]

After an experimental period sometimes considered too short, a patient with Parkinson's disease received a stereotactically implanted adrenal gland autograft for the first time in 1982.[14,102,103] The procedure was then widely used after a group of Mexican neurosurgeons performed a transventricular autograft of adrenal gland tissue in the caudate nucleus.[108,109] This showed that grafting procedures could be done simply, using autograft from the patient with a non-stereotactic procedure. However, the mortality (5%-10%) and the morbidity (24%) rates appeared unacceptable and clinical results were poor; moreover, conflicting results were reported.[71,72,90-92] Nevertheless, several hundred patients were treated by this method,[127] with unconvincing results. In 1989, the first clinical trials were reported using human fetal neurons stereotactically grafted into the striatum.[106] Since then, several series of patients have been carefully selected and postoperatively followed. They all needed immunosuppressive treatment with cyclosporine, except in one study with comparable results.[65] Following the leadership and according to the guidelines of the Swedish group,[104,107] mortality as well as morbidity have been dramatically reduced, clinical evaluation shows better and more stable improvement, and, in a few patients, PET has demonstrated the survival of the graft and its metabolic and physiological activities.[140]

Because of this slow progress, and to overcome obstacles and concerns,[158] other attempts have been made.[166] These have included:

1. the use of autologous sympathetic cervical ganglion, to avoid cyclosporine.[89]
2. amnion transplantation to provide non-neurotransmitter trophic factors that will induce neuronal sprouting.[16]
3. encapsulated cells to prevent immunogenicity.[4,5]
4. genetically engineered cells (*ex vivo* gene therapy with skin fibroblasts or muscle cells) to synthesize enzymes, such as tyrosine hydroxylase, or growth factors.[139]

Gene transfer is also a very recent development, but may provide some hope for transfecting genes in situ to induce the targeted cells to produce dopamine or growth factors. The mechanism itself is still being debated; the release of dopamine does not seem to be involved, or at least does not work alone, and the improvement of clinical effects could be related to trophic factors induced by the surgical trauma, to alterations of the blood brain barrier, or to liberation of neuropeptides.

For the moment, as stated by the investigators themselves, "neural transplantation is still an experimental approach, and not a therapeutic alternative, in Parkinson's disease. Several scientific and technical issues need to be clarified with further animal experiments in parallel with the assessment of different grafting procedures in patients."[105]

Neurosurgical Treatment of Other Movement Disorders

Parkinson's disease is certainly not the only movement disorder,[126] but it has a particularly special place: it is mainly due to the defect of one neurotransmitter produced by a small number of cells located in a restricted area. It can be cured or compensated by the administration of a single drug that is a rather simple molecule. The action of this molecule is essentially to suppress a brake that acts globally on motion. This is probably why, when a treatment is efficient, it can provide >80% improvement, which is almost never observed in other diseases that likely have more complex mechanisms.

Dystonia

The very first attempt at functional surgery was to treat disabling athetosis, which was later classified as a dystonia, although this is still debated. Athetosis due to basal ganglia lesions resulting from neonatal icterus disappeared 15-20 years ago, due to the prevention of this particular severe obstetrical complication.[63] Prior to that time, however, these abnormal movements were severely disabling and required surgical procedures, even if surgery induced hemiplegia. Horsley,[85] Bucy and colleagues,[38-41] and other neurosurgeons had used topectomy in such cases. In the same type of patients, Putnam[136] performed pyramidotomy, either unilaterally or bilaterally.

Another extinct disease is the von Economo-Cruchet lethargic encephalitis, which started in 1917 in Europe and spread throughout the world until 1928. Although patients usually recovered spontaneously, many of them exhibited parkinsonian syndromes. This syndrome differed from idiopathic Parkinson's disease because of a very slow worsening and because of the predominance of movement disorders, mainly dystonia.[1,42] In these patients, different types of stereotactic lesions were applied to treat tremor and dyskinesias; these were observed before the levodopa era and worsened when the drug was administered. Narabayashi et al[119] in 1984 reported improvement or suppression of these dyskinesias after stereotactic lesioning of the ventral lateral thalamic nucleus. Cooper[49] reported a large study including 400 patients with dystonia resulting from local or degenerative disorders. Up to 70% obtained a moderate to marked improvement of symptoms over the long term. The targets he used varied: the ventral lateral nucleus, centrum medianum, and even the pulvinar, but he did not specify what was the most efficient target.

It is now possible to differentiate essential or secondary dystonia with the help of more precise morphological MRI studies of the brain. We thus have to select patients according to the mechanism of the dystonia and the location of the lesion responsible for the dystonia, which could also account for the choice of targets. Two targets have been studied: the GPi and the VPL thalamic nucleus, but their results are inconsistent, and we are not able at the present time to predict the efficacy of lesions or of electrical neuroinhibition based on clinical or anatomical criteria. Essential dystonia usually involves axial muscles. For this reason, the efficacy of deep brain stimulation is thought to be rather low, and the few cases reported are not sufficient to prove its efficacy. Stimulation of the VPL nucleus was effective in one patient with posttraumatic dystonia due to a brain stem lesion. It can thus be assumed that dystonia is not the best indication for deep brain stimulation, whatever the target is.

Spasmodic Torticollis

Spasmodic torticollis is often an idiopathic movement disorder, occurring in young patients. As with all other disabling dyskinesias, patients were referred to neurosurgeons until the efficacy and safety of botulinum toxin injections was demonstrated. Prior to that discovery, bilateral stereotactic lesions of the thalamus were made, with variable effect. Unilateral thalamic lesions were ineffective. Cooper[49] in 1977 reported an improvement in up to 60% of patients, but considered it unethical to offer bilateral thalamotomy, because 40% were not improved or were worsened, with the risk of dysarthria and cognitive dysfunction. More recently, surgery seems to be making a comeback, following the reported good results of posterior rhizotomy.[26]

Conclusion

The history of neurosurgery for movement disorders developed over more than half a century. It has been dominated by the continuing efforts of neurosurgeons and neurologists dedicated to the relief of severely disabling abnormal movements. When medical treatment could not offer an alternative, neurosurgeons tried, with almost no success, to suppress the disorder by altering cerebral function. This led to a panel of ablative procedures, from the cortex to the spinal cord or even the peripheral nerves. Investigators consciously integrated the emerging concepts provided by anatomical studies. Their efforts were temporarily made obsolete when the progress of biochemistry drew neurologists into this field of therapeutics and at the same time triggered a growing interest in the nosological dissection of symptoms, which culminated in the recognition of syndromes. The postmortem study of patients who had been carefully followed, which for a long time remained the main tool for scientific research in neurosciences, provided data that helped to increase knowledge. Surgery for abnormal movements would never have been revived if L-DOPA had not had drawbacks; the appearance of fluctuations and abnormal involuntary movements after a few years of L-DOPA therapy not only reactivated interest in pallidotomy, but forced neurosurgeons to create new and less aggressive methods to treat these patients. The discovery of augmentative procedures, particularly electrical neuroinhibition, has opened a totally new type of surgery characterized by safety and reversibility, which will depend on the recognition of new and powerful targets reached with increasing precision.

References

1. Achart P: **L'encéphalite Léthargique.** Paris: Baillère et fils, 1921
2. Adams JE, Hosobuchi Y, Fields HL: Stimulation of internal capsule for relief of chronic pain. **J Neurosurg 41:**740-744, 1974
3. Aebischer P, Goddard M: Treating Parkinson's disease with lesions of the subthalamic nucleus. **Science 252:**133, 1991
4. Aebischer P, Tresco PA, Winn S, et al: Long-term cross-species brain transplantation of a polymer-encapsulated dopamine-secreting cell line. **Exp Neurol 111:**269-275, 1991
5. Aebischer P, Winn SR, Galletti PM: Transplantation of neural tissue in polymer capsules. **Brain Res 448:** 364-368, 1988
6. Albe-Fessard D: Interactions entre recherches fondamentale et clinique. Deux exemples tirés d'une expérience personnelle. **Can J Neurol Sci 15:**324-332, 1988
7. Albe-Fessard D, Arfel G, Guiot G, et al: Activités électriques caractéristiques de quelques structures cérébrales chez l'homme. **Ann Chir 17:**1185-1214, 1963
8. Albe-Fessard D, Arfel G, Guiot G, et al: Dérivation d'activités spontanées et évoquées dans les structures cérébrales profondes de l'homme. **Rev Neurol 2:** 89-105, 1962
9. Alesch F, Pinter MM, Helscher RJ, et al: Stimulation of the ventral intermediate thalamic nucleus in tremor dominated Parkinson's disease and essential tremor. **Acta Neurochir 136:**75-81, 1995
10. Alexander GE, Crutcher MD: Functional architecture of basal ganglia circuits: neural substrates of parallel processing. **Trends Neurosci 13:**266-271, 1990
11. Andy OJ: Thalamic stimulation for control of movement disorders. **Appl Neurophysiol 46:**107-111, 1983
12. Andy OJ, Jurko MF, Sias FR Jr: Subthalamotomy in treatment of Parkinsonian tremor. **J Neurosurg 20:** 860-870, 1963
13. Aziz TZ, Peggs D, Argarwal E, et al: Subthalamic nucleotomy alleviates parkinsonism in the 1-methyl-4-phenyl-1,2,3,6-tetrahydropyridine (MPTP)-exposed primate. **Br J Neurosurg 6:**575-582, 1992
14. Backlund EO, Granberg PO, Hamberger B, et al: Transplantation of adrenal medullary tissue to striatum in parkinsonism. First clinical trials. **J Neurosurg 62:**169-173, 1985
15. Balagura S, Ralph T: The analgesic effect of electrical stimulation of the diencephalon and mesencephalon. **Brain Res 60:**369-379, 1973
16. Bankiewicz KS, Palmatier M, Plunkett RJ, et al: Reversal of hemiparkinsonian syndrome in nonhuman primates by amnion implantation into caudate nucleus. **J Neurosurg 81:**869-876, 1994
17. Bastian C: The functions of the kinaesthesic area of the brain. **Brain 32:**327-341, 1909
18. Bechtchereva N, Bondartchuk A, Smirnov V, et al: Therapeutic electrostimulations of the brain deep structures. **Vopr Neirokhir 1:**7-12, 1972
19. Benabid AL, Pollak P, Gao D, et al: Chronic electrical stimulation of the ventralis intermedius nucleus of the thalamus as a treatment of movement disorders. **J Neurosurg 84:**203-214, 1996
20. Benabid AL, Pollak P, Gervason C, et al: Long-term suppression of tremor by chronic stimulation of the ventral intermediate thalamic nucleus. **Lancet 337:** 403-406, 1991
21. Benabid AL, Pollak P, Louveau A, et al: Combined (thalamotomy and stimulation) stereotactic surgery of the VIM thalamic nucleus for bilateral Parkinson disease. **Appl Neurophysiol 50:**344-346, 1987
22. Benazzouz A, Gross C, Féger J, et al: Reversal of rigidity and improvement in motor performance by subthalamic high-frequency stimulation in MPTP-treated monkeys. **Eur J Neurosci 5:**382-389, 1993
23. Bergman H, Wichmann T, DeLong MR: Reversal of experimental parkinsonism by lesions of the subthalamic nucleus. **Science 249:**1436-1438, 1990
24. Bertrand C: Functional localization with monopolar stimulation. **J Neurosurg 24:**403-409, 1966
25. Bertrand C: Localization of lesions. **J Neurosurg 24:** 446-448, 1966
26. Bertrand C, Martinez N, Gauthier C: Surgical treatment of parkinsonism: the use of a pneumotaxic guide with recording and stimulation. **Can Med Assoc J 82:**921-923, 1960
27. Birkmayer W, Birkmayer J: The L-Dopa story, in Calme DB (ed): **Parkinsonism and Aging.** New York, NY: Raven Press 1989, pp 1-7
28. Björklund A, Stenevi U: Reconstruction of the nigrostriatal dopamine pathway by intracerebral nigral transplants. **Brain Res 177:**555-560, 1979
29. Björklund A, Stenevi U, Dunnett S, et al: Functional reactivation of the deafferented neostriatum by nigral transplants. **Nature 289:**497-499, 1981
30. Blond S, Caparros-Lefebvre D, Parker F: Control of tremor and involuntary movement disorders by chronic stereotactic stimulation of the ventral intermediate thalamic nucleus. **J Neurosurg 77:**62-68,

1992
31. Blond S, Musolino A, Munari C, et al: Intérêts de la destruction stéréotaxique bifocale en cas de dyskinésies chez des patients ayant une infirmité motrice d'origine cérébrale. **Neurochirurgie 33:**455-461, 1987
32. Bravo GJ, Cooper IS: A clinical and radiological correlation of the lesions produced by chemopallidectomy and thalamectomy. **J Neurol Neurosurg Psychiatry 22:**1-10, 1959
33. Brice J, McLellan L: Suppression of intention tremor by contingent deep-brain stimulation. **Lancet 1:** 1221-1222, 1980
34. Brindley GS, Lewin WS: The sensations produced by electrical stimulation of the visual cortex. **J Physiol 196:**479-493, 1968
35. Broca P: Perte de la parole, ramollissement chronique et destruction partielle du lobe antérieur gauche du cerveau. **Bull Soc Anthropol 11:**235-238, 1861
36. Browder J: Section of the fibers of the anterior limb of the internal capsule in Parkinsonism. **Am J Surg 75:**264-268, 1948
37. Brundin P, Nilsson OG, Strecker RE, et al: Behavioural effects of human fetal dopamine neurons grafted in a rat model of Parkinson's disease. **Exp Brain Res 65:**235-240, 1986
38. Bucy P: Cortical extirpation in the treatment of involuntary movements. **Am J Surg 75:**257-263, 1948
39. Bucy P: Cortical extirpation in the treatment of involuntary movements. **Res Nerv Ment Dis Proc 21:** 551-595, 1942
40. Bucy PC, Buchanan DN: Athetosis. **Brain 55:** 479-492, 1932
41. Bucy PC, Case TJ: Tremor. Physiologic mechanism and abolition by surgical means. **Arch Neurol Psychiatry 41:**721-746, 1939
42. Calne DB, Stern GM, Laurence DR: L-Dopa in postencephalitic parkinsonism. **Lancet 1:**744-747, 1969
43. Caparros-Lefebvre D, Blond S, Vermersch P, et al: Chronic thalamic stimulation improves tremor and levodopa induced dyskinesias in Parkinson's disease. **J Neurol Neurosurg Psychiatry 56:**268-273, 1993
44. Caparros-Lefebvre D, Ruchoux MM, Blond S, et al: Long-term thalamic stimulation in Parkinson's disease: postmortem anatomoclinical study. **Neurology 44:**1856-1860, 1995
45. Changeux JP: **L'Homme Neuronal.** Paris: Fayard, 1983, p 419
46. Charcot J, Pitres A: Contribution à l'étude des localisations dans l'écorce des hémisphères du cerveau. Observations relatives aux paralysies et aux convulsions d'origine corticale. **Rev Mens Méd Chir 1:** 1-18, 113-123, 180-195, 357-376, 437-457, 1877
47. Cooper I: Ligation of the anterior choroidal artery for involuntary movements—parkinsonism. **Psychiatr Q 27:**317-319, 1953
48. Cooper IS: Chemopallidectomy: an investigative technique in geriatric parkinsonians. **Science 121:** 217-218, 1955
49. Cooper IS: Neurosurgical treatment of the dyskinesias, in Keener EB, et al (eds): **Proceedings of the Congress of Neurosurgeons 1976.** Baltimore, Md: Williams & Wilkins, 1977, pp 367-390
50. Cooper IS: Surgical treatment of parkinsonism. **Ann Rev Med 16:**309-330, 1965
51. Cooper IS, Amin I, Chandra R: A surgical investigation of the clinical physiology of the LP-Pulvinar complex in man. **J Neurol Sci 18:**89-110, 1973
52. Cooper IS, Bravo G: Chemopallidectomy and chemothalamectomy. **J Neurosurg 15:**244-256, 1958
53. Cooper IS, Poloukhine N: Chemopallidectomy: neurosurgical technique useful in geriatric parkinsonians. **J Am Geriatr Soc 3:**839-859, 1955
54. DeLong MR: Activity of pallidal neurons during movement. **J Neurophysiol 34:**414-427, 1971
55. Ervin FR, Brown CE, Mark VH: Striatal influence on facial pain. **Confin Neurol 27:**75-86, 1966
56. Fénelon F: Bilan de quatre années de pratique d'une intervention personnelle pour maladie de Parkinson. **Rev Neurol 89:**580-585, 1953
57. Fénelon F: Essai de traitement neuro-chirurgical du syndrome parkinsonien par intervention directe sur les voies extrapyramidales immédiatement sous-striopallidales (anses lenticulaires). **Rev Neurol 83:** 580-585, 1950
58. Fénelon F: Traitement neuro-chirurgical de la maladie de Parkinson par interruption de l'anse lenticulaire. **Presse Med 59:**308-309, 1951
59. Fénelon F, Thiébaut F: Résultats du traitement neuro-chirurgical d'une rigidité parkinsonienne par intervention striopallidale unilatérale. **Rev Neurol 83:**280, 1950
60. Ferrier D: **The Function of the Brain.** London: Smith Elder, 1876
61. Filion M, Tremblay L, Bédard PJ: Abnormal influences of passive limb movement on the activity of globus pallidus neurons in parkinsonian monkeys. **Brain Res 444:**165-176, 1988
62. Foerster O: Resection of the posterior spinal nerve roots in the treatment of gastric crisis and spastic paralysis. **Proc R Soc Med 3:**226-254, 1911
63. Foley J: The athetoid syndrome. A review of a personal series. **J Neurol Neurosurg Psychiatry 46:** 289-298, 1983
64. Frank K, Hambrecht F: Present status of neural prostheses: visual, auditory and motor, in Keener EB (ed): **Clinical Neurosurgery. Proceedings of the Congress of Neurological Surgeons, New Orleans.** Baltimore, Md: Waverly Press, 1976, pp 337-346
65. Freed CR, Breeze RE, Rosenberg NL, et al: Survival of implanted fetal dopamine cells and neurologic improvement 12 to 46 months after transplantation for Parkinson's disease. **N Engl J Med 327:**1549-1555, 1992
66. Freed CR, Breeze RE, Rosenberg NL, et al: Transplantation of human fetal dopamine cells for Parkinson's disease. Results at 1 year. **Arch Neurol 47:** 505-512, 1990
67. Freed WJ, Morihisa JM, Spoor E, et al: Transplanted adrenal chromaffin cells in rat brain reduce lesion-induced rotational behaviour. **Nature 292:**351-352, 1981
68. Freund TF, Bolam JP, Björklund A: Efferent synaptic connections of grafted dopaminergic neurons reinnervating the host neostriatum: a tyrosine hydroxylase immunocytochemical study. **J Neurosci 5:** 603-616, 1985
69. Gaze RM, Gillingham FJ, Kalyanaraman S, et al: Microelectrode recordings from the human thalamus. **Brain 87:**691-706, 1964
70. Gillingham F: surgical management of the dyskine-

sias. **J Neurol Neurosurg Psychiatry 23:**347-348, 1960 (Abstract)

71. Goetz CG, Olanow CW, Koller WC, et al: Multicenter study of autologous adrenal medullary transplantation to the corpus striatum in patients with advanced Parkinson's disease. **N Engl J Med 320:** 337-341, 1989
72. Goetz CG, Tanner CM, Penn RD, et al: Adrenal medullary transplant to the striatum of patients with advanced Parkinson's disease: 1-year motor and psychomotor data. **Neurology 40:**273-276, 1990
73. Guiot G, Brion S: Traitement des mouvements anormaux pour la coagulation pallidale. Technique et résultats. **Rev Neurol 89:**578-580, 1953
74. Guiot G, Derome P, Trigo JC: Le tremblement d'attitude: indication la meilleure de la chirurgie stéréotaxique. **Presse Med 75:**2513-2518, 1967
75. Guiot G, Hardy J, Albe-Fessard D: [Precise delimination of the subcortical structures and identification of thalamic nuclei in man by stereotactic electrophysiology.] **Neurochirurgia 5:**1-18, 1962 (Fr)
76. Guiot G, Pecker J: Tractomie mésencéphalique antérieure pour tremblement parkinsonien. **Rev Neurol 81:**387-389, 1949
77. Guiridi J, Lozano A: A brief history of pallidotomy. **Neurosurgery 41:**1169-1180, 1997
78. Hassler R, Mundinger F, Riechert T: Correlations between clinical and autoptic findings in stereotaxic operations in Parkinsonism. **Confin Neurol 26:** 282-290, 1965
79. Hassler R, Riechert T, Mundinger F, et al: Physiological observations in stereotaxic operations in extrapyramidal motor disturbances. **Brain 83:**337-351, 1960
80. Heath R, Mickle W: Evaluation of seven years experience with depth electrode in human patients, in Ramey ER, O'Doherty DS (eds): **Electrical Studies on the Unanesthetized Brain.** New York, NY: Hoeber, 1960, pp 214-247
81. Heimburger RF: Dentatectomy in the treatment of dyskinetic disorders. **Confin Neurol 29:**101-106, 1967
82. Hitzig E, Fritsch G: Ueber die elektrische Erregbarkeit des Grosshirns. **Arch Anat Physiol und Wissensch Med 37:**300-322, 1870
83. Hodgkin AL, Huxley AF: A quantitative description of membrane current and its application to conduction and excitation in nerve. **J Physiol (Lond) 117:** 500-544, 1952
84. Hoover JE, Strick PL: Multiple output channels in the basal ganglia. **Science 259:**819-821, 1993
85. Horsley V: Remarks on the surgery of the central nervous system. **Br Med J 2:**1286-1292, 1890
86. Horsley V, Beevor C: A minute analysis (experimental) of the various movements produced by stimulating in the monkey different regions of the cortical center of the upper limb as defined by Professor Ferrier. **Trans R Soc London 178:**153-168, 1887
87. Hosobuchi Y, Adams JE, Rutkin B: Chronic thalamic stimulation for the control of facial anesthesia dolorosa. **Arch Neurol 29:**158-161, 1973
88. Isacson O, Brundin P, Kelly PAT, et al: Functional neuronal replacement by grafted striatal neurones in the ibotenic acid-lesioned rat striatum. **Nature 311:** 458-460, 1984
89. Itakura T, Kamei I, Nakai K, et al: Autotransplantation of superior cervical ganglion into the brain. A possible therapy for Parkinson's disease. **J Neurosurg 68:**955-959, 1988
90. Jankovic J, Grossman R, Goodman C, et al: Clinical, biochemical, and neuropathologic findings following transplantation of adrenal medulla to the caudate nucleus for treatment of Parkinson's disease. **Neurology 39:**1227-1234, 1989
91. Jiao S, Ding Y, Zhang W, et al: Adrenal medullary autografts in patients with Parkinson's disease. **N Engl J Med 321:**324-325, 1989 (Letter)
92. Kelly P, Ahlskog J, van Heerden J, et al: Adrenal medullary autograft transplantation into the striatum of patients with Parkinson's disease. **Mayo Clinic Proc 64:**282-290, 1989
93. Kelly PJ, Gillingham FJ: The long-term results of stereotaxic surgery and L-dopa therapy in patients with Parkinson's disease. A 10-year follow-up study. **J Neurosurg 53:**332-337, 1980
94. Klemme RM: Surgical treatment of dystonia, paralysis agitans and athetosis: **Arch Neurol Psychiatry 44:** 926, 1940 (Abstract)
95. Laitinen LV, Bergenheim AT, Hariz MI: Leksell's posteroventral pallidotomy in the treatment of Parkinson's disease. **J Neurosurg 76:**53-61, 1992
96. Lamarre Y, Joffroy A: Experimental tremor in monkeys activity of thalamic and precentral cortical neurons in the absence of peripheral feedback. **Adv Neurol 24:**109-112, 1979
97. Langston JW, Irwin I, Langston EB, et al: 1-Methyl-4-phenylpyridinium ion (MPP+): identification of a metabolite of MPTP, a toxin selective to the substantia nigra. **Neurosci Lett 48:**87-92, 1984
98. Le Beau J, Dondey M: Premières observations humaines de repérage de structures cérébrales profondes par refroidissement localisé et réversible au cours des interventions stéréotaxiques. **Neurochirurgia 7:**24-33, 1964
99. Lenz FA, Kwan HC, Dostrovsky JO, et al: Single unit analysis of the human ventral thalamic nuclear group. Activity correlated with movement. **Brain 113:**1795-1821, 1990
100. Lenz FA, Tasker RR, Kwan HC: Single unit analysis of the human ventral thalamic nuclear group correlation of thalamic "tremor cells" with the 3-6 Hz component of parkinsonian tremor. **J Neurosci 8:** 754-764, 1988
101. Limousin P, Pollak P, Benazzouz A, et al: Effect on parkinsonian signs and symptoms of bilateral subthalamic nucleus stimulation. **Lancet 345:**91-95, 1995
102. Lindvall O: Transplantation into human brain: present status and future possibilities. **J Neurol Neurosurg Psychiatry 52 (Suppl):**39-54, 1989
103. Lindvall O, Backlund EO, Farde L, et al: Transplantation in Parkinson's disease: two cases of adrenal medullary grafts to the putamen. **Ann Neurol 22:** 457-468, 1987
104. Lindvall O, Brundin P, Widner H, et al: Grafts of fetal dopamine neurons survive and improve motor function in Parkinson's disease. **Science 247:**574-577, 1990
105. Lindvall O, Gustavii B, Åstedt B, et al: Fetal dopamine-rich mesencephalic grafts in Parkinson's disease. **Lancet 2:**1483-1484, 1988 (Letter)
106. Lindvall O, Rehncrona S, Brundin P, et al: Human fetal dopamine neurons grafted into the striatum in

two patients with severe Parkinson's disease. A detailed account of methodology and a 6-month follow-up. **Arch Neurol 46:**615-631, 1989

107. Lindvall O, Widner H, Rehncrona S, et al: Transplantation of fetal dopamine neurons in Parkinson's disease: one-year clinical and neurophysiological observations in two patients with putaminal implants. **Ann Neurol 31:**155-165, 1992
108. Madrazo J, Drucker-Colín R, Díaz V, et al: Open microsurgical autograft of adrenal medulla to the right caudate nucleus in two patients with intractable Parkinson's disease. **N Engl J Med 316:** 831-834, 1987
109. Madrazo I, Léon V, Torres C, et al: Transplantation of fetal substantia nigra and adrenal medulla to the caudate nucleus in two patients with Parkinson's disease. **N Engl J Med 318:**51, 1988 (Letter)
110. Mahalik TJ, Finger TE, Stromberg I, et al: Substantia nigra transplants into denervated striatum of the rat ultrastructure of graft and host interconnections. **J Comp Neurol 240:**60-70, 1985
111. Marsden CD, Parkes JD, Quinn N: Fluctuations of disability in Parkinson's disease—clinical aspects, in Marsden CD, Fahn S (eds). **Movement Disorders.** Boston, Mass: Butterworth, 1981, pp 96-122
112. Mazars G, Merienne L, Cioloca C: Control of dyskinesias due to sensory deafferentation by means of thalamic stimulation. **Acta Neurochir Suppl 30:** 239-243, 1980
113. Meyers HR: Surgical procedure for postencephalitic tremor, with notes on the physiology of the premotor fibers. **Arch Neurol Psychiatry 44:**455-459, 1940
114. Meyers R: Historical background and personal experiences in the surgical relief of hyperkinesia and hypertonus, in Fields WS (ed): **Pathogenesis and Treatment of Parkinsonism.** Springfield, Ill: Charles C Thomas, 1958, pp 229-270
115. Meyers R: The modification of alternating tremors, rigidity and festination by surgery of the basal ganglia. **Res Nerv Ment Dis Proc 21:**602-665, 1942
116. Meyers R: The human frontocorticopontine tract: functional inconsequence of its surgical interruption. **Neurology 1:**341-356, 1951
117. Meyers R, Fry WJ, Fry FJ, et al: Early experiences with ultrasonic irradiation of the pallidofugal and nigral complexes in hyperkinetic and hypertonic disorders. **J Neurosurg 16:**32-54, 1959
118. Narabayashi H, Okuma T: Procaine oil blocking of the globus pallidus for treatment of rigidity and tremor of parkinsonism: preliminary report. **Proc Jap Acad 29:**134, 1953
119. Narabayashi H, Yokochi F, Nakajiina Y: Levodopa-induced dyskinesia and thalamotomy. **J Neurol Neurosurg Psychiatry 47:**831-839, 1984
120. Nashold B, Slaughter DG: **Some Observations on Tremor. Third Symposium on Parkinson's Disease.** New York, NY: Livingstone, 1969
121. N'Guyen JP, Geny C, Pollon B, et al: Improvement of action tremor by motor cortex stimulation. A case report. **Mov Disord** (In press, 1997)
122. Ohye C, Maeda T, Narabayashi H: Physiologically defined VIM nucleus. Its special reference to control of tremor. **Appl Neurophysiol 39:**285-295, 1976
123. Oliver LC: Surgery in Parkinson's disease. Division of the lateral pyramidal tract for tremor. Report on forty-eight operations. **Lancet 1:**910-913, 1949
124. Parent A, Hazrati LN: Functional anatomy of the basal ganglia. I. The cortico-basal ganglia-thalamo-cortical loop. **Brain Res Brain Res Rev 20:**91-127, 1995
125. Parent A, Hazrati LN: Functional anatomy of the basal ganglia. II. The place of subthalamic nucleus and external pallidum in basal ganglia circuitry. **Brain Res Brain Res Rev 20:**128-154, 1995
126. Parkinson J: **Essay on the Shaking Palsy.** London: Sherwood, Nealy and Jones, 1917, p 16
127. Penn RD, Goetz CG, Tanner CM: The adrenal medullary transplant operation for Parkinson's disease: clinical observations in five patients. **Neurosurgery 22:**999-1004, 1988
128. Percheron G, Fénelon G, Leroux-Hugon V, et al: Histoire du système des ganglions de la base. La lente émergence d'un système cérébral majeur. **Rev Neurol 150:**543-554, 1994
129. Percheron G, Filion M, Tremblay L: The role of the medial pallidum in the pathophysiology of akinesia in primates, in Narabayashi H, Nagatsu T, Yanagisawa N (eds): **Parkinson's Disease.** New York, NY: Raven Press, 1993, pp 84-87
130. Percheron G, François C, Talbi B, et al: The primate motor thalamus. **Brain Res Rev 146:**93-181, 1996
131. Percheron G, François C, Yelnik J, et al: The basal ganglia related system of primates: definition, description and informational analysis, in Percheron G, McKenzie JS, Feger J (eds): **The Basal Ganglia IV. New Ideas and Data on Structure and Function.** New York, NY: Plenum Press, 1994, pp 3-20
132. Percheron G, Parent A, Crossman A, et al: Substrat anatomo-physiologique de l'akinésie chez le primate. **Rev Neurol 146:**575-584, 1990
133. Percheron G, Yelnik J, François C, et al: Analyse informationnelle du système lié aux ganglions de la base. **Rev Neurol 150:**614-626, 1994
134. Piallat B, Benazzouz A, Benabid AL: Subthalamic nucleus lesion in rats prevents dopaminergic nigral neurodegeneration after striatal 6-OHDA injection: behavioural and immunohistochemical studies. **Eur J Neurosci 8:**1408-1414, 1996
135. Putnam TJ: Results of treatment of athetosis by section of extrapyramidal tracts in the spinal cord. **Arch Neurol Psychiatry 39:**258-275, 1938
136. Putnam TJ: Treatment of athetosis and dystonia by section of the extrapyramidal motor tracts. **Arch Neurol Psychiatry 29:**504-521, 1933
137. Redfern RM: History of stereotactic surgery for Parkinson's disease. **Br J Neurosurg 3:**271-304, 1989
138. Rose G, Gerhardt G, Strömberg I, et al: Monoamine release from dopamine-depleted rat caudate nucleus reinnervated by substantia nigra transplants: an *in vivo* electrochemical study. **Brain Res 341:**92-100, 1985
139. Sauer H, Rosenblad C, Björklund A: Glial cell line-derived neurotrophic factor but not transforming growth factor ß3 prevents delayed degeneration of nigral dopaminergic neurons following striatal 6-hydroxydopamine lesion. **Proc Natl Acad Sci USA 92:**8935-8939, 1995
140. Sawle GV, Bloomfield PM, Björklund A, et al: Transplantation of fetal dopamine neurons in Parkinson's disease: PET (^{18}F)-6-L-fluorodopa studies in two patients with putaminal implants. **Ann Neurol 31:** 166-173, 1991

141. Schmidt RH, Ingvar M, Lindvall O, et al: Functional activity of substantia nigra grafts reinnervating the striatum: neurotransmitter metabolism and (^{14}C)2-deoxy-D-glucose autoradiography. **J Neurochem 38:** 737-748, 1982
142. Siegfried J: Effets de la stimulation du noyau sensitif du thalamus sur les dyskinésies et la spasticité. **Rev Neurol 142:** 380-383, 1986
143. Siegfried J: Therapeutic stereotactic procedures on the thalamus for motor movement disorders. **Acta Neurochir 124:**14-18, 1993
144. Siegfried J, Lippitz B: Bilateral chronic electrostimulation of ventroposterolateral pallidum: a new therapeutic approach for alleviating all parkinsonian symptoms. **Neurosurgery 35:**1126-1130, 1994
145. Spatz M: **Spezialle Physiologie des Zentralnervensystems des Wirbe-Tierce.** Berlin: J Springer, 1927, pp 318-417
146. Spiegel E, Wycis H: Stereoencephalotomy, in **Clinical and Physiological Applications. Part II.** New York, NY: Grune & Stratton 1962, p 176
147. Spiegel EA: Development of stereoencephalotomy for extrapyramidal diseases. **J Neurosurg 24:** 433-439, 1966
148. Spiegel EA, Wycis HT: Pallido-ansotomy: anatomic-physiologic foundation and histopathologic control, in Field WS (ed): **Pathogenesis and Treatment of Parkinsonism.** Springfield, Ill: Charles C Thomas, 1958, pp 86-105
149. Spiegel EA, Wycis HT, Marks M, et al: Stereotaxtic apparatus for operations on the human brain. **Science 106:**349-350, 1947
150. Stenevi U, Björklund A, Svendgaard NA: Transplantation of central and peripheral monoamine neurons to the adult rat brain: techniques and conditions for survival. **Brain Res 114:**1-20, 1976
151. Svennilson E, Torvik A, Lowe R, et al: Treatment of parkinsonism by stereotactic thermolesions in the pallidal region. A clinical evaluation of 81 cases. **Acta Psychiatr Neurol Scand 35:**358-377, 1960
152. Talairach J, Hecaen H, David M, et al: Recherches sur la coagulation thérapeutique des structures sous-corticales chez l'homme. **Rev Neurol 81:**4-24, 1949
153. Talairach J, Tournoux P, Szikla G, et al: [Surgical treatment of Parkinson's disease. Methodologic remarks and surgical technic.] **Int J Neurol 2:**76-91, 1961 (Fr)
154. Tasker R: Effets sensitifs et moteurs de la stimulation thalamique chez l'homme. Applications cliniques. **Rev Neurol 142:**316-326, 1986
155. Thompson WG: Successful brain grafting. **N Y Med J 51:**701-702, 1890
156. Tóth S: The effect of the removal of the nucleus dentatus on the parkinsonian syndrome. **J Neurol Neurosurg Psychiatry 24:**143-147, 1961
157. Trétiakoff C: **Contribution à L'Étude de L'Anatomie Pathologique, du Locus Niger de Soemmering.** Soutenue à Paris, 1919 (Thesis)
158. Turner DA, Kearney W: Scientific and ethical concerns in neural fetal tissue transplantation. **Neurosurgery 33:**1031-1037, 1993
159. Upton ARM, Cooper IS: Some neurophysiological effects of cerebellar stimulation in man. **Can J Neurol Sci 3:**237-254, 1976
160. von Economo: Die Nachkrandheiten der encephalitis lethargica, ihr wesen und ihne behanlung. **Ther d Gegenw 69:**529, 1928
161. Walter RD, Adey WR, Rand R, et al: Observations on recording and stimulating globus pallidus and thalamus in man. **Electroencephalogr Clin Neurophysiol 13:**308, 1961 (Abstract)
162. Wertheimer P, David M: Naissance et croissance de la neurochirurgie. **Neurochirurgie 25:**3-10, 1979
163. Woolsey CN, Erickson TC, Gilson WE: Localization in somatic sensory and motor areas of human cerebral cortex as determined by direct recording of evoked potentials and electrical stimulation. **J Neurosurg 51:**476-506, 1979
164. Yasui N, Narabayashi H, Kondo T, et al: Slight cerebellar signs in stereotactic thalamotomy and subthalamotomy for Parkinsonism. **Appl Neurophysiol 39:**315-320, 1976
165. Zervas NT, Horner FA, Pickren KS: The treatment of dyskinesia by stereotaxtic dentatectomy. **Confin Neurol 29:**93-100, 1967
166. Zurn AD, Tseng J, Aebischer P: Symptomatic cell therapies: cells as biological minipumps. **Eur Neurol 36:**396-408, 1996

CHAPTER 3

Clinical Characteristics of Parkinson's Disease: Diagnosis and Assessment

Isabelle M. Germano, MD, and C. Warren Olanow, MD, FRCP(C)

In 1917, James Parkinson[20] described the syndrome of "shaking palsy" and the symptoms of the disease that would eventually bear his name. Although Parkinson's disease is a distinct clinical entity, parkinsonism is a generic term that encompasses a number of different clinical syndromes that can be secondary to many disease states or can be a part of a variety of primary neurodegenerative disorders.

Parkinson's disease accounts for approximately 75% of all cases of parkinsonism. It affects persons of all races and of either gender (with a slight predominance of males), and is seen in all geographic distributions in the world. Parkinson's disease is estimated to affect approximately 1%-2% of the population over the age of 55 years. Between 5% and 10% of cases have a positive family history with an autosomal dominant pattern of inheritance, and there is a greater risk of developing Parkinson's disease in first degree relatives than in the general population.

Parkinson's disease is characterized by four cardinal manifestations: tremor, rigidity, bradykinesia, and gait disturbance with postural instability. The onset is often insidious, and subtle changes in motor function or personality may occur years prior to diagnosis.[1] As the disease evolves, the more typical signs and symptoms emerge. With continued progression, patients begin to develop additional features, including autonomic dysfunction and dementia. Pathologically, Parkinson's disease is characterized by a loss of neurons in the pars compacta of the substantia nigra (SNc), a reduction in striatal dopamine, and the presence of intracellular cytoplasmic inclusions known as Lewy bodies.

In early cases, virtually all patients respond to levodopa (L-DOPA) therapy and experience meaningful clinical improvement; this observation has proven useful for diagnosis. In a study emanating from the London Brain Bank, approximately 25% of patients diagnosed as having Parkinson's disease were incorrectly diagnosed and the diagnosis was not pathologically confirmed.[13] In a retrospective review aimed at determining which features most accurately predict Parkinson's disease pathology, Hughes and co-workers[12] found the highest correlation with the following features: 1) asymmetric presentation; 2) resting tremor; and 3) a good response to L-DOPA. Still, this did not capture all patients, reflecting the diverse manner in which Parkinson's disease can present. Nonetheless, as a general rule, if a parkinsonian patient does not respond to an adequate trial of L-DOPA, it is reasonable to question the diagnosis.[19]

On the other hand, with disease progression, the course of Parkinson's disease is characterized by the development of adverse effects associated with L-DOPA and the development of new features that do not respond to L-DOPA. After 5-10 years of treatment, more than one half of patients experience dyskinesia (involuntary movements, generally of a choreiform type), motor fluctuations (alternating good and bad responses to L-DOPA known as the "on" and "off" periods), and neuropsychiatric problems, including hallucinations and confusion. Additionally, patients may also develop dementia, postural instability, freezing episodes, and autonomic dysfunction that do not respond to L-DOPA and may actually be aggravated by the drug. These new features may reflect degeneration of nondopaminergic components of the central nervous system. Thus, despite the advances made with medical therapy, many Parkinson's disease patients end up with advanced disease that cannot be satisfactorily controlled with currently available medical treatments. These patients cannot manage their activities of daily living (ADL) and are confined to bed or a wheelchair.

THE CARDINAL FEATURES OF PARKINSON'S DISEASE

The four cardinal features of Parkinson's disease are listed in Table 1 and described individually below.

TABLE 1

CARDINAL MANIFESTATIONS OF PARKINSON'S DISEASE

- Resting tremor
- Rigidity
- Bradykinesia
- Gait disturbance with postural instability

Tremor

The tremor of Parkinson's disease is its most recognized feature. It is the presenting complaint in approximately 60%-70% of patients and is seen in 70%-80% of patients. Tremor usually occurs early in the course of the disease, affecting only a single limb. The tremor frequently spreads to involve both limbs on one side, as well as to the limbs on the opposite side of the body. Occasionally, tremor affects the lips and chin as well. Unlike other parkinsonian features, tremor tends to abate in the more advanced stages of the disease. While tremor is often the defining component of Parkinson's disease, it is frequently more a cosmetic than a disabling problem. Patients with tremor as the dominant feature of Parkinson's disease tend to have a more benign or slow-progressing course.[14] In contrast, some patients with well-documented Parkinson's disease never develop tremor, although this tends to augur for more rapid progress.

The most common tremor seen in Parkinson's disease consists of alternating contractions of agonist and antagonist muscle groups and tends to occur at rest, with a frequency of 4-5 cycles per second. In the early stages, it may be mild and intermittent, and have a postural component. It usually begins in the distal part of one arm and subsequently spreads to the ipsilateral leg, and may eventually generalize to involve all limbs, as well as the jaw and lower facial muscles. Tremor frequently responds to L-DOPA or other anti-parkinsonian medications, although it is not uncommon for tremor to persist despite these medications.

Early on, it may be difficult to distinguish Parkinson's disease tremor from essential tremor, which is also most pronounced on assuming a posture. Differentiating features include the kinetic component to the tremor in essential tremor and the tendency for the postural tremor in Parkinson's disease to begin after a short latency rather than immediately. Essential tremor is also associated with a positive family history in 50% of cases, has a much longer and more benign course, and tends to be improved with alcohol.[15] Parkinson's disease tremor tends to disappear during sleep and is increased with stress.

Rigidity

Passive resistance to movement or rigidity is another of the characteristic features of Parkinson's disease. The increase in resistance may be continuous throughout the range of movement (known as "lead-pipe rigidity") or intermittent or ratchety as the limb is passively moved through its range of movement (known as "cogwheel rigidity"). The limbs tend to be most affected, but rigidity can also affect neck muscles. When the axial rigidity is greater than the appendicular rigidity, the possibility of an atypical parkinsonism should be considered. Some have considered that the cogwheel effect may be due to an underlying tremor that is not appreciated clinically. Care should be taken to ensure that tremor is not mistaken for cogwheel rigidity. Rigidity can be elicited by the Jendrassik's maneuver, during which tone is measured by moving a limb back and forth while the patient is asked to pat the leg or open and close the other hand. The onset of rigidity is thought to be due to activation of the gamma-efferent system and is useful in detecting tone in patients with very early disease. Similar to the tremor of Parkinson's disease, rigidity can be increased with stress. Rigidity is more likely to be a disabling feature for parkinsonian patients than is tremor.

It is important to differentiate rigidity from spasticity. The latter consists of resistance to movement due to a lesion of the corticospinal tract that inhibits local reflex activity. Spasticity is characterized by a "clasp-knife" phenomenon in which an initial increase in tone suddenly gives away and tone is relatively normal throughout the remainder of the range of movement. Clinically, spasticity is easier to elicit with rapid movements, while rigidity is best detected by moving the limb through its range of movement more slowly. Spasticity is also associated with other features, such as hyperreflexia, extensor plantar responses, and motor weakness, that are not typically seen in parkinsonism, and a silent electromyogram at rest.

Bradykinesia

Bradykinesia, or slowness of movement, consists of slowness in initiating (reaction time) or performing (movement time) active movements. As such, bradykinesia is a common and often disabling feature of Parkinson's disease. Bradykinesia is a characteristic feature of Parkinson's disease and can be associated with facial masking, decreased eye blinking, and difficulty rising from a chair and performing sequential motor acts. The patients have difficulty in initiating movement and performing rapid alternating movements so that the time required to complete a task is increased. As a consequence, patients who have bradykinesia often begin to experience impairment in performing their ADL.

Neurophysiological tests indicate that reaction time is more severely affected than movement time in Parkinson's disease, and changes in these parameters can be seen prior to the determination that the patient has bradykinesia. Bradykinesia can occur in the absence of rigidity and tremor and vice versa. Although the correct muscles are activated and the relationship between agonists and antagonists is appropriate, the initial surge or motor activity is inadequate and movements are fragmented into a series of incremental steps.

Bradykinesia and rigidity are often associated with a reduction in spontaneous limb movement, leading to the development of bursitis and other arthritic changes. These problems are common, and may in fact be the presenting features of Parkinson's disease. If a patient older than 50 years of age presents with bursitis in more than one joint on the same side of the body, the diagnosis of Parkinson's disease should be considered.

Gait Dysfunction and Postural Instability

Changes in gait and imbalance are a major cause of disability in patients with Parkinson's disease. The mildly symptomatic patient with unilateral disease may exhibit only a slight reduction in arm swing when walking and a tendency to drag the leg on the affected side. As the disease progresses, gait may become impaired and postural stability compromised. Parkinsonian patients have a characteristic gait that is comprised of short shuffling steps with a flexed posture, flexion of the limbs, and decreased arm swing. They tend to lose their balance and may

TABLE 2

ADDITIONAL MANIFESTATIONS OF PARKINSON'S DISEASE

Incoordination	Edema
Micrographia	Scoliosis
Blurred vision	Kyphosis
Impaired upgaze	Pain and sensory symptoms
Blepharospasm	Seborrhea
Glabellar reflex	Constipation
Dysarthria	Urinary urgency, hesitancy, and frequency
Dysphagia reflex	Loss of libido
Sialorrhea	Impotence
Masked face	Freezing
Hand and foot deformities	Dementia
Dystonia	Depression

tend to run forward as though they are trying to catch up to their center of gravity. This is known as a festinating gait.

Parkinson's disease patients have particular difficulty turning. They hold their bodies rigid and take several steps to make a turn. This is referred to as "turning en bloc." Turning and initiating gait, particularly when walking through doorways, may be hampered by sudden freezing of movement and a hesitation in getting started. Interestingly, there are a number of sensory cues that patients can use to overcome these problems, suggesting that the circuitry underlying normal movements and gait is still relatively preserved. As the disease progresses, normal postural reflex mechanisms are lost, causing tilting of the trunk and the tendency for patients to experience propulsion and retropulsion that can be demonstrated by gently pushing or pulling the patient. This can result in falling and an increased risk of fractures. Canes and walkers may be helpful, but eventually patients cannot walk independently and are confined to bed or a wheelchair. Disturbances of gait and balance are therefore a major source of disability for Parkinson's disease patients.

ADDITIONAL MANIFESTATIONS OF PARKINSON'S DISEASE

In addition to the four cardinal features of Parkinson's disease, there are a series of other features that evolve as independent features or as part of the cardinal features and may occur at various stages of Parkinson's disease.[25] Together with the cardinal features, they contribute to patient disability. These features are summarized in Table 2 and some are briefly discussed below.

Micrographia

In cases of micrographia, the handwriting becomes small and illegible. Micrographia is a characteristic feature of parkinsonism but does not necessarily imply Parkinson's disease. Micrographia may be related to impairment in manual dexterity, although it can be seen prior to any obvious clinical deficit.

Preclinical Impairment in Manual Dexterity

Impaired dexterity can affect routine daily tasks, such as dressing and shaving, prior to a formal diagnosis of Parkinson's disease. This may occur in the absence of any overt neurological signs. There are many cases in which clear documentation exists of motor performance prior to the emergence of clinical features sufficient to make a diagnosis of Parkinson's disease. Akinesia of facial muscles can result in a masked face (i.e., a face without expression, with a fixed and vacant stare), another common early feature.

Visual Complaints and Ocular Findings

Visual complaints and ocular findings are

common in patients with Parkinson's disease. Patients often complain of blurred vision, although there is no demonstrable abnormality in the visual system. Blepharitis is common because of the dry eyes secondary to reduced blinking.

Hypophonia and Sialorrhea

A patient with Parkinson's disease may slur words or experience hypophonia, i.e., a diminution in speech volume. Furthermore, they may experience sialorrhea, i.e., excessive drooling and dysphagia. In the extreme, these symptoms can result in malnutrition and aspiration pneumonia.

Musculoskeletal Changes

Ulnar deviation of the hand with flexion of metacarpal, phalangeal, and distal interphalangeal joints and hyperextension of the proximal interphalangeal joints is common. Abnormal truncal posturing with tilt to one side is common. Occasionally, patients experience kyphosis or scoliosis. Bursitis, as described above, is a common early feature.

Pain and Sensory Symptoms

Pain and sensory symptoms are frequently observed in patients with Parkinson's disease. The pain consists of muscle cramps, stiffness, radiculopathy, and arthralgia.[8] Paresthesia is noted in approximately 40% of patients.

Dermatological Lesions

Seborrhea involving the scalp, neck, and occasionally the extremities is very common in Parkinson's disease. Patients are often noted to have an oily forehead.

Autonomic Dysfunction

Gastrointestinal dysfunction, particularly constipation, is a common and often disturbing problem in Parkinson's disease.[6] Urinary dysfunction and impotence are important genitourinary problems in Parkinson's disease patients. These are frequently mistaken for prostate dysfunction and patients often undergo unnecessary surgery. Orthostatic hypotension that may be worsened by medication can be troublesome, but if it is severe, the possibility of a multisystem atrophy should be considered.[10]

Freezing Phenomenon

The freezing phenomenon consists of brief (seconds to minutes) arrests in performing or initiating a movement. It may occur independent of rigidity or bradykinesia and may be seen in the on or off stage during L-DOPA therapy.

Neuropsychiatric Problems

Cognitive changes with dementia are seen in approximately one third of Parkinson's disease patients.[2,9] Executive functions tend to be affected, but Parkinson's disease patients can develop a dementia that is indistinguishable from Alzheimer's disease. Hallucinations are often an early feature of this problem. A large number of Parkinson's disease patients also experience depression. It remains unclear whether this is a component of the monoamine depletion or is secondary to having a chronic illness.

Levodopa Complications

The pharmaceutical treatment of Parkinson's disease results in amelioration of many parkinsonian features, as described in Chapter 7, "Pharmacological Treatment of Parkinson's Disease and Dystonia." However, the introduction of L-DOPA has brought about the recognition of clinical features that reflect the consequences of L-DOPA treatment.[4] Chronic L-DOPA treatment is associated with the development of involuntary movements or dyskinesia. These are usually choreiform (dance-like) in nature but can resemble dystonia, myoclonus, and other movement disorders. Diagnosis is facilitated by identifying that these movements are caused by L-DOPA and disappear when L-DOPA is withheld. Patients can also experience motor fluctuations in which the parkinsonian status fluctuates between on and off periods. On time refers to the period of good motor function and relief from parkinsonian symptoms due to therapeu-

TABLE 3

COMMON PITFALLS IN THE DIAGNOSIS OF PARKINSON'S DISEASE

Symptoms	Differential Diagnosis	Parkinson's Disease
Tremor	Benign essential tremor	Resting tremor (not action)
Dementia	Alzheimer's disease	Extrapyramidal signs predominate
Joint deformities	Rheumatoid arthritis	Hand & foot deformities are striatal
Falling	Syncope, tumor	No focal weakness; cogwheel effect present
Dysphagia/fatiguability	Miasthenia gravis	These extrapyramidal manifestations are associated with the four cardinal symptoms

tic effects of the anti-parkinsonian medications. It is often associated with dyskinesia (see above). On the other hand, off time refers to the period of poor motor function and increase in parkinsonian symptoms that results from the loss of the medication's effect. In the early stages of the disease, patients experience a long-lasting benefit following a dose of L-DOPA. With disease progression, the duration of benefit declines. When the medication provides benefit that lasts for <4 hours, they are said to be experiencing "wearing-off." In the more advanced stages, the duration of an L-DOPA dose falls to that of its plasma half-life (approximately 60-90 minutes) and patients appear to fluctuate independently of their plasma L-DOPA level. This is sometimes referred to as the true on-off phenomenon or "yo-yoing." When evaluating patients with advanced Parkinson's disease, it is important to evaluate them in both the on and off states, as well as to record the percentage of off time and on time with and without dyskinesia.

ASSESSMENT OF PARKINSON'S DISEASE PATIENTS AND RATING SCALES

The correct diagnosis of Parkinson's disease is crucial in formulating a reasonable therapeutic approach, predicting the long-term prognosis, and entering a patient into a clinical trial. There are no specific laboratory tests that are diagnostic of Parkinson's disease, so the history and neurological examination remain fundamental. Magnetic resonance imaging studies may be useful in distinguishing patients with secondary or atypical parkinsonism.[18] Positron emission tomography (PET) studies using fluorodopa (F-DOPA) demonstrate decreased striatal uptake, particularly in the posterior putamen.[3] This is found in virtually all Parkinson's disease patients, but unfortunately the procedure is expensive and is not widely available (see Chapter 6, "Functional Brain Imaging of Parkinson's Disease"). The major challenges in approaching a patient with suspected Parkinson's disease include distinguishing changes related to aging and differentiating Parkinson's disease from other parkinsonian disorders. Some common differential diagnoses are summarized in Table 3.

A thorough history is crucial when diagnosing Parkinson's disease. Establishing the onset of symptoms in Parkinson's disease may be difficult; nevertheless, the chronology of symptoms is important to establish. Tremor is the first symptom in the majority of patients with Parkinson's disease. Thus, a history of dementia predating the onset of motor symptoms is more suggestive of Alzheimer's disease. The neurological examination of patients with suspected Parkinson's disease should be focused on the specific functions relevant to the extrapyramidal system. In particular a careful examination of the following systems should be performed: mental status, speech, oculomotor, motor, gait, and autonomic functions.

When assessing patients for medical or surgical trials of new interventions, it is crucial to have a standardized scale for evaluating patient status at baseline and then at various predetermined time points throughout the trial. Physi-

TABLE 4

UNIFIED PARKINSON'S DISEASE RATING SCALE

Subscales	Point Value Range
I. Mentation, Behavior, and Mood	0-16
1. Intellectual impairment	
2. Thought disorder	
3. Depression	
4. Motivation/initiative	
II. Activities of Daily Living	0-52
5. Speech	
6. Salivation	
7. Swallowing	
8. Handwriting	
9. Cutting food and handling utensils	
10. Dressing	
11. Hygiene	
12. Turning in bed and adjusting bedclothes	
13. Falling (unrelated to freezing)	
14. Freezing when walking	
15. Walking	
16. Tremor	
17. Sensory complaints related to parkinsonism	
III. Motor Examination	0-108
18. Speech	
19. Facial expression	
20. Tremor at rest	
21. Action or postural tremor of hands	
22. Rigidity	
23. Finger taps	
24. Hand movements	
25. Rapid alternating movements of the hands	
26. Leg agility	
27. Rising from chair	
28. Posture	
29. Gait	
30. Postural stability	
31. Body bradykinesia and hypokinesia	
IV. Complications of Therapy (in the past week)	0-23
32. Duration of dyskinesias	
33. Disability from dyskinesias	
34. Pain from dyskinesias	
35. Early morning dystonia	
36. Predictable off periods	
37. Unpredictable off periods	
38. Sudden onset off periods	
39. Proportion of day spent in the off state	
40. Anorexia, nausea, vomiting	
41. Sleep disturbance	
42. Symptomatic orthostasis	
Total	0-199

cians evaluating Parkinson's disease patients undergoing transplantation therapies developed the Core Assessment Program for Intracerebral Transplantation (CAPIT) rating scale to provide uniformity across centers and to allow results in different centers and with different techniques to be compared.[16,17] The core of this evaluation is the Unified Parkinson's Disease Rating Scale (UPDRS), which is a standardized, validated method of assessing Parkinson's disease, with proven interrater reliability[5,7,22] (Table 4). Other components of the CAPIT include the Hoehn and Yahr staging scale (Table 5), a home diary assessment of percentage of time during the waking day that the patient is in the off, on with dyskinesia, and on without dyskinesia states; an L-DOPA challenge test, which measures the duration of benefit following a single dose of L-DOPA; a series of timed motor tasks; and a standardized videotape recording of the patient during both on and off states. When possible, PET evaluations are helpful in assessing disease progression or survival of implanted dopamine neurons. The tests performed are summarized in Table 6.

TABLE 5

HOEHN AND YAHR STAGING SCALE

Stage	Definition
1.0	Unilateral involvement only
1.5	Unilateral and axial involvement
2.0	Bilateral involvement without impairment of balance
2.5	Mild bilateral involvement with recovery on retropulsion (pull) test
3.0	Mild to moderate bilateral involvement, some postural instability but physically independent
4.0	Severe disability, still able to stand to walk unassisted
5.0	Wheelchair-bound or bedridden unless aided

TABLE 6

Tests for Evaluating Parkinson's Disease Patients

Clinical Rating Scales

- UPDRS in both on and off states
- Hoehn & Yahr stage[11] in both on and off states
- Schwab and England disability scale[23]
- Dyskinesia rating scale
- Self-assessment diary quantifying waking hours in off, on with dyskinesia, and on without dyskinesia stages during the week prior to each visit

Timed Motor Tests

- Pronation-supination test: time in seconds to perform 20 cycles of alternating tapping of the knee with the palm and the dorsal surface of hand
- Hand/arm movement between two points: time in seconds to perform 10 cycles of tapping the index finger between two points placed 30 cm (12 in) apart horizontally
- Finger dexterity: time in seconds to perform 10 complete cycles of tapping the thumb with each finger in rapid succession; there has been recent criticism of this component because it does not distinguish impairment due to parkinsonism and dyskinesia[16]
- Stand-walk-sit test: time in seconds to rise from a chair and stand, walk 7 M (23 ft), turn, walk back to the chair, and sit

Levodopa Test

- After a 12-hour fast, the patient undergoes a modified UPDRS examination immediately before and then at 30, 60, 120, 180, 240, and 300 minutes after receiving his/her standard early morning dose of L-DOPA/carbidopa. The duration of time that the patient responds to L-DOPA and the area under the dose response curve are measures of disease severity.

Videotape Evaluations

- Standardized videotape analyses performed during the on and off stages

PET Studies

- Striatal F-DOPA-PET provides a measure of tracer uptake and storage in presynaptic nigrostriatal terminals and correlates with clincial deficits and the number of pigmented nigral neurons in Parkinson's disease patients.[21,24]
- Fluorodeoxyglucose (FDG)-PET provides a measure of resting-state regional glucose metabolism and allows for quantification of the Parkinson's disease-related pattern. This pattern is characterized by increased metabolism in the internal segment of the globus pallidus and thalamus, coupled with decreased metabolism in the premotor cortex and supplementary motor area.[3]

The core of the clinical assessment is the UPDRS and basic knowledge of its component parts is needed to understand reports on clinical outcome. The UPDRS includes six sections (see Table 4 for sections I-IV). Questions in Sections I-III are scored using a five-point scale that ranges from 0-4, with higher scores representing increasing qualitative measures of impairment and disability.

Section I contains four questions to assess mentation, behavior, and mood. The items include intellectual impairment, thought disorder, depression, and motivation/initiative. Each item is scored on a scale from 0 (none/normal) to 4 (severe, complete loss), and the total score for the four items ranges from 0 to 16.

Section II contains 13 questions to assess ADL. The items include speech, salivation, swallowing, handwriting, cutting food and handling utensils, dressing, hygiene, turning in bed and adjusting bed clothes, falling (unrelated to freezing), freezing when walking, walking, tremor, and sensory complaints related to parkinsonism. Each item is scored from 0 (normal) to 4 (disabled), and the total score for the 13 items ranges from 0 to 52.

Section III is the motor examination portion of the UPDRS. Individual questions evaluate speech, facial expression, tremor at rest (for face, hands, and feet), action or postural tremor of hands, rigidity (neck, upper and lower extremities), finger taps, hand movements, rapid alternating movements of the hands, leg agility, rising from a chair, posture, gait, postural stability, and body bradykinesia and hypokinesia. Each item is scored on a scale from 0 (normal) to 4 (severe, marked, or unable), and the total score ranges from 0 to 108.

Section IV evaluates complications of drug therapy and includes question about dyskinesias (duration, disability, pain, and presence of early morning dystonia), clinical fluctuations (predictable on/off periods and predictable off periods associated with ingestion of medications, sudden off periods, and portion of the waking day in an off period), and other complications (anorexia, nausea, or vomiting; sleep disturbances; and symptomatic orthostasis). Four items (32, 33, 34, and 39) are scored on a scale from 0 to 4, and seven items (35, 36, 37, 38, 40, 41, and 42) are scored either 0 (no) or 1 (yes). The total possible score ranges from 0 to 23.

Section V of the UPDRS is a modification of the Hoehn and Yahr scale.[11] This scale reflects the patient's ability to perform routine ADL. It is a subjective rating tool consisting of eight arbitrarily designated stages of disease severity, with scores ranging from 0 (no signs of disease) to 5 (wheelchair-bound or bedridden unless aided).

Section VI consists of one question for the physician and/or patient to score the functional activity according to the Schwab and England Scale.[23] The physician or patient provides a score between 0% and 100%, where 0% represents the highest level of impairment and disability and 100% represents a fully normal and independent state.

Conclusion

The clinical diagnosis of Parkinson's disease is made by evaluating the patient's history, neurological examination, and response to dopamine replacement therapy. There are no blood tests that are diagnostic of Parkinson's disease, and brain CT and MRI are typically unrevealing. Causes of secondary parkinsonism must be ruled out before the diagnosis of idiopathic Parkinson's disease can be made. The four cardinal symptoms of Parkinson's disease may occur in combination with many other manifestations. Prior to a recommendation for surgery, it is crucial that the correct clinical diagnosis of Parkinson's disease be made by an expert team. Furthermore, it is essential that a baseline evaluation using standardized rating scales be performed to allow determination of the effects of surgery.

References

1. Brooks DJ: The early diagnosis of Parkinson's disease. **Ann Neurol** (In press)
2. Brown RG, Marsden CD: How common is dementia in Parkinson's disease? **Lancet 2:**1262-1265, 1984
3. Eidelberg D, Moeller JR, Dhawan V, et al: The metabolic topography of parkinsonism. **J Cereb Blood Flow Metab 14:**783-801, 1994
4. Fahn S: Adverse effects of levodopa, in Olanow CW, Lieberman AN (eds): **The Scientific Basis for the Treatment of Parkinson's Disease.** Park Ridge, NJ: Parthenon Publishing, 1992, pp 89-112
5. Fahn S, Elton RL, Members of the UPDRS Development Committee: Unified Parkinson's disease rating scale, in Fahn S, Marsden CD, Calne DB, et al (eds): **Recent Developments in Parkinson's Disease.** New York, NY: Raven Press, 1986, pp 153-163
6. Goetz CG, Lutge W, Tanner CM: Autonomic dysfunction in Parkinson's disease. **Neurology 36:**73-75, 1986
7. Goetz CG, Stebbins GT, Shale HM, et al: Utility of an objective dyskinesia rating scale for Parkinson's disease: inter- and intrarater reliability assessment. **Mov Disord 9:**390-394, 1994
8. Goetz CG, Tanner CM, Levy M, et al: Pain in Parkinson's disease. **Mov Disord 1:**45-50, 1986
9. Gotham AM, Brown RG, Marsden CD: Depression in Parkinson's disease: a quantitative and qualitative analysis. **J Neurol Neurosurg Psychiatry 49:**381-389, 1986
10. Graham JG, Oppenheimer DR: Orthostatic hypotension and nicotine sensitivity in a case of multiple system atrophy. **J Neurol Neurosurg Psychiatry 32:** 28-34, 1969
11. Hoehn MM, Yahr MD: Parkinsonism: onset, progression, and mortality. **Neurology 17:**427-442, 1967
12. Hughes AJ, Ben-Shlomo Y, Daniel SE, et al: What features improve the accuracy of clinical diagnosis in Parkinson's disease: a clinicopathologic study. **Neurology 42:**1142-1146, 1992
13. Hughes AJ, Daniel SE, Kilford L, et al: Accuracy of clinical diagnoses of idiopathic Parkinson's disease: a clinico-pathologic study of 100 cases. **J Neurol Neurosurg Psychiatry 55:**181-184, 1992
14. Jankovic J, McDermott M, Carter J, et al: Variable expression of Parkinson's disease: a base-line analysis of the DATATOP cohort. **Neurology 40:**1529-1534, 1990
15. Koller WC, Busenbark KL: Essential tremor, in Watts RL, Koller WC (eds): **Movement Disorders: Neurologic Principles and Practice.** New York, NY: McGraw-Hill, 1997, pp 365-386
16. Lang AE, Benabid AI, Koller WC, et al: The core assessment program for intracerebral transplantation. **Mov Disord 10:**527-528, 1995
17. Langston JW, Widner H, Goetz CG, et al: Core assessment program for intracerebral transplantations

(CAPIT). **Mov Disord 7**:2-13, 1992
18. Olanow CW: Magnetic resonance imaging in parkinsonism. **Neurol Clin 10**:405-420, 1992
19. Olanow CW, Koller WC: Algorithm (decision tree) for the treatment of Parkinson's disease. **Neurology (Suppl)** (In press)
20. Parkinson J: **Essay on the Shaking Palsy.** London: Sherwood, Neely & Jones, 1817
21. Pate BD, Kawamata T, Yamada T, et al: Correlation of striatal fluorodopa uptake in the MPTP monkey with dopaminergic indices. **Ann Neurol 34**:331-338, 1993
22. Richards M, Marder K, Cote L, et al: Interrater reliability of the Unified Parkinson's Disease Rating Scale motor examination. **Mov Disord 9**:89-91, 1994
23. Schwab RS, England AC: Projection technique for evaluating surgery in Parkinson's disease, in Gillingham FJ, Donaldson IML (eds): **Third Symposium on Parkinson's Disease.** Edinburgh: E & S Livingstone, 1969, pp 152-157
24. Snow BJ, Tooyama I, McGeer EG, et al: Human positron emission tomographic [18F]fluorodopa studies correlate with dopamine cell counts and levels. **Ann Neurol 34**:324-330, 1993
25. Zetusky WJ, Jankovic J, Pirozzolo FJ: The heterogeneity of Parkinson's disease: clinical and prognostic implications. **Neurology 35**:522-526, 1985

CHAPTER 4

Pathophysiology of Movement Disorders and Basal Ganglia

Thomas Wichmann, MD, and Mahlon R. DeLong, MD

Movement disorders of basal ganglia origin generally fall into either the hypokinetic group, characterized by a paucity of movement, as in Parkinson's disease, or into the hyperkinetic group, characterized by involuntary movements, as in chorea, ballismus, and dystonia. Over the past decade, there have been major insights into the anatomy and function of the basal ganglia and into the pathophysiology of these disorders.

Anatomy of the Basal Ganglia

The basal ganglia are components of larger segregated circuits, which also involve parts of the cortex and thalamus.[1,4,5] These circuits appear to be anatomically organized in a manner similar to each other. In the monkey, functionally segregated motor, oculomotor, associative, and limbic circuits have been identified. Each of them originates from specific cortical areas, passes through separate portions of the basal ganglia and thalamus, and then projects back onto the original cortical area, in a closed-loop manner. The striatum functions as the major "input" stage of the basal ganglia portion of each of these circuits, whereas the internal segment of the globus pallidus (GPi) and the pars reticulata of the substantia nigra (SNr) serve as output stations. Input to the basal ganglia also arises from the thalamus and the brain stem. Intrinsic connections between the striatum and the output nuclei are summarized in Figure 1.

Movement disorders appear to result from disturbances in the motor circuit. This circuit takes origin from the pre- and postcentral sensorimotor fields and engages the motor territories of the basal ganglia and the ventral anterior and ventral lateral thalamus. Cortical projections from the sensorimotor fields terminate largely in the postcommissural putamen, the motor portion of the striatum (see Figure 1). Putamenal output is in turn directed toward motor portions of the GPi and SNr via two pathways: a direct, monosynaptic pathway from the putamen to the GPi/SNr, and an indirect pathway passing through the motor areas of the external pallidal segment (GPe) and the subthalamic nucleus (STN). There are also direct reciprocal connections between the GPe and the GPi/SNr

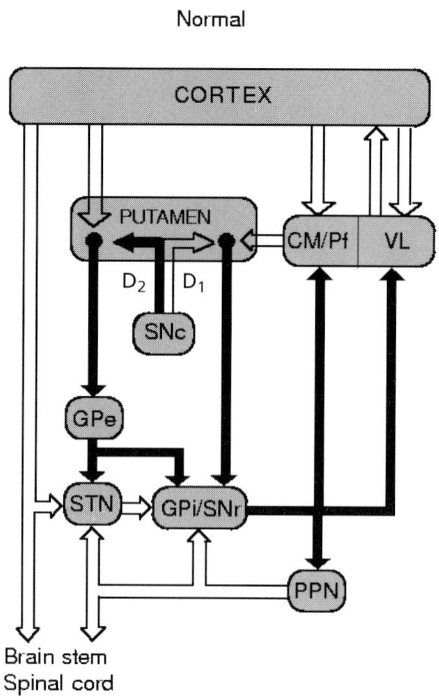

Figure 1: Schematic diagram of the basal ganglia-thalamocortical circuitry under normal conditions. Inhibitory connections are shown as *filled arrows,* excitatory connections as *open arrows.* D_1 = dopamine D_1 receptors; D_2 = dopamine D_2 receptors; CM/Pf = centromedian and parafascicular nuclei of the thalamus; PPN = pedunculopontine nucleus; VL = ventral lateral thalamus.

that circumvent the STN.[75] GPi/SNr motor output is directed not only to the ventral anterior and ventral lateral thalamus, where it influences the activity of thalamocortical projection neurons, but also to the pedunculopontine nucleus in the midbrain. The role of this latter projection remains uncertain, but it appears to provide a pathway over which output neurons may more directly access bulbar and spinal cord centers, circumventing the cortex. Recent studies suggest that the striatum also receives input from the thalamic centromedian and parafascicular nuclei.[43,50,136,137,141,142] These thalamic projections may terminate on neurons of the direct pathway,[141,142] whereas cortical input may preferentially target striatal neurons of the indirect pathway. Cortical inputs to the STN provide yet another entry point for sensorimotor integration in the basal ganglia. With the exception of the glutamatergic (and thus excitatory) projection between the STN and the GPi/SNr, the intrinsic connections of the basal ganglia, as well as their output to the thalamus, superior colliculus, and midbrain, are all inhibitory and gamma-aminobutyric acid (GABA)ergic.

Dopamine appears to play a central role in the regulation of basal ganglia activity. According to the prevailing model, release of dopamine from terminals of the nigrostriatal projection, which arises from the pars compacta of the substantia nigra (SNc), facilitates transmission at the striatal level over the direct pathway via activation of D_1 receptors, and inhibits transmission over the indirect pathway via activation of D_2 receptors.[60,61] Both D_1 and D_2 receptors are located on dendritic spines of striatal output neurons. This anatomical configuration enables striatal dopamine to modulate corticostriatal and thalamostriatal transmission. The net effect of dopamine release in the striatum appears to be a reduction in basal ganglia output from the GPi and SNr (see Figure 1) and a dampening of the transmission of phasic cortical inputs through the basal ganglia. By disinhibition, this reduction leads to increased activity of thalamocortical projection neurons and a facilitation of movement. A reduction in the release of striatal dopamine, as occurs in parkinsonism, should increase basal ganglia outflow and inhibit movement.

In addition, basal ganglia output appears to be modulated by extrastriatal release of dopamine. For example, the SNc sends dopaminergic projections to the STN and GPi, and dopamine may reach the SNr via dendritic release.[28,56,100] In these nuclei, dopamine appears to act on receptors located presynaptically, as well as postsynaptically on output neurons. The functional consequences of dopamine receptor activation at extrastriatal sites are not known with certainty, but considerable interest and speculation have been expressed in this matter.[29,64,65,130]

Functional Considerations

By virtue of their projections, the basal ganglia are positioned to modulate the activity of large portions of the frontal cortex that are concerned with the control of movement and with limbic and associative functions. The anatomical similarities between the different circuits suggest that the operation of the basal ganglia is also similar in each circuit, and that conclusions drawn from the study of one may be applicable to the others. Among the circuits passing through the basal ganglia, the physiology of the motor circuit is best understood and is described below.

Motor Functions of the Basal Ganglia

The basal ganglia are implicated in a wide variety of motor functions, including the planning, initiation, and execution of movements. Inferences about their role in motor control have been based largely on considerations of deficits arising from functional or structural abnormalities affecting these nuclei. This approach is often misleading because abnormal basal ganglia output may produce abnormal signs simply by nonspecific disruption of the normal operations of thalamocortical and brain stem mechanisms. Furthermore, movement disorders such as Parkinson's disease affect not only the basal ganglia, but also cortical and other subcortical regions,[53,54,62,90] rendering the reduction of the pathophysiology of these diseases to abnormalities in the basal ganglia alone too simplistic. For instance, although a role of the basal ganglia in initiation of movement is suggested by the paucity of movement and impairment of movement initiation (akinesia) in Parkinson's disease, experimental support for this role is lacking. Similarly, a role of the basal ganglia in movement execution, as suggested by the slowness of movements (bradykinesia) present in Parkinson's disease, is still questionable because data based on lesions in animals and humans are inconsistent regarding this point.[40,82,83,93,106,113,134,145] A role of the basal ganglia in the control of sequential or simultaneous movements has been inferred from the fact that parkinsonian patients perform poorly in motor tasks that involve such movements.[15,16,35,57,109] These patients also rely more heavily on external cues when executing these movements than do normal controls, suggesting that the basal ganglia-thalamocortical circuitry may have a role in the generation or use of internally cued sequential or simultaneous movements.[35,57,109] Similarly, observations of deficits in parkinsonian patients have been used to argue for a role of the basal ganglia in the execution of learned movements.[66,84,108,135] The evidence that this occurs under normal conditions is also incomplete at present.

Arguing against a prominent role of the basal ganglia in the normal control of movement is the fact that lesions of the basal ganglia outflow nuclei (i.e., pallidotomy) have relatively minor long-term effects on motor performance.[40,41,82,113,152] For instance, the models predict that reduced basal ganglia output should lead to excess movement (see below). Pallidal lesions in normal or parkinsonian monkeys or in parkinsonian patients, however, have not been associated with involuntary movement, other than occasional transient dyskinesias[41,98,148] (see Mink and Thach[113] for further discussion).

On the other hand, evidence for involvement of the basal ganglia in the control of movement comes both from electrophysiological studies in which the discharge of single basal ganglia neurons during motor performance was recorded and from neuroimaging studies, especially positron emission tomography (PET). For instance, studies of neuronal activity have indeed shown that many neurons in the basal ganglia exhibit discharge correlated with certain aspects of limb or eye movements.[7-9,32,38,58,69,76-79,115,157] Recent discussions regarding the nature of the motor function of the basal ganglia have focused on such issues as to what degree these structures contribute to the processing of cortical information, and also whether they have a role in the control of physical parameters of movement, the extent of movement, or the formation of motor memory. All of these questions are actively under consideration.

Active processing of cortical information in the basal ganglia would depend on at least some degree of convergence and integration of sensory and motor inputs within the basal ganglia. The basal ganglia almost certainly integrates cortical inputs to some degree, simply because the number of cortical neurons projecting to the striatum is larger than the number of striatal recipient neurons, and the number of output neurons in the striatum, in turn, is larger than the number of recipient neurons in the GPi/SNr. Pallidal neurons have large dendritic fields that are traversed by a multitude of striatal efferent fibers,[55,128] an arrangement that may form the anatomical basis for convergence at this level. However, anatomical and recording studies have also shown that the overriding principle of basal ganglia function is that of parallel organization with segregation between different pathways. For instance, electrophysiological recording studies have shown that neurons with certain functional characteristics, such as skeletomotor or oculomotor functions, are spatially separate from neurons with different functional characteristics. Even within the skeletomotor representation, neuronal activity is highly specific to individual body parts. Segregation and convergence may coexist, with segregation of functionally specialized areas in the basal ganglia and a certain degree of convergence within such areas.

Much of the argument regarding convergence and segregation in the basal ganglia has arisen from the fact that anatomical data show a degree of dispersion and convergence within these nuclei that is far greater than that demonstrated physiologically. This discrepancy points to the possibility that not all anatomical "channels" of information are actually open and used under physiological conditions; i.e., segregation is a phenomenon that is actively maintained under normal conditions. A good example of segregation even within the motor circuit is that most neurons respond to only a narrow range of input stimuli, such as movements around a single joint.[7-9,32,38,58,69,115,157] The motor circuit itself can perhaps be subdivided into anatomically and functionally segregated subcircuits, emanating from different cortical areas.[81,117,160] The dynamic dimension of segregation is apparent from the observation that neuronal activity in monkeys depleted of dopamine is much less specific, with many motor-related neurons in both segments of the globus pallidus and in the STN responding to examination of multiple joints, sometimes on both sides of the body.[18,52,110,121,153] Dopamine may therefore help to maintain segregation between different circuits passing through the basal ganglia.

Regardless of the exact degree of segregation, tonic high-frequency inhibitory output of GPi/SNr motor areas to the thalamus probably restrains the overall amount of movement. Facilitation of a particular cortically initiated movement is likely the result of a phasic reduction in basal ganglia output, leading to a (brief) disinhibition of thalamocortical neurons.[30] Given the polarities of connections in the direct and indirect pathways of the motor circuit, it can be appreciated that phasic activation of the direct pathway acts as a brake, whereas the activation of the indirect pathway acts like an accelerator or facilitator for movement.[94] On a smaller scale, the motor function of the basal ganglia may depend on the temporal or spatial pattern with which the impulses are transmitted via the direct and indirect pathways. The *temporal* interplay between the activity of direct and indirect inputs to the basal ganglia output nuclei may give the basal ganglia a role in influencing movement characteristics, such as amplitude or velocity. This would be most meaningful if the motor circuit acted to compare proprioceptive feedback with efferent copies of motor commands from precentral motor areas. With this mechanism, the motor circuit could scale movements by constraining motor commands issued to the periphery to lie within desired limits. The *spatial* distribution of impulses transmitted via the direct and indirect pathways in the GPi/SNr is a critical element in a second hypothesis which proposes that the basal ganglia focuses movement,[74,111-113] by facilitating intended movements and inhibiting related but unwanted movements involving the same or nearby joints, thereby stabilizing and selecting individual movements. Given the rather late onset of phasic discharge of most basal ganglia neurons in relation to movements,[7-9,32,38,58,69,115,157] it is likely that most of the basal ganglia operation influences ongoing movements. However, neuronal activity correlated with aspects of motor preparation or motor "set" has also been found in the basal ganglia.[3,6,88,139]

Movement Disorders

More progress has recently been made in understanding the pathophysiological mechanisms underlying the major movement disorders of basal ganglia origin than in the elucidation of the role of the basal ganglia in the control of normal movement. In general, hypo- and hyperkinetic disorders result from disruption of the balance between the activity of the direct and indirect pathways, which appears to characterize the normal state. In general, hypokinetic movement disorders appear to arise from a relative preponderance of activity of the indirect pathway, leading to an increase of (inhibitory) basal ganglia output to the thalamus and brain stem. Conversely, hyperkinetic disorders may result from a decrease of activity in the indirect pathway, leading to reduced basal ganglia output. The role of the direct pathway in these disorders remains uncertain.

Hypokinetic Movement Disorders

Pathophysiological Model

Parkinsonism is a clinical syndrome characterized by varying degrees of akinesia, bradykinesia, rigidity, and tremor. The term "akinesia" is defined as poverty of movement, secondary to impaired movement initiation, whereas "bradykinesia" refers to slowness of movement. Rigidity is characterized by an increased resistance to passive stretch, often associated with a ratchety "cogwheel" sensation due to subclinical tremor. Parkinsonian tremor consists of low-frequency (4- to 6-Hz) oscillations, occurring mainly at rest. The pathophysiological common denominator of all forms of parkinsonism is the reduction of striatal dopaminergic transmission, resulting from either structural or functional disruption of nigrostriatal pathways. The study of the pathophysiological mechanisms linking nigral cell degeneration and clinical parkinsonism has been greatly facilitated by the introduction of an animal model that reproduces many of the pathological and behavioral abnormalities of human parkinsonism, i.e., the primate treated with 1-methyl-4-phenyl-1,2,3,6-tetrahydropyridine (MPTP).[1,17,39,110]

Recent experiments in this model utilizing single-cell recordings in the basal ganglia and studies of metabolic activity (with 2-deoxyglucose) suggest that loss of dopaminergic input to the striatum leads to an activation of the indirect pathway and decreased activity in the direct pathway (Figure 2). These changes result in increased basal ganglia output to the thalamus, leading to increased inhibition of thalamocortical neurons. In accordance with this, microelectrode recording of single-cell activity has shown that the activity of GPe neurons is decreased, whereas the activity of STN and GPi neurons is increased relative to pre-MPTP levels (Figure 3A).[18,51,52,110] These changes may disproportionately affect the motor circuit. For instance, pathology studies and [^{18}F]fluorodopa (F-DOPA)-PET results[20] obtained in preclinical and early clinical parkinsonian patients have shown that in all stages of parkinsonism, dopamine depletion is consistently greatest in the sensorimotor territory of the striatum—the putamen. The preferential involvement of the motor circuit in parkinsonian pathophysiology is also supported by the finding that lesions of the motor territory within the globus pallidus and the STN have striking effects on parkinsonian signs, including

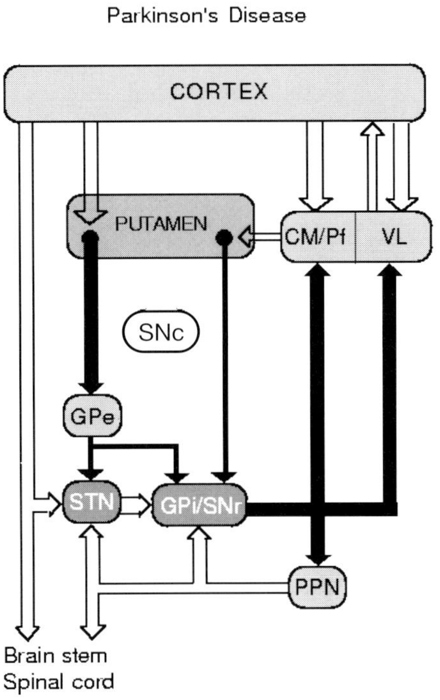

Figure 2: Activity changes in the basal ganglia-thalamocortical circuitry in Parkinson's disease. Degeneration of the nigrostriatal pathway leads to differential changes in the two striatopallidal projections, indicated by the thickness of the connecting arrows (compare to Figure 1). Basal ganglia output to the thalamus is increased. Changes at the cortical or brain stem level are unexplored, and therefore not shown in this figure. For abbreviations, see Figure 1 legend.

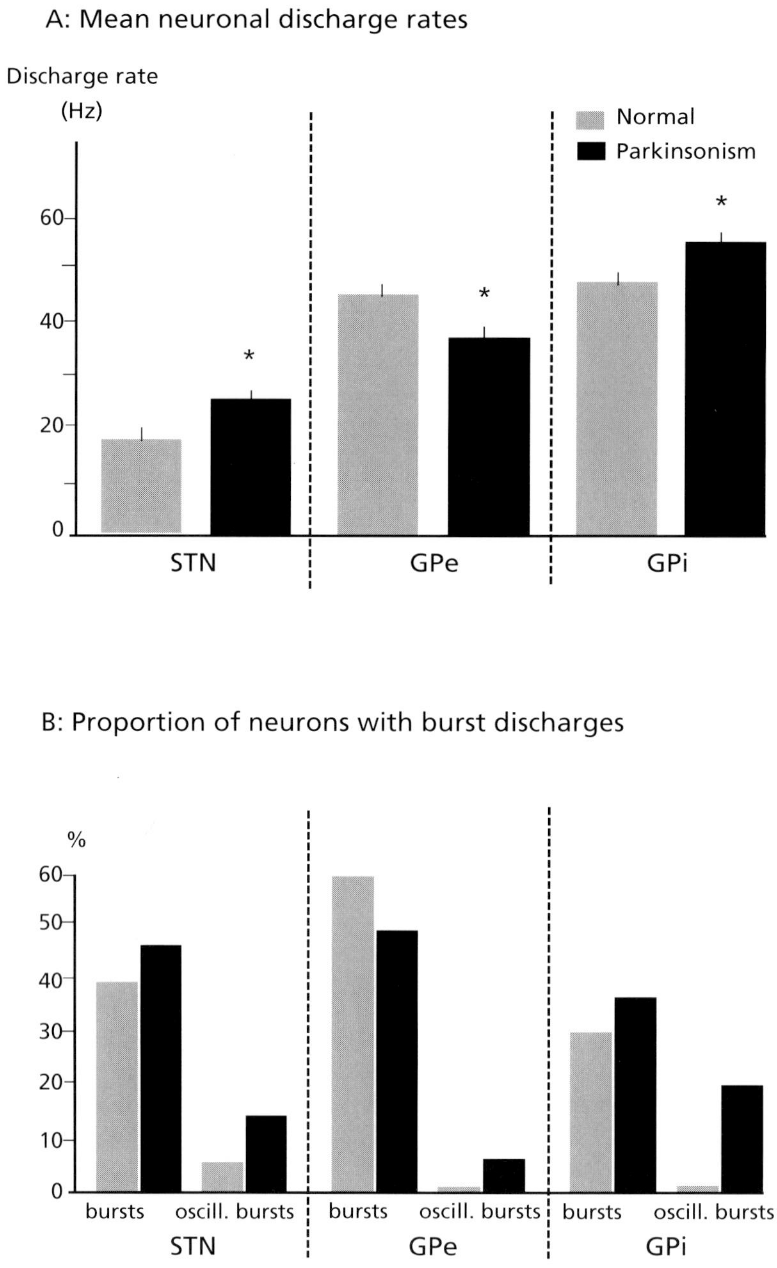

Figure 3: Example of activity changes seen in primates rendered parkinsonian by treatment with the dopaminergic neurotoxin MPTP. Shown are the results obtained in three African green monkeys that were systemically treated with MPTP. All three animals were subjected to electrophysiological extracellular single-cell recording in the GPe, GPi, and STN before (light gray columns) and after (dark columns) MPTP. **A)** Changes in the average discharge rate of neurons in the STN, GPe, and GPi. The average discharge frequency in the GPe is decreased, whereas the rates in the STN and GPi are increased. Asterisks = $P<0.05$ (Student's t-test). **B)** Total proportion of cells that showed burst discharges, as well as the proportion of cells with oscillatory burst discharges (as identified by autocorrelation analysis). The most significant change after treatment with MPTP was an increase in oscillatory burst discharges in all three structures. For details of methods and results, see Bergman et al.[18]

akinesia, bradykinesia, and rigidity[10-13,17,46,85,96,123,148] (Vitek JL, Baron M, Kaneoke Y, et al: Microelectrode-guided pallidotomy is an effective treatment for medically intractable Parkinson's disease. Presented at American Academy of Neurology Annual Meeting, 1994).

In addition to these changes in *tonic* basal ganglia activity, *phasic* neuronal responses to joint manipulation in the STN, GPi, and thalamus[18,52,110,153] have been found to occur more often, to be more pronounced, and to show widened receptive fields after treatment with MPTP. Spontaneous burst discharges, often of an oscillatory nature with bursts occurring at the parkinsonian tremor frequency, are also more frequently seen (Figure 3B).[18] Finally, there is a marked change in the synchrony of discharge in the basal ganglia. Cross-correlation studies have revealed that a substantial proportion of neighboring neurons in the globus pallidus and the STN discharge in unison in MPTP-treated primates.[18] This is in contrast to the virtual absence of synchronized discharge of such neurons in normal monkeys.[157]

As a consequence of the encouraging results of lesions of the basal ganglia output structures on parkinsonian signs in MPTP-treated primates, stereotactic lesioning of these nuclei has gained widespread acceptance as a treatment for Parkinson's disease in humans.[12,46,85,96,97,147] Electrophysiological recording during these procedures has revealed that, as in MPTP-induced parkinsonism in primates, neuronal discharge rates in the GPi are increased relative to the GPe and are characterized by frequent burst discharges and a high degree of synchronous discharge of neighboring neurons (although studies in normal controls are not feasible, of course).[45,105,144,149,150,154]

The fact that GPi lesions[13,46,85,96,97,147] and high-frequency stimulation of the STN (presumably leading to inactivation of the nucleus) remarkably ameliorate parkinsonism, drug-induced dyskinesias, and motor fluctuations[14,103,132] also supports the concept that Parkinson's disease is associated with increased basal ganglia output. PET studies have demonstrated that the decreased cortical activation seen in parkinsonian patients is at least partially resolved after stereotactic pallidotomy, concomitant with recovery of motor function.[27,46,123]

Akinesia, Bradykinesia, and Rigidity

The changes in tonic and phasic activity of basal ganglia output (see above) are postulated to result in akinesia, bradykinesia, and rigidity via influences on target nuclei in the thalamus and brain stem. Increased tonic inhibition of thalamocortical neurons by excessive output from the GPi/SNr may, for example, reduce the responsiveness of cortical mechanisms involved in motor control and may prevent the faithful transmission to the cortex of superimposed phasic reductions in activity that occur during movement execution, which may interfere with the normal scaling of movement. Increased tonic inhibition of thalamocortical neurons by increased basal ganglia output in parkinsonism may also render precentral motor areas less responsive to other inputs normally involved in initiating movement or may interfere with "set" functions that have been shown to be highly dependent on the integrity of basal ganglia pathways.[2] In addition, increased gain in the feedback from proprioceptors, reflected by increased phasic activity in the basal ganglia, may signal excessive movement or velocity to precentral motor areas, leading to slowing or premature arrest of ongoing movements and to greater reliance upon external clues during movement.

Evidence for the involvement of abnormal activity in cortical areas that belong to the motor circuit and are presumably related to motor planning comes from studies of the *Bereitschaftspotential* (readiness potential), a slow negative cortical potential that precedes self-paced movements and is thought to reflect the neural activity in supplementary motor cortex.[37] The early portion of the *Bereitschaftspotential* is smaller in parkinsonian patients than in age-matched controls,[44,123] suggesting a deficit in the normal function of the supplementary motor area in the early stages of preparation for self-initiated movements. PET studies of cerebral blood flow in human patients have revealed that dopamine loss in the striatum leads to decreased blood flow (thus, by inference, reduced synaptic activity) in the supplementary motor area, motor cortex, and dorsolateral prefrontal cortex.[20,21,25,46,47,49,123]

The concept that increased inhibition of thalamocortical neurons by increased output from the GPi/SNr results in akinesia is probably too simplistic, because lesions of the areas of the thalamus that receive basal ganglia input (i.e., ventral anterior and ventral lateral areas) do not appear to result in akinesia.[72,118-120] Abnormal basal ganglia output to targets other than the thalamus, such as the pedunculopontine nucleus, has therefore been suggested to play a role in the development of akinesia.[86,140] A troubling concern with this suggestion, however, is that anatomically the projections from the pedunculopontine nucleus are again directed largely to the basal ganglia and thalamus.[87,99,138]

As an alternative to having specific effects on cortical processing, the increased tonic and phasic discharge in the basal ganglia may simply increase the signal-to-noise ratio in the thalamocortical projection to a variable and unpredictable degree, thereby disturbing cortical processing in a nonspecific manner.[159] This view would better account for the absence of clear-cut motor side effects after pallidotomy or thalamotomy,[22,118,124,146] and may also better explain the paradox of why pallidal lesions and stimulation are both effective treatments in parkinsonian patients. According to this view, both procedures may ameliorate parkinsonian motor signs by reducing (lesions) or stabilizing (stimulation) the amount of subcortical noise with which cortical motor areas would have to cope.

Abnormalities of neuronal activity in the basal ganglia and cortex lead to prominent effects at the spinal cord level that likely contribute to the development of rigidity. For instance, α-motoneuron excitability appears to be increased,[107] possibly via abnormal processing of information transmitted to the spinal cord by Ia afferents.[23,133] This may be due to increased inhibition of Ib interneurons by altered basal ganglia output (mediated via pontine and reticulospinal projections).[42] Abnormal α-motoneuron excitability may also be due in part to a fixed and abnormally high gain in long-latency reflexes, as was found in parkinsonian subjects.[101] The abnormal phasic responses generated within the basal ganglia[18,52,110] or abnormally large inputs to the striatum from motor or somatosensory cortex could be responsible for increased production of long-latency reflexes (acting through the motor circuit projection to the supplementary motor area).

Although the pathophysiological changes in basal ganglia discharge underlying akinesia, bradykinesia, and rigidity are thought to be the same in general terms (i.e., changes of tonic or phasic basal ganglia output), the expression of these signs may depend on abnormalities in different motor subcircuits. Conceivably, akinesia, a defect in movement preparation and initiation, may be related to abnormal discharge in the subcircuit most consistently associated with movement preparation, i.e., the subcircuit emanating from the supplementary motor area and mesial cortical motor areas. In contrast, bradykinesia and rigidity may result from abnormalities in the subcircuit arising from primary motor cortex.[81]

Tremor

Although tremor in Parkinson's disease has been largely considered to result from oscillatory discharge in the thalamus, it has more recently been linked to abnormal discharge in the basal ganglia.[150,155] This possibility is in large part based on the observations that surgical interruption of pallidal outflow, either by disruption of pallidal efferents or by lesions of the GPi, can produce lasting relief of tremor in parkinsonian patients[73,143,148] and that lesions of the STN in MPTP-treated African green monkeys reduce tremor significantly.[17] This may be explainable by increased tonic basal ganglia output to the thalamus, which may promote oscillatory activity through increased hyperpolarization in that nucleus.[24,104] This tendency for rhythmic oscillations of thalamocortical neurons may be further enhanced by periodic bursting in the reticular thalamus during moments of immobility. Alternatively, it has been speculated that loss of dopamine in the basal ganglia output nuclei (GPi/ SNr) rather than in the striatum may be important in the generation of tremor.[36,158] In support of this, it appears that primate species (African green monkeys) that lose dopamine supply to the GPi after treatment with MPTP tend to develop tremor, whereas species (macaques) that appear to have preserved dopamine input to the GPi do not.[18,19,158] The local loss of dopamine may lead to unmasking of pacemaker-like properties[116] in the basal ganglia nuclei themselves, which have been demonstrated by intracellular recordings from the GPi in brain slices from adult guinea pigs when the recorded cells were abruptly depolarized from a hyperpolarized membrane potential.[116] Furthermore, bursts of spikes synchronous with tremor have also been recorded in the STN and GPi of MPTP-treated monkeys[18,52,155] and in parkinsonian patients undergoing pallidotomy.[18,154,155] Oscillations generated in motor areas of the basal ganglia output nuclei or the thalamus will eventually lead to rhythmic activity in thalamocortical cells, which in turn may lead to oscillations in corticospinal projection neurons. In parkinsonian patients undergoing stereotactic thalamotomy, neurons discharging at the parkinsonian tremor frequency have indeed been detected in areas of the thalamus that receive basal ganglia input.[91,102,126]

Nonmotor Phenomena

Parkinson's disease clearly encompasses more than motor phenomena. Although a detailed discussion of the pathogenesis of nonmotor signs of parkinsonism is beyond the scope of this chapter, it is likely that these abnormalities develop as a consequence of abnormal discharge in nonmotor circuits of the basal ganglia, which may be affected by dopamine loss in much the same way as the motor circuit. For instance, oculomotor abnormalities appear to be the result of dopaminergic loss in the "oculomotor" basal ganglia-thalamocortical circuit.[129] Similarly, some of the cognitive and psychiatric disturbances seen in parkinsonian patients are reminiscent of syndromes seen with lesions of the dorsolateral prefrontal cortex (problems with executive functions) or of the anterior cingulate gyrus (apathy, personality changes). These symptoms may be the result of loss of dopamine in the dorsolateral or ventral caudate nucleus, respectively.[33] Finally, disturbance of the normal function of cortical-basal ganglia-thalamocortical circuits has also been implicated in the occurrence of obsessive-compulsive symptoms in some parkinsonian patients, as well as in patients with other diseases of presumed basal ganglia origin, such as Tourette's syndrome.[34,48,80,125]

Hyperkinetic Movement Disorders

Just as Parkinson's and Huntington's diseases represent opposite extremes clinically, so do the underlying pathophysiological mechanisms. The main hyperkinetic symptoms—chorea, ballismus, and dystonia—all appear to be characterized by reduced basal ganglia output to the thalamus, leading to disinhibition of thalamocortical neurons, which in turn leads to the development of involuntary movements. The term "chorea" refers to discrete, involuntary, arrhythmic, jerky movements, whereas "ballismus" refers to more proximal involuntary movements of larger amplitude. The term "dystonia" refers to slower, more sustained movements and abnormal postures with co-contraction of agonist and antagonist muscles due to loss of reciprocal inhibition.

Hemiballismus

Hemiballismus results most often from lesions involving the STN.[26,31,68,70,92,156] In terms of the anatomical model outlined above, such lesions interrupt the indirect pathway, leaving activity along the direct pathway unopposed. Electrophysiological experiments in primates have demonstrated that fiber-sparing STN lesions result in reduced neuronal activity in both the GPi and the GPe, concomitant with the development of chorea, and that the proportion of cells that respond to somatosensory examination is greatly reduced in both nuclei under these conditions.[67] These findings of reduced tonic and phasic discharge in the GPi in hemiballismus have been confirmed in a patient with this disorder who underwent pallidotomy because of intractable involuntary movements (JL Vitek, RAE Bakay, MR DeLong, unpublished observations, 1996). Recently, it was also shown in an MPTP-treated animal that STN lesions lead to increases in discharge in thalamic areas that receive input from the basal ganglia, presumably due to reduced (inhibitory) GPi/SNr output to the thalamus following the loss of excitatory drive from the STN on GPi/SNr neurons (Y Kaneoke et al, unpublished data, 1996).

Chorea

Huntington's disease is the classic basal ganglia disorder characterized by chorea (Figure 4). The motor symptoms appear to be largely due to degeneration of specific striatal neurons, which follows a characteristic time course. It appears that initially striatal output neurons of the indirect pathway (projecting to the GPe) are preferentially affected, leading to reduced inhi-

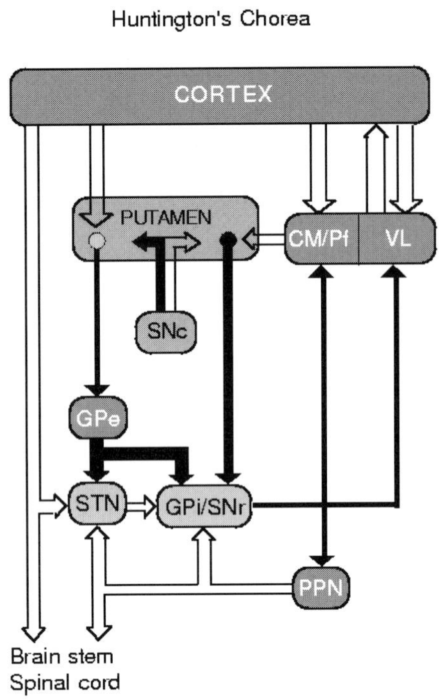

Figure 4: Activity changes in the basal ganglia-thalamocortical circuitry in early Huntington's chorea. Early degeneration of the striatal projection to the GPe leads to reduced basal ganglia output to the thalamus; reduced basal ganglia output is the hallmark of all hyperkinetic disorders. For abbreviations, see Figure 1 legend.

bition of neurons in that nucleus. This subsequently results in increased inhibition of STN neurons, decreased GPi output, and disinhibition of the thalamus, the hallmark of hyperkinetic disorders. In later stages of the disease, inhibitory striatal output neurons to the GPi also degenerate, which results in disinhibition of GPi neurons. It is postulated that increased activity of GPi neurons reduces the amount of chorea and leads to the development of parkinsonian features in late stages of the disease.

Drug-Induced Dyskinesias

The chronic administration of dopaminergic drugs to parkinsonian patients may lead to the development of dyskinesias by shifting the balance between direct and indirect pathways toward the direct pathway, resulting in decreased basal ganglia output. Dopamine receptor activation may result in activation of the direct pathway (via dopamine D_1 receptors) and inhibition of the putamen-GPe connection (part of the indirect pathway, via D_2 receptors). Both changes will again lead to reduced basal ganglia output and presumably to increased activity of thalamocortical neurons. It is unknown why this phenomenon occurs predominantly after previous damage to the nigrostriatal system (Parkinson's disease) and prolonged pulsatile exposure to dopaminergic agonists. Compensatory changes in dopamine receptor number or binding characteristics in response to dopamine depletion may be essential for this phenomenon.[59]

Dystonia

The pathophysiology of dystonia is less well understood than that of the other hyperkinetic disorders. The term "dystonia" describes both a symptom and a disease (or diseases) that may arise from a variety of probably unrelated disease processes of basal ganglia, cerebellar,[63,89,151] and brain stem origin.[89,95] Dystonia secondary to basal ganglia dysfunction often develops after focal striatal lesions, particularly of the putamen, frequently weeks or months after the inciting lesion, suggesting that it results from secondary changes rather than from the primary lesion. Conceivably, changes in the affinity or number of dopamine receptors in the remainder of the striatum, or a reorganization of striatal topography may be the basis for this phenomenon. Dystonia is often seen in the context of parkinsonism, with a subgroup of patients responding to treatment with levodopa (L-DOPA) (so-called "dopa-responsive dystonia").[122,127] In most cases, however, damage to the nigrostriatal tract is probably not necessary for the development of dystonia.[131] Dystonia may develop in individuals with Parkinson's disease treated with L-DOPA and in normal individuals exposed to neuroleptics (tardive dystonia). There is no consensus regarding whether stimulation of D_1 receptors, D_2 receptors, or both is needed for dystonia to occur.

Mitchell et al[114] have shown in 2-deoxyglucose studies that synaptic activity in the GPi and STN is increased in MPTP-treated monkeys that were rendered dystonic by repeated injections of dopaminergic agonists. This result, in conjunction with studies in monkeys rendered dystonic by small ibotenic acid lesions of the putamen, in which the concentration of metenkephalin in the GPe (indicating the activity of the putamen-GPe pathway) was reduced,[71] suggests that a reduction in activity of the putamen-GPe connection, resulting in increased inhibition of both the STN and the GPi, may be involved in the development of dystonia of striatal origin. In addition, overactivity in the direct pathway may also contribute significantly to decreased GPi output, although direct evidence for this is lacking. Recent direct recording from GPi neurons in patients with dystonia during the course of pallidotomy has revealed lowered levels of tonic discharge, but with increased phasic responses to proprioceptive input, further supporting this hypothesis.

Given these considerations, the pathophysiology of chorea and that of dystonia of basal ganglia origin are similar at the level of gross changes in the neuronal activity of the basal ganglia output nuclei. It seems plausible that while in ballismus and chorea the reduction of STN input is the key factor in reducing GPi discharge, in dystonia the lowered rates in the GPi result from overactivity in the direct pathway from the putamen to the GPi. The preservation of neuronal responses to proprioceptive input in the GPi in dystonic individuals suggests that the STN input is present and perhaps even increased in dystonia. It is possible that there is increased coupling of discharge in dystonia, leading to agonist/antagonist co-contraction and "overflow" of muscle contraction.

Summary

The evidence from animal experiments and from ablative procedures in humans has lent strong support to a model of normal function of the basal ganglia in movement, and the pathophysiological considerations outlined above. The models, however, clearly fall short of "explaining" the role of the basal ganglia in voluntary movement and movement disorders, primarily because of the unavailability of feasible methods to clearly establish the physiological function of the basal ganglia. Nonetheless, impressive advances in the understanding and treatment of these disorders have been made in recent years.

References

1. Albin RL, Young AB, Penney JB: The functional anatomy of basal ganglia disorders. **Trends Neurosci 12:**366-375, 1989
2. Alexander GE, Crutcher MD: Functional architecture of basal ganglia circuits: neural substrates of parallel processing. **Trends Neurosci 13:**266-271, 1990
3. Alexander GE, Crutcher MD: Preparation for movement: neural representations of intended direction in three motor areas of the monkey. **J Neurophysiol 64:** 133-150, 1990
4. Alexander GE, Crutcher MD, DeLong MR: Basal ganglia-thalamocortical circuits: parallel substrates for motor, oculomotor, "prefrontal" and "limbic" functions. **Prog Brain Res 85:**119-146, 1990
5. Alexander GE, DeLong MR, Strick PL: Parallel organization of functionally segregated circuits linking basal ganglia and cortex. **Annu Rev Neurosci 9:** 357-381, 1986
6. Anderson M, Inase M, Buford J, et al: Movement and preparatory activity of neurons in pallidal-receiving areas of the monkey thalamus, in Mano N, Hamada I, DeLong MR (eds): **Role of Cerebellum and Basal Ganglia in Voluntary Movement.** Amsterdam: Elsevier, 1993, pp 163-170
7. Anderson ME: Discharge patterns of basal ganglia neurons during active maintenance of postural stability and adjustment to chair tilt. **Brain Res 143:** 325-338, 1977
8. Anderson ME, Turner RS: A quantitative analysis of pallidal discharge during targeted reaching movement in the monkey. **Exp Brain Res 86:**623-632, 1991
9. Anderson RJ, Aldridge JW, Murphy JT: Function of caudate neurons during limb movements in awake primates. **Brain Res 173:**489-501, 1979
10. Aziz TZ, Peggs D, Sambrook MA, et al: Lesion of the subthalamic nucleus for the alleviation of 1-methyl-4-phenyl-1,2,3,6-tetrahydropyridine (MPTP)-induced parkinsonism in the primate. **Mov Disord 6:** 288-292, 1991
11. Bakay RAE, DeLong MR, Vitek JL: Posteroventral pallidotomy for Parkinson's disease. **J Neurosurg 77:** 487-488, 1992 (Letter)
12. Baron MS, Vitek JL, Bakay RAE, et al: Treatment of advanced Parkinson's disease by GPi pallidotomy: 1 year pilot-study results. **Ann Neurol 40:**355-366, 1996
13. Baron M, Vitek J, Turner R, et al: Lesions in the sensorimotor region of the internal segment of the globus pallidus (GPi) in parkinsonian patients are effective in alleviating the cardinal signs of Parkinson's disease. **Soc Neurosci 19:**1584, 1993
14. Benazzouz A, Gross C, Féger J, et al: Reversal of rigidity and improvement in motor performance by subthalamic high-frequency stimulation in MPTP-treated monkeys. **Eur J Neurosci 5:**382-389, 1993
15. Benecke R, Rothwell JC, Dick JPR, et al: Disturbance of sequential movements in patients with Parkinson's disease. **Brain 110:**361-379, 1987
16. Bennett KMB, Marchetti M, Iovine R, et al: The drinking action of Parkinson's disease subjects. **Brain 118:**959-970, 1995
17. Bergman H, Wichmann T, DeLong MR: Reversal of experimental parkinsonism by lesions of the subthalamic nucleus. **Science 249:**1436-1438, 1990

18. Bergman H, Wichmann T, Karmon B, et al: The primate subthalamic nucleus. II. Neuronal activity in the MPTP model of parkinsonism. **J Neurophysiol 72:**507-520, 1994
19. Bernheimer H, Birkmayer W, Hornykiewicz O, et al: Brain dopamine and the syndromes of Parkinson and Huntington. Clinical, morphological and neurochemical correlations. **J Neurol Sci 20:**415-455, 1973
20. Brooks DJ: Detection of preclinical Parkinson's disease with PET. **Neurology 41 (Suppl 2):**24-27, 1991
21. Brooks DJ: Functional imaging in relation to parkinsonian syndromes. **J Neurol Sci 115:**1-17, 1993
22. Burchiel KJ: Thalamotomy for movement disorders. **Neurosurg Clin N Am 6:**55-71, 1995
23. Burke D, Gandevia SC, McKeon B: Monosynaptic and oligosynaptic contributions to human ankle jerk and H-reflex. **J Neurophysiol 52:**435-448, 1984
24. Buzsáki G, Smith A, Berger S, et al: Petit mal epilepsy and parkinsonian tremor: hypothesis of a common pacemaker. **Neuroscience 36:**1-14, 1990
25. Calne DB, Snow BJ: PET imaging in Parkinsonism. **Adv Neurol 60:**484-487, 1993
26. Carpenter MB, Whittier JR, Mettler FA: Analysis of choreoid hyperkinesia in the rhesus monkey. Surgical and pharmacological analysis of hyperkinesia resulting from lesions in the subthalamic nucleus of Luys. **J Comp Neurol 92:**293-332, 1950
27. Ceballos-Baumann AO, Obeso JA, Vitek JL, et al: Restoration of thalamocortical activity after posteroventral pallidotomy in Parkinson's disease. **Lancet 344:**814, 1994 (Letter)
28. Cheramy A, Leviel V, Glowinski J: Dendritic release of dopamine in the substantia nigra. **Nature 289:** 537-542, 1981
29. Chesselet MF, Delfs JMD: Basal ganglia and movement disorders: an update. **Trends Neurosci 19:** 417-422, 1996
30. Chevalier G, Deniau JM: Disinhibition as a basic process in the expression of striatal functions. **Trends Neurosci 13:**277-280, 1990
31. Crossman AR, Sambrook MA, Jackson A: Experimental hemachorea/hemiballismus in the monkey. Study on the intracerebral site of action in a drug-induced dyskinesia. **Brain 107:**579-596, 1984
32. Crutcher MD, DeLong MR: Single cell studies of the primate putamen. II. Relations to direction of movement and pattern of muscular activity. **Exp Brain Res 53:**244-258, 1984
33. Cummings JL: Frontal-subcortical circuits and human behavior. **Arch Neurol 50:**873-880, 1993
34. Cummings JL, Cunningham K: Obsessive-compulsive disorder in Huntington's disease. **Biol Psychiatry 31:**263-270, 1992
35. Cunnington R, Iansek R, Bradshaw JL, et al: Movement-related potentials in Parkinson's disease. Presence and predictability of temporal and spatial cues. **Brain 118:**935-950, 1995
36. Dacko S, Smith MG, Schneider JS: Immunohistochemical study of the pallidal complex in symptomatic and asymptomatic MPTP-treated monkeys, normal human, and Parkinson's disease patients. **Soc Neurosci Abstr 16:**428, 1990 (Abstract)
37. Deecke L: Cerebral potentials related to voluntary actions: parkinsonism and normal subjects, in Delwaide PJ, Agnoli A (eds): **Clinical Neurophysiology in Parkinsonism: Contribution to Assessment and Pathophysiology.** Amsterdam: Elsevier, 1985, pp 91-105
38. DeLong MR: Activity of pallidal neurons during movement. **J Neurophysiol 34:**414-427, 1971
39. DeLong MR: Primate models of movement disorders of basal ganglia origin. **Trends Neurosci 13:** 281-285, 1990
40. DeLong MR, Coyle JT: Globus pallidus lesions in the monkey produced by kainic acid: histologic and behavioral effects. **Appl Neurophysiol 42:**95-97, 1979
41. DeLong MR, Georgopoulos AP: Motor functions of the basal ganglia, in Brookhart JM, Mountcastle VB, Brooks VB, et al (eds): **Handbook of Physiology. The Nervous System. Motor Control.** Bethesda, Md: American Physiological Society, 1981, pp 1017-1061
42. Delwaide PJ, Pepin JL, Maertens de Noordhout A: Short-latency autogenic inhibition in patients with parkinsonian rigidity. **Ann Neurol 30:**83-89, 1991
43. Deschênes M, Bourassa J, Parent A: Two different types of thalamic fibers innervate the rat striatum. **Brain Res 701:**288-292, 1995
44. Dick JPR, Rothwell JC, Day BL, et al: The Bereitschaftspotential is abnormal in Parkinson's disease. **Brain 112:**233-244, 1989
45. Dogali M, Berić A, Sterio D, et al: Anatomic and physiological considerations in pallidotomy for Parkinson's disease. **Acta Neurochir Suppl 64:**9-12, 1995
46. Dogali M, Fazzini E, Kolodny E, et al: Stereotactic ventral pallidotomy for Parkinson's disease. **Neurology 45:**753-761, 1995
47. Eidelberg D: Positron emission tomography studies in parkinsonism. **Neurol Clin 10:**421-433, 1992
48. Eidelberg D, Moeller JR, Antonini A, et al: The metabolic anatomy of Tourette's syndrome. **Neurology 48:** 927-934, 1997
49. Eidelberg D, Moeller JR, Dhawan V, et al: The metabolic topography of Parkinsonism. **J Cereb Blood Flow Metab 14:**783-801, 1994
50. Féger J, Bevan M, Crossman AR: The projections from the parafascicular thalamic nucleus to the subthalamic nucleus and the striatum arise from separate neuronal populations: a comparison with the corticostriatal and corticosubthalamic efferents in a retrograde double-labelling study. **Neuroscience 60:** 125-132, 1994
51. Filion M, Tremblay L: Abnormal spontaneous activity of globus pallidus neurons in monkeys with MPTP-induced parkinsonism. **Brain Res 547:** 142-151, 1991
52. Filion M, Tremblay L, Bédard PJ: Abnormal influences of passive limb movement on the activity of globus pallidus neurons in parkinsonian monkeys. **Brain Res 444:**165-176, 1988
53. Forno LS, DeLanney LE, Irwin I, et al: Similarities and differences between MPTP-induced parkinsonism and Parkinson's disease. Neuropathologic considerations. **Adv Neurol 60:**600-608, 1993
54. Forno LS, Langston JW, DeLanney LE, et al: Locus ceruleus lesions and eosinophilic inclusions in MPTP-treated monkeys. **Ann Neurol 20:**449-455, 1986
55. François C, Percheron G, Yelnik J, et al: A golgi analysis of the primate globus pallidus. I. Inconstant processes of large neurons, other neuronal types, and afferent axons. **J Comp Neurol 227:**182-199, 1984

56. Gauchy C, Desban M, Glowinski J, et al: NMDA regulation of dopamine release from proximal and distal dendrites in the cat substantia nigra. **Brain Res 635:** 249-256, 1994
57. Georgiou N, Bradshaw JL, Iansek R, et al: Reduction in external cues and movement sequencing in Parkinson's disease. **J Neurol Neurosurg Psychiatry 57:** 368-370, 1994
58. Georgopoulos AP, DeLong MR, Crutcher MD: Relations between parameters of step-tracking movements and single cell discharge in the globus pallidus and subthalamic nucleus of the behaving monkey. **J Neurosci 3:**1586-1598, 1983
59. Gerfen CR: Dopamine receptor function in the basal ganglia. **Clin Neuropharmacol 18:**S162-S177, 1995
60. Gerfen CR, Engber TM, Mahan LC, et al: D_1 and D_2 dopamine receptor-regulated gene expression of striatonigral and striatopallidal neurons. **Science 250:**1429-1432, 1990
61. Gerfen CR, Keefe KA, Gauda EB: D1 and D2 dopamine receptor function in the striatum: coactivation of D1 and D2-dopamine receptors on separate populations of neurons results in potentiated immediate early gene response in D1-containing neurons. **J Neurosci 15:**8167-8176, 1995
62. Gibb WR: Neuropathology of Parkinson's disease and related syndromes. **Neurol Clin 10:**361-376, 1992
63. Gille M, Jacquemin C, Kiame G, et al: Myélinolyse centropontine avec ataxie cérébelleuse et dystonie. **Rev Neurol 149:**344-346, 1993
64. Gnanalingham KK, Robertson RG: The effects of chronic continuous versus intermittent levodopa treatments on striatal and extrastriatal D_1 and D_2 dopamine receptors and dopamine uptake sites in the 6-hydroxydopamine lesioned rat—an autoradiographic study. **Brain Res 640:**185-194, 1994
65. Gnanalingham KK, Smith LA, Hunter AJ, et al: Alterations in striatal and extrastriatal D-1 and D-2 dopamine receptors in the MPTP-treated common marmoset: an autoradiographic study. **Synapse 14:** 184-194, 1993
66. Graybiel AM: Building action repertoires: memory and learning functions of the basal ganglia. **Curr Opin Neurobiol 5:**733-741, 1995
67. Hamada I, DeLong MR: Excitotoxic acid lesions of the primate subthalamic nucleus result in reduced pallidal neuronal activity during active holding. **J Neurophysiol 68:**1859-1866, 1992
68. Hamada I, DeLong MR: Excitotoxic acid lesions of the primate subthalamic nucleus result in transient dyskinesias of the contralateral limbs. **J Neurophysiol 68:**1850-1858, 1992
69. Hamada I, DeLong MR, Mano NI: Activity of identified wrist-related pallidal neurons during step and ramp wrist movements in the monkey. **J Neurophysiol 64:**1892-1906, 1990
70. Hammond C, Feger J, Bioulac B, et al: Experimental hemiballism in the monkey produced by unilateral kainic acid lesion in corpus Luysii. **Brain Res 171:** 577-580, 1979
71. Hantraye P, Riche D, Maziere M, et al: A primate model of Huntington's disease: behavioral and anatomical studies of unilateral excitotoxic lesions of the caudate-putamen in the baboon. **Exp Neurol 108:**91-104, 1990
72. Hassler R, Mundinger F, Riechert T: **Stereotaxis in Parkinsonian Syndromes.** New York, NY: Springer-Verlag, 1979
73. Hassler R, Reichert T, Mundinger F, et al: Physiological observations in stereotaxic operations in extrapyramidal motor disturbances. **Brain 83:**337-350, 1960
74. Hazrati LN, Parent A: Convergence of subthalamic and striatal efferents at pallidal level in primates: an anterograde double-labeling study with biocytin and PHA-L. **Brain Res 569:**336-340, 1992
75. Hazrati LN, Parent A, Mitchell S, et al: Evidence for interconnections between the two segments of the globus pallidus in primates: a PHA-L anterograde tracing study. **Brain Res 533:**171-175, 1990
76. Hikosaka O, Matsumara M, Kojima J, et al: Role of basal ganglia in initiation and suppression of saccadic eye movements, in Mano N, Hamada I, DeLong MR (eds): **Role of the Cerebellum and Basal Ganglia in Voluntary Movement.** Amsterdam: Elsevier, 1993, pp 213-220
77. Hikosaka O, Sakamoto M: Cell activity in monkey caudate nucleus preceding saccadic eye movements. **Exp Brain Res 63:**659-662, 1986
78. Hikosaka O, Sakamoto M, Usui S: Functional properties of monkey caudate neurons. I. Activities related to saccadic eye movements. **J Neurophysiol 61:** 780-798, 1989
79. Hikosaka O, Wurtz RH: Visual and oculomotor functions of monkey substantia nigra pars reticulata. III. Memory-contingent visual and saccade responses. **J Neurophysiol 49:**1268-1284, 1983
80. Hollander E, Cohen L, Richards M, et al: A pilot study of the neuropsychology of obsessive-compulsive disorder and Parkinson's disease: basal ganglia disorders. **J Neuropsychiatry Clin Neurosci 5:** 104-107, 1993
81. Hoover JE, Strick PL: Multiple output channels in the basal ganglia. **Science 259:**819-821, 1993
82. Horak FB, Anderson ME: Influence of globus pallidus on arm movements in monkeys. I. Effects of kainic-induced lesions. **J Neurophysiol 52:**290-304, 1984
83. Hore J, Vilis T: Arm movement performance during reversible basal ganglia lesions in the monkey. **Exp Brain Res 39:**217-228, 1980
84. Houk JC, Wise SP: Distributed modular architecture linking basal ganglia, cerebellum, and cerebral cortex: their role in planning and controlling action. **Cereb Cortex 5:**95-110, 1995
85. Iacono RP, Lonser RR: Reversal of Parkinson's akinesia by pallidotomy. **Lancet 343:**418-419, 1994 (Letter)
86. Inglis WL, Winn P: The pedunculopontine tegmental nucleus: where the striatum meets the reticular formation. **Prog Neurobiol 47:**1-29, 1995
87. Jackson A, Crossman AR: Nucleus tegmenti pedunculopontinus: efferent connections with special reference to the basal ganglia, studied in the rat by anterograde and retrograde transport of horseradish peroxidase. **Neuroscience 10:**725-765, 1983
88. Jaeger D, Gilman S, Aldridge JW: Primate basal ganglia activity in a precued reaching task: preparation for movement. **Exp Brain Res 95:**51-64, 1993
89. Janati A, Metzer WS, Archer RL, et al: Blepharospasm associated with olivopontocerebellar atrophy. **J Clin Neuro Ophthalmol 9:**281-284, 1989
90. Jellinger KA: Pathology of Parkinson's disease.

Changes other than the nigrostriatal pathway. **Mol Chem Neuropathol 14:**153-197, 1991

91. Jones MW, Tasker RR: The relationship of documented destruction of specific cell types to complications and effectiveness in thalamotomy for tremor in Parkinson's disease. **Stereotact Funct Neurosurg 54/55:**207-211, 1990
92. Kase CS, Maulsby GO, deJuan E, et al: Hemichorea-hemiballism and lacunar infarction in the basal ganglia. **Neurology 31:**452-455, 1981
93. Kato M, Kimura M: Effects of reversible blockade of basal ganglia on a voluntary arm movement. **J Neurophysiol 68:**1516-1534, 1992
94. Kita H:Physiology of two disynaptic pathways from the sensorimotor cortex to the basal ganglia output nuclei, in Percheron G, McKenzie JS, Feger J (eds): **The Basal Ganglia IV. New Ideas and Data on Structure and Function.** New York, NY: Plenum, 1994, pp 263-276
95. Krauss JK, Mohadjer M, Braus DF, et al: Dystonia following head trauma: a report of nine patients and review of the literature. **Mov Disord 7:**263-272, 1992
96. Laitinen LV: Pallidotomy for Parkinson's disease. **Neurosurg Clin N Am 6:**105-112, 1995
97. Laitinen LV, Bergenheim AT, Hariz MI: Leksell's posteroventral pallidotomy in the treatment of Parkinson's disease. **J Neurosurg 76:**53-61, 1992
98. Laitinen LV, Bergenheim AT, Hariz MI: Ventroposterolateral pallidotomy can abolish all parkinsonian symptoms. **Stereotact Funct Neurosurg 58:**14-21, 1992
99. Lavoie B, Parent A: Pedunculopontine nucleus in the squirrel monkey: projections to the basal ganglia as revealed by anterograde tract-tracing methods. **J Comp Neurol 344:**210-231, 1994
100. Lavoie B, Smith Y, Parent A: Dopaminergic innervation of the basal ganglia in the squirrel monkey as revealed by tyrosine hydroxylase immunohistochemistry. **J Comp Neurol 289:**36-52, 1989
101. Lee RG, Murphy JT, Tatton WG: Long-latency myotatic reflexes in man: mechanisms, functional significance, and changes in patients with Parkinson's disease or hemiplegia. **Adv Neurol 29:**489-507, 1983
102. Lenz FA, Normand SL, Kwan HC, et al: Statistical prediction of the optimal site for thalamotomy in parkinsonian tremor. **Mov Disord 10:**318-328, 1995
103. Limousin P, Pollak P, Benazzouz A, et al: Effect on parkinsonian signs and symptoms of bilateral subthalamic nucleus stimulation. **Lancet 345:**91-95, 1995
104. Llinás RR: The intrinsic electrophysiological properties of mammalian neurons: insights into central nervous system function. **Science 242:**1654-1664, 1988
105. Lozano A, Hutchison W, Kiss Z, et al: Methods for microelectrode-guided posteroventral pallidotomy. **J Neurosurg 84:**194-202, 1996
106. MacLean PD: Effects of lesions of globus pallidus on species-typical display behavior of squirrel monkeys. **Brain Res 149:**175-196, 1978
107. Marsden CD: The mysterious motor function of the basal ganglia: the Robert Wartenburg lecture. **Neurology 32:**514-539, 1982
108. Marsden CD: Which motor disorder in Parkinson's disease indicates the true motor function of the basal ganglia? **Ciba Found Symp 107:**225-241, 1984
109. Martin KE, Phillips JG, Iansek R, et al: Inaccuracy and instability of sequential movements in Parkinson's disease. **Exp Brain Res 102:**131-140, 1994
110. Miller WC, DeLong MR: Altered tonic activity of neurons in the globus pallidus and subthalamic nucleus in the primate MPTP model of parkinsonism, in Carpenter MB, Jayaraman A (eds): **The Basal Ganglia II: Structure and Function: Current Concepts.** New York, NY: Plenum, 1987, pp 415-427
111. Mink JW, Thach WT: Basal ganglia motor control. I. Nonexclusive relation of pallidal discharge to five movement modes. **J Neurophysiol 65:**273-300, 1991
112. Mink JW, Thach WT: Basal ganglia motor control. II. Late pallidal timing relative to movement onset and inconsistent pallidal coding of movement parameters. **J Neurophysiol 65:**301-329, 1991
113. Mink JW, Thach WT: Basal ganglia motor control. III. Pallidal ablation: normal reaction time, muscle cocontraction, and slow movement. **J Neurophysiol 65:**330-351, 1991
114. Mitchell IJ, Luquin R, Boyce S, et al: Neural mechanisms of dystonia: evidence from a 2-deoxyglucose uptake study in a primate model of dopamine agonist-induced dystonia. **Mov Disord 5:**49-54, 1990
115. Mitchell SJ, Richardson RT, Baker FH, et al: The primate globus pallidus: neuronal activity related to direction of movement. **Exp Brain Res 68:**491-505, 1987
116. Nambu A, Llinas R: Electrophysiology of the globus pallidus neurons: an in vitro study in guinea pig brain slices. **Soc Neurosci Abstr 16:**428, 1990 (Abstract)
117. Nambu A, Yoshida S, Jinnai K: Discharge patterns of pallidal neurons with input from various cortical areas during movement in the monkey. **Brain Res 519:**183-191, 1990
118. Narabayashi H: Sterotaxic Vim thalamotomy for treatment of tremor. **Eur Neurol 29 (Suppl 1):** S29-S32, 1989
119. Narabayashi H: Surgical treatment in the levodopa era, in Stern G (ed): **Parkinson's Disease.** London: Chapman & Hall, 1990, pp 597-646
120. Narabayashi H, Maeda T, Yokochi F: Long-term follow-up study of nucleus ventralis intermedius and ventrolateralis thalamotomy using a microelectrode technique in parkinsonism. **Appl Neurophysiol 50:** 330-337, 1987
121. Nini A, Feingold A, Slovin H, et al: Neurons in the globus pallidus do not show correlated activity in the normal monkey, but phase-locked oscillations appear in the MPTP model of Parkinsonism. **J Neurophysiol 74:**1800-1805, 1995
122. Nygaard TG: Dopa-responsive dystonia. **Curr Opin Neurol 8:**310-313, 1995
123. Obeso JA, Rothwell JC, Ceballos-Baumann A, et al: The mechanism of action of pallidotomy in Parkinson's disease (PD): physiological and imaging studies. **Soc Neurosci Abstr 21:**1982, 1995 (Abstract)
124. Page RD, Sambrook MA, Crossman AR: Thalamotomy for the alleviation of levodopa-induced dyskinesia: experimental studies in the 1-methyl-4-phenyl-1,2,3,6-tetrahydropyridine-treated parkinsonian monkey. **Neuroscience 55:**147-165, 1993
125. Palumbo D, Maughan A, Kurlan R: Hypothesis III. Tourette syndrome is only one of several causes of a developmental basal ganglia syndrome. **Arch Neurol 54:**475-483, 1997
126. Paré D, Curro'Dossi R, Steriade M: Neuronal basis

of the parkinsonian resting tremor: a hypothesis and its implications for treatment. **Neuroscience 35:** 217-226, 1990

127. Patel K, Roskrow T, Davis JS, et al: Dopa responsive dystonia. **Arch Dis Child 73:**256-257, 1995
128. Percheron G, Yelnik J, François C: A golgi analysis of the primate globus pallidus. III. Spatial organization of the striato-pallidal complex. **J Comp Neurol 227:** 214-227, 1984
129. Pifl C, Bertel O, Schingnitz G, et al: Extrastriatal dopamine in symptomatic and asymptomatic rhesus monkeys treated with 1-methyl-4-phenyl-1,2,3,6-tetrahydropyridine (MPTP). **Neurochem Int 17:**263-270, 1990
130. Pifl C, Schingnitz G, Hornykiewicz O: Effect of 1-methyl-4-phenyl-1,2,3,6-tetrahydropyridine on the regional distribution of brain monoamines in the rhesus monkey. **Neuroscience 44:**591-605, 1991
131. Playford ED, Fletcher NA, Sawle GV, et al: Striatal [^{18}F]dopa uptake in familial idiopathic dystonia. **Brain 116:**1191-1199, 1993
132. Pollak P, Benabid AL, Limousin P, et al: Subthalamic nucleus stimulation alleviates akinesia and rigidity in parkinsonian patients. **Adv Neurol 69:**591-594, 1996
133. Pollock LJ, Davis L: Muscle tone in parkinsonian states. **Arch Neurol Psychiatry 23:**303-319, 1930
134. Ranson SW, Berry C: Observations on monkeys with bilateral lesions of the globus pallidus. **Arch Neurol Psychiatry 46:**504-508, 1941
135. Rolls ET: Neurophysiology and cognitive functions of the striatum. **Rev Neurol 150:**648-660, 1994
136. Sadikot AF, Parent A, Francois C: Efferent connections of the centromedian and parafascicular thalamic nuclei in the squirrel monkey: a PHA-L study of subcortical projections. **J Comp Neurol 315:** 137-159, 1992
137. Sadikot AF, Parent A, Smith Y, et al: Efferent connections of the centromedian and parafascicular thalamic nuclei in the squirrel monkey: a light and electron microscopic study of the thalamostriatal projection in relation to striatal heterogeneity. **J Comp Neurol 320:**228-242, 1992
138. Scarnati E, Gasbarri A, Campana E, et al: The organization of nucleus tegmenti pedunculopontinus neurons projecting to basal ganglia and thalamus: a retrograde fluorescent double labeling study in the rat. **Neurosci Lett 79:**11-16, 1987
139. Schultz W, Romo R: Role of primate basal ganglia and frontal cortex in the internal generation of movements. I. Preparatory activity in the anterior striatum. **Exp Brain Res 91:**363-384, 1992
140. Shima F, Ishido K, Sun SJ, et al: Surgical control of akinesia in Parkinson's disease. **Eur Neurol 36 (Suppl 1):**55-61, 1996
141. Sidibé M, Smith Y: Differential synaptic innervation of striatofugal neurones projecting to the internal or external segments of the globus pallidus by thalamic afferents in the squirrel monkey. **J Comp Neurol 365:**445-465, 1996
142. Sidibé M, Smith Y: Synaptic interactions between thalamic afferents and striatal interneurons in monkeys. **Soc Neurosci Abstr 22:**411, 1996 (Abstract)
143. Spiegel EA, Wycis HT: Ansotomy in paralysis agitans. **Arch Neurol Psychiatry 71:**598-614, 1954
144. Sterio D, Berić A, Dogali M, et al: Neurophysiological properties of pallidal neurons in Parkinson's disease. **Ann Neurol 35:**586-591, 1994
145. Strub RL: Frontal lobe syndrome in a patient with bilateral globus pallidus lesions. **Arch Neurol 46:** 1024-1027, 1986
146. Struppler A, Gurfinkel V, Mathis J, et al: Motor performance in parkinsonism following stereotactic thalamotomy. **Adv Neurol 60:**403-407, 1993
147. Sutton JP, Couldwell W, Lew MF, et al: Ventroposterior medial pallidotomy in patients with advanced Parkinson's disease. **Neurosurgery 36:**1112-1117, 1995
148. Svennilson E, Torvik A, Lowe R, et al: Treatment of Parkinsonism by stereotactic thermolesions in the pallidal region. A clinical evaluation of 81 cases. **Acta Psychiatr Neurol Scand 35:**358-377, 1960
149. Taha JM, Favre J, Baumann TK, et al: Characteristics and somatotopic organization of kinesthetic cells in the globus pallidus of patients with Parkinson's disease. **J Neurosurg 85:**1005-1012, 1996
150. Taha JM, Favre J, Baumann TK, et al: Tremor control after pallidotomy in patients with Parkinson's disease: correlation with microrecording findings. **J Neurosurg 86:**642-647, 1997
151. Tranchant C, Maquet J, Eber AM, et al: Angiome caverneux cérébelleux, dystonie cervicale et diaschisis cortical croisé. **Rev Neurol 147:**599-602, 1991
152. Trouche E, Beaubaton D, Amato G, et al: Changes in reaction time after pallidal or nigral lesion in the monkey. **Adv Neurol 40:**29-38, 1984
153. Vitek JL, Ashe J, DeLong MR, et al: Altered somatosensory response properties of neurons in the "motor" thalamus of MPTP treated parkinsonian monkeys. **Soc Neurosci Abstr 16:**425, 1990 (Abstract)
154. Vitek JL, Kaneoke Y, Turner R, et al: Neuronal activity in the internal (GPi) and external (GPe) segments of the globus pallidus (GP) of parkinsonian patients is similar to that in the MPTP-treated primate model of parkinsonism. **Soc Neurosci Abstr 19:**1584, 1993 (Abstract)
155. Vitek JL, Wichmann T, DeLong MR: Current concepts of basal ganglia neurophysiology with respect to tremorgenesis, in Findley LJ, Koller W (eds): **Handbook of Tremor Disorders.** New York, NY: Marcel Dekker, 1994, pp 37-50
156. Whittier JR, Mettler FA: Studies on the subthalamus of the rhesus monkey. II. Hyperkinesia and other physiologic effects of subthalamic lesions with special references to the subthalamic nucleus of Luys. **J Comp Neurol 90:**319-372, 1949
157. Wichmann T, Bergman H, DeLong MR: The primate subthalamic nucleus. I. Functional properties in intact animals. **J Neurophysiol 72:**494-506, 1994
158. Wichmann T, Bergman H, DeLong MR: The primate subthalamic nucleus. III. Changes in motor behavior and neuronal activity in the internal pallidum induced by subthalamic inactivation in the MPTP model of parkinsonism. **J Neurophysiol 72:** 521-530, 1994
159. Wichmann T, DeLong MR: Functional and pathophysiological models of the basal ganglia. **Curr Opin Neurobiol 6:**751-758, 1996
160. Yoshida S, Nambu A, Jinnai K: The distribution of the globus pallidus neurons with input from various cortical areas in the monkeys. **Brain Res 611:** 170-174, 1993

CHAPTER 5

ADVANCES IN THE NEUROPATHOLOGY OF PARKINSON'S DISEASE

DANIEL P. PERL, MD

For the neuropathologist, establishing the diagnosis of Parkinson's disease has been based on morphological observations made in the first half of the 20th century, which are only recently being re-examined using modern tools of neuropathology and neurobiology. Further, insights from our understanding of other neurodegenerative diseases have provided important areas for investigation.

For the diagnostic neuropathologist, the principal histopathological alterations present in cases of Parkinson's disease include neuronal loss in the pars compacta of the substantia nigra accompanied by Lewy bodies in a variable percentage of the remaining neurons. However, it is readily acknowledged that the degree and distribution of cell loss in the nigra remains incompletely studied and the extent of Lewy body formation required to establish a diagnosis of this condition remains to be specifically established.

NEURONAL LOSS IN THE SUBSTANTIA NIGRA

Clearly, the loss of pigmented neurons in the substantia nigra is most closely related to the striatal dopaminergic deficit that underlies this condition (Figure 1). However, relatively little work has been done to document the extent of such loss with respect to the magnitude of motor symptoms and other clinical manifestations of the disease. In addition, cell loss in the substantia nigra is said to occur in association with normal aging, yet the degree to which the neurodegenerative process must be superimposed over such losses in order to initiate symptoms remains poorly studied. It is frequently mentioned that a loss of 60% to 70% of nigra neurons must occur before extrapyramidal symptoms are identified. However, such a statement is based on rather informal clinical impressions and simplified assessments of neuronal loss. The neuronal loss in the substantia nigra is not uniform within the nucleus, and studies indicate that its ventrolateral aspects are most vulnerable to loss.[5,8,11]

Recently, there has been a dramatic change in the approach to quantitative morphological studies through the introduction of the principles of stereology and the recognition that prior nonbiased sampling approaches to quantitation may reach inappropriate conclusions.[1,12,24,26] Techniques that sample only "representative" areas are incapable of differentiating between a reduction in the number of neurons, a shrink-

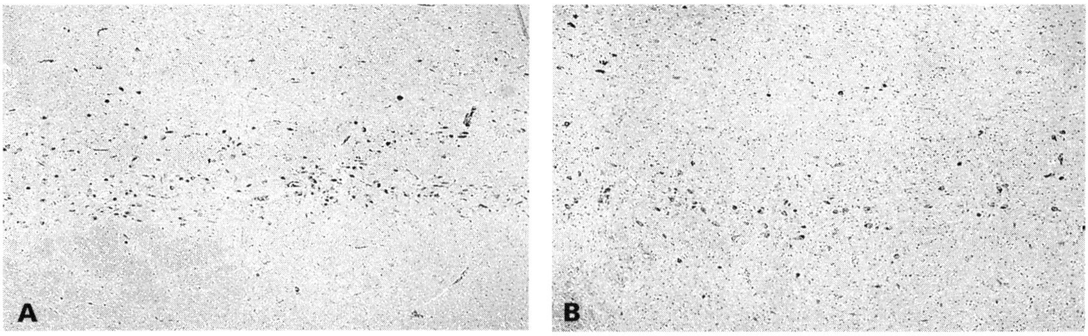

Figure 1: Microphotograph of the substantia nigra in a patient without **(A)** and a patient with **(B)** Parkinson's disease. Note the paucity of neuromelanin-containing neurons *(dark cells)* in B. (Hematoxylin-eosin, original magnification X 50.)

age of neurons, or a differential change between subregions of a structure. Unfortunately, other than a few unique exceptions (see, for example, Pakkenberg et al[22]), most prior attempts to quantitate the number of substantia nigra neurons have used such representative section techniques; indeed, most investigators have chosen only a single level for histological sampling and quantification of the intactness of the nigral neuronal populations.

Lewy Bodies

The Lewy body was first identified by Frederic H. Lewy[18] in 1912, in the substantia innominata (basal forebrain) and the dorsal motor nucleus of the vagus in cases of Parkinson's disease. It was Tretiakoff[25] who in 1919 first recognized the presence of these inclusions in the substantia nigra. Lewy bodies are large, spherical, eosinophilic, intracytoplasmic inclusions (Figure 2). When such inclusions are present within the substantia nigra, along with evidence of neuron loss in this nucleus, there is a very high correlation with a clinical diagnosis of Parkinson's disease.[10] On the other hand, when a clinical diagnosis of Parkinson's disease is made, the likelihood of finding substantia nigra degeneration accompanied by Lewy bodies is not nearly as high. Two studies that reviewed the postmortem evaluations in a series of cases thought clinically to be Parkinson's disease showed that only about 75% demonstrated the presence of Lewy body pathology.[15,23]

Lewy bodies, ranging in size from 4 to 30 μm in diameter, have a brightly eosinophilic core and are classically surrounded by a paler concentric band or bands at the periphery. Lewy bodies are typically solitary within each neuron; however, multiple inclusions within the same neuron may, on occasion, be encountered. In the pigmented nigra neurons, the Lewy bodies push the neuromelanin granules aside and typically occupy a majority of the perikary. In addition to the above-mentioned locations, Lewy bodies may be found in the hypothalamus, locus ceruleus, nucleus basalis of Meynert, raphe nuclei, and autonomic ganglia. Involvement of the latter structures is commonly accompanied by significant autonomic dysfunction.[20]

Ultrastructural examination of Lewy bodies has shown them to be composed of a radially arranged array of straight filaments measuring 8-10 nm in diameter.[4] At the edge of the inclusion, the filaments are associated with an electron-dense granular material as well as vesicular profiles. The Lewy body is not membrane-bound, and the paired helical filaments associated with the neurofibrillary tangles of Alzheimer's disease are not encountered with Lewy bodies.

Immunohistochemical studies have demonstrated that the core of the Lewy body reacts strongly to the lightweight component of the neurofilament triplet proteins; however, the medium-weight and heavyweight neurofilament subunits also appear to be present. In a detailed epitope mapping study, Hill and coworkers[14] demonstrated compartmentalization of the neurofilament constituents of the inclusion, with the

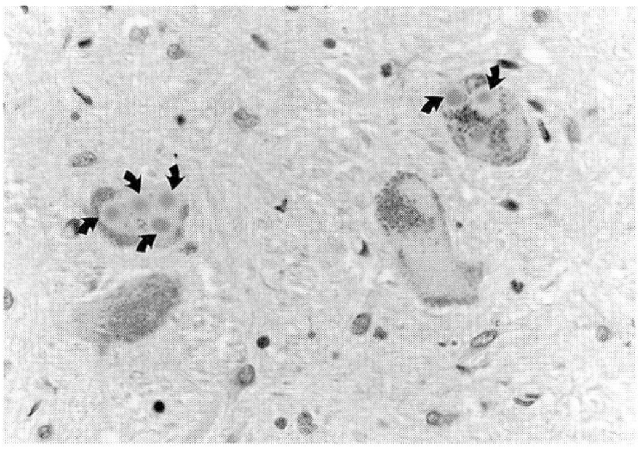

Figure 2: Brain microphotograph showing large spherical intracytoplasmic inclusions, i.e., Lewy bodies *(arrows)* in a patient with Parkinson's disease (hematoxylin-eosin, original magnification X 400).

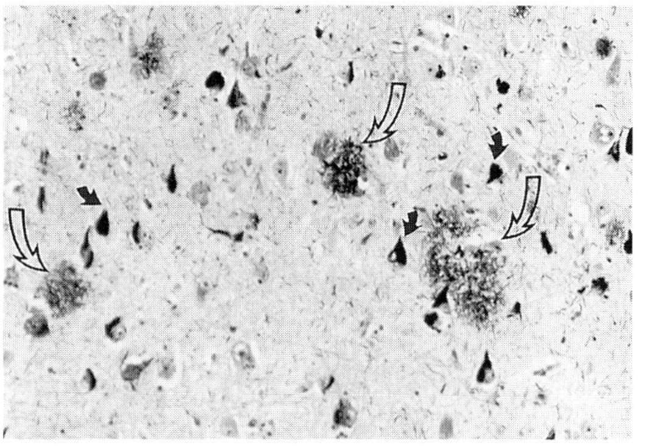

Figure 3: Brain microphotograph showing neurofibrillary tangles within neurons *(black arrows)* and senile plaques *(open arrows)* in a patient with Parkinson's disease (hematoxylin-eosin, original magnification X 250).

N-terminal domain of the neurofilament rod portion being localized to the core of the Lewy body. The C-terminal portions, where most of the phosphorylation sites of these neurofilament subunits are located, are localized to the more peripheral portions of the Lewy body. An important advance was the recognition that Lewy bodies characteristically show positive staining with ubiquitin antibodies.[17] Using such staining approaches, it was found that many cases of Parkinson's disease show the presence of significant numbers of ubiquitin-positive inclusion bodies in the neocortex (see below).

Although the Lewy body is virtually required for a diagnosis of Parkinson's disease, it is by no means seen exclusively in this clinical setting. For example, Lewy bodies have been described in some cases of subacute sclerosing panencephalitis (with long-term survival), Hallervorden-Spatz disease, and ataxia telangiectasia.[19] The significance of the appearance of this inclusion in these varied clinical settings remains unclear, but likely represents the relatively limited repertoire of responses of the neuron to neurodegenerative processes.

Overlap With Alzheimer's Disease

In the neuropathological evaluation of Alzheimer's disease, it is now recognized that, in addition to the neurofibrillary tangles and senile plaques in the hippocampus and neocortex (Figure 3), the changes of Parkinson's disease (nigral neuronal loss and Lewy body formation) are also encountered. In a number of studies it has been shown that approximately 25% of clinically recognized Alzheimer's disease cases showed neuropathological evidence of Parkinson's disease in the midbrain in addition to the changes associated with Alzheimer's disease.[3,13,16] It is currently unclear whether such cases of combined Alzheimer's disease and Parkinson's disease pathologies represent the co-existence of these two relatively common age-related neurodegenerative diseases in the same patient. This is not likely because the lifetime cumulative risk of developing Parkinson's disease is only about 4%. More likely, this superimposition of the two disorders represents shared pathogenetic mechanisms for the two disorders or perhaps an underlying shared genetic susceptibility.

This concept is made even more difficult because the vast majority of such cases also show evidence of Lewy body formation in the pyramidal neurons of the neocortex.[15] The recognition of the existence of such cases has led to the introduction of a number of new diagnostic terms, such as senile dementia, Lewy body type; Lewy body dementia; diffuse cortical Lewy body disease; and dementia with Lewy bodies.[21] Such cases are now readily recognized by neuropathologists through the application of anti-ubiquitin immunohistochemistry on neocortical sections. These preparations reveal prominent ubiquitin-staining spherical inclusion bodies within the cytoplasm of neocortical neurons. Again, the extent and distribution of such changes required to establish the presence of these clinical entities is now being debated and some researchers are even establishing specific diagnostic criteria for Lewy body dementia.[13,21] However, the basic question of the nature of such cases and their relationship to the core pathology of both Alzheimer's disease and Parkinson's disease remains far from clear. Until we understand the nature of such lesions and the underlying etiopathogenetic mechanisms responsible for their formation, such nosological questions will remain unresolved.

Incidental Lewy Bodies

In the neuropathological examination of large numbers of brains derived from elderly individuals, one will find, on occasion, cases in which a few isolated Lewy bodies are identified within the substantia nigra and/or the locus ceruleus, in the absence of any previous clinical evidence of Parkinson's disease. When this occurs, one generally gets the impression that there has not been any appreciable loss of substantia nigra neurons. However, the author is not aware of any attempt to rigorously count nigral neurons in such cases, so this remains an impression only, without confirming scientifically valid data. Nevertheless, diagnostic neuropathologists generally referred to these patients as incidental Lewy body cases.

The frequency of incidental Lewy body cases increases with age and it has been estimated that 10% of individuals in their ninth decade show the presence of these inclusion bodies in the substantia nigra.[7,9] Some authors have suggested that in this setting, the presence of a few Lewy bodies in the absence of significant neuronal degeneration in the pigmented nuclei represents a "normal" aging change. Others, however, have considered such cases to represent an early, presymptomatic phase of Parkinson's disease in which either the patient failed to develop any observable symptoms, or any neurological impairment was so subtle as to not have attracted clinical attention. Nevertheless, the consideration that these cases may represent an initial phase of Parkinson's disease has led some to use such brain specimens to investigate early pathogenetic features of the disorder.[2,6]

Obviously, it is impossible to tell whether such an individual, if allowed to survive for additional years, would have gone on to accumulate sufficient neurodegenerative changes to finally manifest overt symptoms leading to a clinical diagnosis. However, it should be acknowledged that clinically recognized Parkinson's disease is fairly common, and as a slowly progressive disease process, it is likely that it would take a number of years to develop sufficient damage to the substantia nigra for impairment to be of a magnitude to be recognized clinically. Therefore, there is likely a considerable presymptomatic, preclinical period (certainly many years, perhaps a decade or more) for any Parkinson's disease patient. It would be expected that some individuals would die of other causes during that period. Are such individuals those that end up being diagnosed as incidental Lewy body cases? This is likely; however, there is no certainty about that question.

Studies for the Future

The etiology and pathogenesis of Parkinson's disease remains unclear, although increasing evidence indicates that oxidative stress represents an important step in the pathogenetic sequence. However, whether that step is an early event or a late one is currently unknown. Hopefully, information gained from the study of rare genetic forms of Parkinson's disease will provide important clues with relevance to the more common sporadic forms of the disease. Animal models of Parkinson's disease are incomplete and really do not fully mimic the condition as it is seen in humans. The unraveling of genetic forms of the disease will hopefully, in a fashion similar to that accomplished with amyotrophic lateral sclerosis, lead to transgenic models that more closely model the human disorder. Finally, the use of properly obtained human postmortem tissues derived from Parkinson's disease patients can be employed more vigorously to apply modern neurobiological tools for the study of the disease.

It is clear that the coming decade will provide important new insights into the nature of this common age-related condition.

REFERENCES

1. Coggeshall RE, Lekan HA: Methods for determining numbers of cells and synapses: a case for more uniform standards of review. **J Comp Neurol 364:**6-15, 1996
2. Dexter DT, Sian J, Rose S, et al: Indices of oxidative stress and mitochondrial function in individuals with incidental Lewy body disease. **Ann Neurol 35:**38-44, 1994
3. Ditter SM, Mirra SS: Neuropathologic and clinical features of Parkinson's disease in Alzheimer's disease patients. **Neurology 37:**754-760, 1987
4. Duffy PE, Tennyson VM: Phase and electron microscopic observations of Lewy bodies and melanin granules in the substantia nigra and locus caeruleus in Parkinson's disease. **J Neuropathol Exp Neurol 24:** 398-414, 1965
5. Fearnley JM, Lees AJ: Ageing and Parkinson's disease: substantia nigra regional selectivity. **Brain 114:** 2283-2301, 1991
6. Fernandez A, de Ceballos ML, Rose S, et al: Alterations in peptide levels in Parkinson's disease and incidental Lewy body disease. **Brain 119:**823-830, 1996
7. Forno LS, Alvord EC, et al: The pathology of parkinsonism: I. Some new observations and correlations, in Plum F, McDowell F (ed): **Recent Advances in Parkinsonism. Contemporary Neurology Series.** Philadelphia, Pa: FA Davis, 1971, pp 120-130
8. German DC, Manaye K, Smith WK, et al: Midbrain dopaminergic cell loss in Parkinson's disease: computer visualization. **Ann Neurol 26:**507-514, 1989
9. Gibb WRG, Lees AJ: The relevance of the Lewy body to the pathogenesis of idiopathic Parkinson's disease. **J Neurol Neurosurg Psychiatry 51:**745-752, 1988
10. Gibb WRG, Lees AJ: The significance of the Lewy body in the diagnosis of idiopathic Parkinson's disease. **Neuropathol Appl Neurobiol 15:**27-44, 1989
11. Goto S, Hirano A, Matsumoto S: Subdivisional involvement of nigrostriatal loop in idiopathic Parkinson's disease and striatonigral degeneration. **Ann Neurol 26:**766-770, 1989
12. Gundersen HJ, Bagger P, Bendtsen TF, et al: The new stereology tools: disector, fractionator, nucleator and point sampled intercepts and their use in pathological research and diagnosis. **APMIS 96:**857-881, 1988
13. Hansen L, Salmon D, Galasko D, et al: The Lewy body variant of Alzheimer's disease: a clinical and pathologic entity. **Neurology 40:**1-8, 1990
14. Hill WD, Lee VMY, Hurtig HI, et al: Epitopes located in spatially separate domains of each neurofilament subunit are present in Parkinson's disease Lewy bodies. **J Comp Neurol 309:**150-160, 1991
15. Hughes AJ, Daniel SE, Kilford L, et al: Accuracy of clinical diagnosis of idiopathic Parkinson's disease: a clinico-pathological study of 100 cases. **J Neurol Neurosurg Psychiatry 55:**181-184, 1992
16. Hulette C, Mirra S, Wilkinson W, et al: The Consortium to Establish a Registry for Alzheimer's Disease (CERAD). Part IX. A prospective cliniconeuropathologic study of Parkinson's features in Alzheimer's disease. **Neurology 45:**1991-1995, 1995
17. Kuzuhara S, Mori H, Izumiyama N, et al: Lewy bodies are ubiquitinated. A light and electron microscopic immunocytochemical study. **Acta Neuropathol 75:**345-353, 1988
18. Lewy FH: Paralysis agitans 1. Pathologisch Anatomic, in **Handbuch der Neurologie III.** Berlin: Springer Verlag, 1912, pp 920-933
19. Lowe J: Lewy Bodies, in Calne DB (ed): **Neurodegenerative Diseases.** Philadelphia, Pa: WB Saunders, 1994, pp 51-69
20. Lowe J, Lennox G, Leigh PN: Disorders of movement and system degenerations, in Graham, DI, Lantos PI (eds): **Greenfield's Neuropathology, Volume II.** London: E Arnold, 1997, pp 281-366
21. McKieth IG, Galasko D, Kosaka K, et al: Consensus guidelines for the clinical and pathologic diagnosis of dementia with Lewy bodies (DLB): report of the consortium on DLB international workshop. **Neurology 47:**1113-1124, 1996
22. Pakkenberg B, Møller A, Gundersen HJG, et al: The absolute number of nerve cells in substantia nigra in normal subjects and in patients with Parkinson's disease estimated with an unbiased stereological method. **J Neurol Neurosurg Psychiatry 54:**30-33, 1991
23. Rajput AH, Rozdilsky B, Rajput A: Accuracy of clinical diagnosis in parkinsonism—a prospective study. **Can J Neurol Sci 18:**275-278, 1991
24. Sterio DC: The unbiased estimation of number and sizes of arbitrary particles using the disector. **J Microsc 134:**127-136, 1984
25. Trétiakoff C: Contribution à L'étude de L'anatomie Pathologique du Locus Niger de Soemmering. Université de Paris, 1919 (Thesis)
26. West MJ: New stereological methods for counting neurons. **Neurobiol Aging 14:**275-285, 1993

CHAPTER 6

FUNCTIONAL BRAIN IMAGING OF PARKINSON'S DISEASE

KEN KAZUMATA, MD, LAUREN V. MORAN, BA, AND DAVID EIDELBERG, MD

Functional brain imaging with positron emission tomography (PET) has provided novel insights into the pathophysiology of Parkinson's disease and other movement disorders. PET is a quantitative technique employed to localize and measure physiological and biochemical processes in the brain and other organs. In a PET experiment, a subject is given a small dose of positron-emitting radioactivity in the form of a compound of biological interest (Table 1). The spatial and temporal distribution of the radiotracer is measured quantitatively in the course of the PET imaging study, providing a tomographic representation of regional radioactivity accumulation. Regional cerebral blood flow (rCBF) is measured with $[^{15}O]H_2O$ or CO_2, and regional rates of cerebral glucose metabolism (rCMRG) are assessed with $[^{18}F]$fluorodeoxyglucose (FDG). Additionally, PET techniques have been used to assess presynaptic dopaminergic function using $[^{18}F]$fluorodopa (F-DOPA),[12,85] as well as a variety of dopamine transporter binding ligands, such as cocaine,[60] methylphenidate,[87] CFT 2ß-carbomethoxy-3ß-(4-fluorophenyl-[N-^{11}C-methyl]tropane (WIN) 35-428,[32] and 2ß-carbomethyl-3ß-(4-iodophenyl)tropane (ßCIT)[42,53] and its alkylated esters.[14,45]

In this chapter, recent PET studies in patients with Parkinson's disease are reviewed, focusing on the potential application of PET tracers in assessing the outcome of surgical interventions for parkinsonism, including implantation of fetal mesencephalic tissue, pallidotomy, thalamotomy, and deep brain high-frequency stimulation.

THE DOPAMINE SYSTEM

Quantitative Assessment of Dopaminergic Function

F-DOPA is the most extensively used radiotracer applied to the study of Parkinson's disease. PET using F-DOPA measures dopaminergic function by quantifying the rate of tracer uptake and decarboxylation in presynaptic nigrostriatal terminals. F-DOPA is rapidly metabolized in the plasma by catechol-O-methyltransferase (COMT) to 3-O-methyl-fluorodopa (3OMFD) after injection and is transported across the

TABLE 1

POPULAR RADIOTRACERS IN ASSESSING MOVEMENT DISORDERS*

Biological Behavior	Tracer	Application
Regional synaptic activity		
rCMRG	[^{18}F]FDG	Differential diagnosis (parkinsonism), selection of candidates for stereotactic surgery, research
rCBF	[^{15}O]H_2O	Research
Marker of the presynaptic dopaminergic terminal		
Dopamine precursor	[^{18}F]F-DOPA, [^{18}F]tyrosine	Diagnosis of parkinsonism, assessment of severity, progression and post-transplantation changes
Dopamine transporter (re-uptake site)	[^{11}C]-, [^{18}F]-, or [^{123}I]-labeled cocaine derivatives	
Marker of the postsynaptic dopaminergic terminal		
D_2 receptor	[^{11}C]raclopride, [^{11}C] or [^{18}F]n-methyl spiperone	Research, diagnosis of Parkinson's disease, Huntington's disease, and other disorders

* FDG = fluorodeoxyglucose; rCBF = regional cerebral blood flow; rCMRG = regional cerebral metabolic rate of glucose.

blood-brain barrier (BBB) by the large neutral amino acid. It is subsequently decarboxylated to [^{18}F]dopamine by the enzyme dopa decarboxylase (DDC) and accumulates in striatal dopaminergic vesicles. Simple target-to-background calculations are obtained by dividing striatal count rates in a neutral brain region, such as the occipital cortex, to provide a useful means of comparing regional measures of uptake without blood sampling. Alternatively, multiple time graphical analysis has been applied extensively to estimate kinetic rate constants from striatal F-DOPA uptake based upon the time course of striatal and plasma F-DOPA radioactivity (K_i).[73] Compartmental models have also been developed to estimate specific kinetic rate constants for striatal DDC activity (k_3).[16,40,52]

A number of prior studies have indicated that the assessment of nigrostriatal dopaminergic function using F-DOPA-PET yields quantitative parameters that can correlate with independent disease severity measures and that can reliably discriminate early-stage Parkinson's disease patients from normal control subjects.[19,22,43,45,56] The relationship between F-DOPA uptake and the number of dopaminergic neurons was investigated in both human and animal experimental models of parkinsonism.[72,82] Brooks et al[12] reported reductions of F-DOPA uptake in the putamen and caudate in patients with idiopathic Parkinson's disease, corresponding to 45% and 85%, respectively, of normal values. Importantly, asymmetries in putamenal F-DOPA uptake have been correlated with the corresponding asymmetries in clinical manifestations.[4,19,56] Additionally, significant negative correlations have been found between striatal radiotracer uptake rate constants and quantitative disease severity ratings.[4,19,45,85] In a recent study using a high-resolution PET scanner, the authors have also reported a significant correlation between the striatal-to-occipital ratio and disease severity ratings.[45]

The development of radiotracers that bind to the striatal dopamine transporter has led to another means for directly imaging the nigrostriatal dopaminergic system with PET or single photon emission computed tomography (SPECT). The most extensively studied agents in this category are the cocaine analogues, such as ßCIT, and its fluoroalkyl esters, including [^{18}F] N-2-fluoropropyl-2ß-carbomethoxy-3ß-(4-iodophenyl)nortropane (FP-ßCIT)[1,42] (Figure 1). Dopamine transporter is expressed on dopaminergic nigral terminals, and quantification of

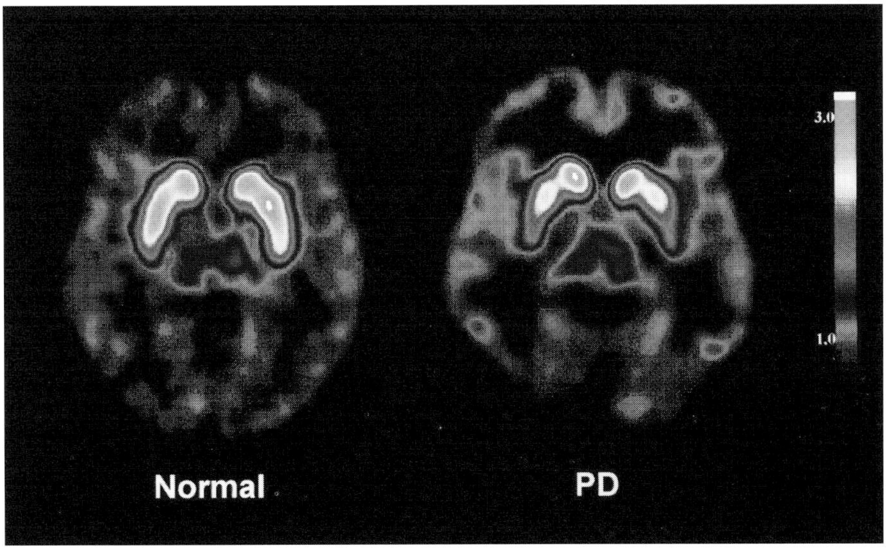

Figure 1: Dopamine transporter binding measured by the uptake of FP-ßCIT, a cocaine analogue, as seen on FP-ßCIT-PET images in a normal volunteer and a mildly affected Parkinson's disease patient. An asymmetrical reduction in putamenal uptake is evident in the Parkinson's disease patient.

striatal dopamine transporter appears to be directly related to the extent of nigral cell degeneration.[89] Imaging of dopamine transporter may have advantages over F-DOPA for several reasons:

1. As dopaminergic neurons decline in normal senescence, F-DOPA uptake may be maintained at a constant level by the up-regulation of DDC activity, thus potentially making F-DOPA-PET insensitive to age-related decrements in presynaptic dopaminergic function. Because dopamine transporter may not be as subject to up-regulation as DDC,[49] the former may be a more sensitive marker for nigrostriatal cell loss in parkinsonism and normal aging.[45]
2. Transport of 3OMFD across the BBB may affect quantification of DDC activity, thus confounding results achieved using F-DOPA-PET.[32,42,45]
3. Finally, the signal-to-noise ratio is potentially higher for dopamine transporter imaging than for F-DOPA-PET.[43,45] A number of recent SPECT studies have demonstrated the utility of ßCIT and FP-ßCIT as effective markers of nigrostriatal dopaminergic degeneration in parkinsonism.[5,45,64,70,81] SPECT imaging with these tracers reliably differentiates Parkinson's disease subjects from normal volunteers, and the degree of striatal binding correlates with clinical measures of Parkinson's disease severity. In contrast to F-DOPA-PET,[36] FP-ßCIT-SPECT studies have shown a decline of dopaminergic function with normal aging.[45,86] The authors' laboratory has recently reported that PET imaging with FP-ßCIT can provide images with higher resolution and better quantification than SPECT images acquired with the same ligand.[14]

Application of Dopaminergic Imaging in Mesencephalic Fetal Implantation

The implantation of fetal mesencephalon may prove to be useful in the treatment of Parkinson's disease.[10,27] In vivo assessment of presynaptic nigrostriatal dopaminergic function with F-DOPA-PET may be used to monitor graft survival and development after transplantation. To date only a limited number of patients have been studied using PET. One patient exhibited sustained postoperative increases in F-DOPA uptake in the grafted putamen 33 months after transplantation.[29] Sawle et al[77] subsequently reported two Parkinson's disease patients who underwent unilateral implantation into the putamen and had F-DOPA-PET imaging before and 12-13 months following surgery. These patients had substantial increases in F-DOPA uptake in the grafted putamen and decreases in the nongrafted striatum, presumably associated with disease progression. In one of these patients, clinical improvement continued 3 years after transplantation and was accompanied by a further increase in F-DOPA uptake in the grafted putamen. In the other patient, there was no further increase in F-DOPA uptake or improvement in clinical symptoms between 1 and 3 years after transplantation.[57-59] Widner et al[88] reported two patients with1-methyl-4-phenyl-1, 2,3,6-tetrahydropyridine (MPTP)-induced parkinsonism treated with bilateral implantation in the caudate and putamen. These patients showed significant clinical improvement 6 months after transplantation, as well as appreciable bilateral increases in striatal F-DOPA uptake. Recently, Remy et al[75] reported increases in F-DOPA uptake in five patients with unilateral implantation in the putamen; changes in the F-DOPA uptake rate constant were significantly correlated with clinical improvement measures.

The authors have recently performed fetal mesencephalic tissue implantation in six patients with Parkinson's disease. Ventral mesencephalic tissue was acquired from aborted human fetuses at 6-9 weeks postconception and transplanted into the putamen bilaterally. F-DOPA-PET imaging performed 1 year postimplantation showed a significant increase in F-DOPA uptake in both putamina, corresponding approximately to a 15% increase compared to normal values (Figure 2). These findings suggest that F-DOPA-PET may be a useful tool in monitoring graft survival and development after fetal mesencephalic transplantation.

The following mechanisms are presumed to underlie growth of the dopaminergic graft: 1) synaptic reinnervation;[10] 2) diffusion of neurotransmitter from the graft; 3) sprouting host dopaminergic neurons by local trophic effects; and 4) alteration of the BBB by revascularization.[33,76] In previous investigations, both the striatal-to-occipital ratio and K_i F-DOPA-PET indices have been employed to quantify changes in striatal radiotracer uptake following fetal implantation procedures.[75,77] A number of caveats must be considered in the investigation of these published findings. F-DOPA crosses the BBB in competition with other neutral amino acids.[38,44,56] Thus, any alteration of plasma amino acid content (including changes in peripheral levodopa [L-DOPA] levels) may alter F-DOPA transport and can confound F-DOPA-PET quantifiers of dopaminergic function. In addition, the assessment of graft survival and growth using F-DOPA-PET may potentially be overestimated by postoperative increases in net transport of F-DOPA across the BBB.[65,78]

Indeed, evidence indicates that both permeability and surface area can increase after tissue transplantation. Fluorescence histochemical measurements of monoamine uptake into central neurons suggest that the BBB to monoamines may not be fully developed in infant rats.[61] The influx rate of amino acids is greater during the first weeks of life and subsequently falls to the level found in adult rats at 8-10 weeks of age.[6] Guttman et al[36] reported five patients who underwent adrenal medulla implantation and who had pre- and postoperative F-DOPA-PET scans. In two patients, increased permeability of the BBB was shown at the implanted sites using gallium ethylenediamine-tetra-acetic acid ([^{68}Ga] EDTA) and PET. By contrast, Dusart et al[18] demonstrated two different types of angiogenesis in the thalamus after transplantation of dissociated fetal tissue. Although these authors observed mature angiogenesis in the grafted site, reactive angiogenesis with an immature BBB developed in lesions without engraftment. These results indicate that angiogenesis may also induce significant increases in F-DOPA uptake without necessarily implicating reinnervation from the grafted tissues.

Postmortem results from two patients who underwent fetal mesencephalic implantation and postoperative F-DOPA-PET have been reported. Kordower and colleagues[50] reported one patient who showed substantial clinical improvement and progressive increases in F-DOPA uptake in the grafted putamen. Pathological examination 18 months following surgery revealed

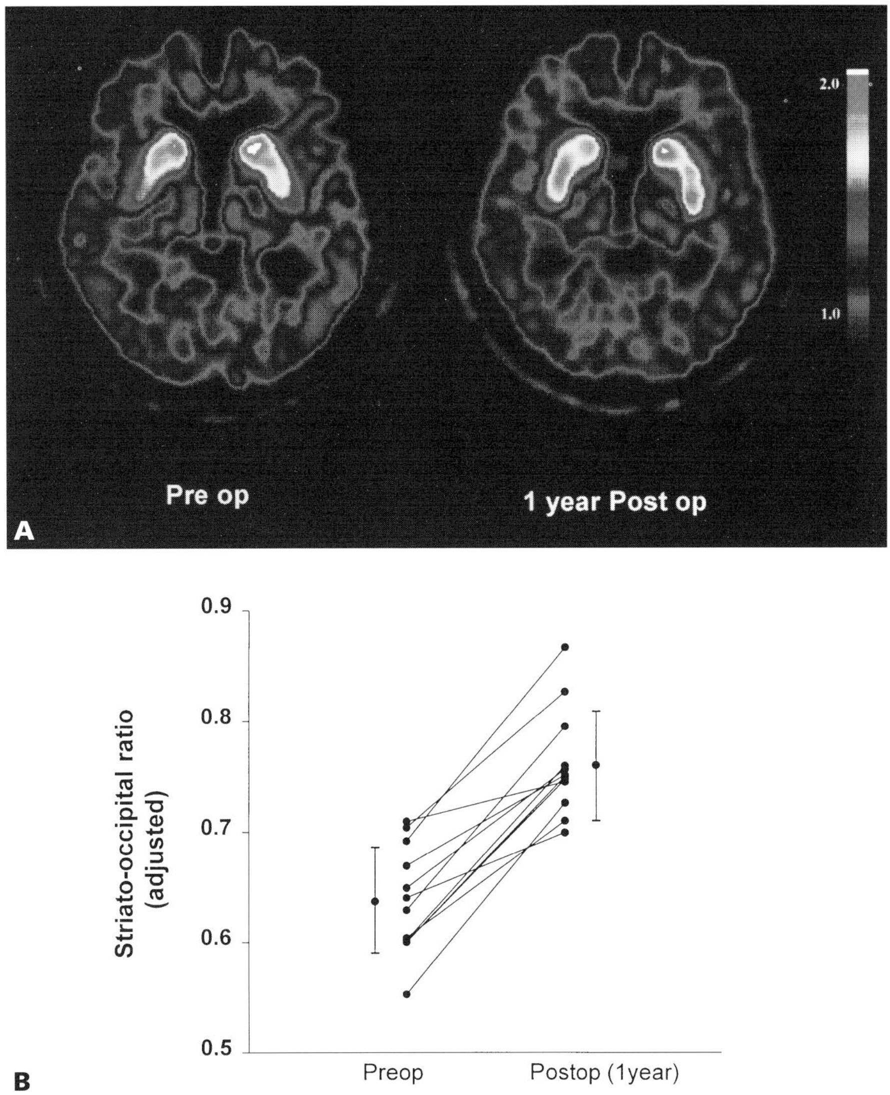

Figure 2: A) F-DOPA-PET scans obtained before and 1 year following the implantation of fetal mesencephalic tissue in a patient with Parkinson's disease. Preoperatively, there is evidence of a significant reduction in bilateral F-DOPA uptake, predominantly in the posterior putamen. An increase in radiotracer uptake in the putamen is evident 1 year following tissue implantation into this region. **B)** Comparison of striato-occipital ratio measurements determined with F-DOPA-PET before and 1 year following fetal mesencephalic tissue implantation for Parkinson's disease. A significant increase in radiotracer uptake is evident postoperatively.

evidence of graft survival and dopaminergic reinnervation of the striatum, but no evidence of sprouting of host dopaminergic neurons. Another patient underwent intrastriatal and intraventricular implantation of fetal dopaminergic tissue. F-DOPA-PET scanning 15 months following surgery (8 months before death) disclosed increased radiotracer uptake in the pericaudate area and in the putamen—sites where implantation had been performed. Postmortem examination revealed only gliosis and inflammatory response in these areas.[28]

Further technological development is required to optimize fetal implantation surgery as a therapeutic option in advanced parkinsonism. The safety and efficacy of these procedures is currently unknown and is a topic of several controlled clinical studies. Whether changes in striatal F-DOPA uptake accurately reflect graft survival is also the subject of ongoing investigation. Alternative dopaminergic imaging methods may afford a complementary tool for the assessment of outcome following fetal implantation. Specifically, adjunctive imaging of striatal dopamine transporter activity before and after implantation procedures may lead to a broader understanding of the effects of neural implantation on the nigrostriatal dopamine system.

Brain Metabolism and Blood Flow

Network Quantification

In most degenerative neurological conditions, local cerebral blood flow and metabolism are coupled processes and relate to synaptic activity within a given brain region. The measurements of local rates of metabolism or regional activation responses may not fully describe the complexities of neural systems involved in a neurodegenerative process and their modulation with treatment. These networks may be represented as patterns of covariation among spatially distributed brain regions and can be altered by behavioral activation or the presence of disease.

Neurodegenerative processes such as parkinsonism can be quantitatively assessed using FDG and PET to measure regional rates of glucose utilization. The authors have employed a statistical model of regional metabolic covariation to identify abnormal brain topographies in Parkinson's disease and related disorders.[19-23] This algorithm, known as the Scaled Subprofile Model (SSM),[3,68,69] is a form of principal component analysis that identifies patterns of regional covariation in brain metabolism data. Through modifications of the functional imaging data prior to performing the principal component analysis, SSM analysis both characterizes the regional covariance structure of subject groups and measures the expression of the obtained regional covariance patterns in individual subjects (subject scores). In this way, SSM provides a means of comparing the expression of these patterns in different populations and of examining their relationship with independent clinical descriptions, such as disease severity and subject age.

In Parkinson's disease patients, SSM analysis revealed a reproducible pattern of regional metabolism characterized by increased lentiform and thalamic metabolism associated with reduced metabolism in the lateral frontal, paracentral, and parieto-occipital areas.[19-22,24,25] In addition, the degree of individual expression of this covariance pattern correlates with disease severity ratings and independent PET measurements of striatal F-DOPA uptake in Parkinson's disease patients.[19-22] These results agree with experimental animal models, in which parkinsonian signs are associated with excessive pallidofugal inhibitory outflow with concomitant suppression of brain function in primary and associated motor cortical regions.[2,66] A reduction of nigrostriatal dopaminergic activity leads to increased functional activity in the putamen and the subthalamic nucleus.[9,51,80,83,90] Increased activity in the subthalamic nucleus results in overactivity of the pallidothalamic pathway with concomitant suppression of thalamocortical excitatory inputs (Figure 3). Indeed, the authors have recently noted a significant correlation between the expression of SSM metabolic brain networks and neuronal activity of the internal segment of the globus pallidus (GPi) in 18 Parkinson's disease patients who underwent single-unit recordings during pallidotomy.[25,84]

Stereotactic Pallidotomy: Operative Changes in Network Modulation

Leksell's posterolateral ventral pallidotomy has been shown to significantly improve akinetic symptoms in Parkinson's disease, as well as to relieve dyskinesia associated with L-DOPA administration.[7,8,17,54,63] The pathophysiology of pallidal ablation for the relief of parkinsonism is not completely understood. The ameliorative effects of pallidotomy have been attributed to the reduc-

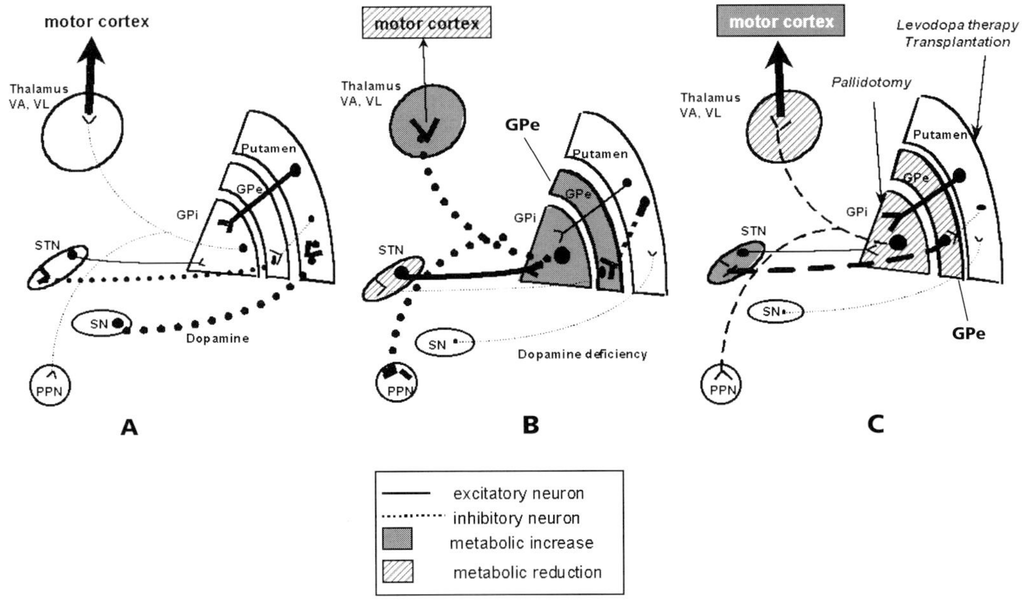

Figure 3: Schematic drawing illustrating synaptic activity and regional metabolism in normal brain **(A)**; consequent to the dopaminergic depletion in Parkinson's disease **(B)**; and following surgical and pharmacological interventions **(C)**. GPi = internal segment of the globus pallidus; GPe = external segment of the globus pallidus; STN = subthalamic nucleus; PPN = pedunculopontine nucleus; SN = substantia nigra pars compacta; VA = ventral anterior thalamic nucleus; VL = ventral lateral thalamic nucleus.

tion of excessive inhibitory outflow from the GPi.

The authors originally reported eight Parkinson's disease patients undergoing pallidotomy who had FDG-PET preoperatively and 6 months postoperatively.[24] The authors applied SSM analysis to rCMRG difference values to identify patterns of regional change occurring with surgery. The topography identified in this analysis closely resembled the Parkinson's disease-related profile identified previously and was characterized by operative decreases in the hypermetabolism of the lentiform nucleus on the surgical side covarying with bilateral increases in supplementary motor area metabolism (Figure 4). Subject scores for this operative difference profile were highly correlated with changes in contralateral limb CAPIT (Core Assessment Program for Intracerebral Transplantation) scores.[55] These findings indicate that functionally and anatomically interconnected brain regions remote from the lesion site are modulated by pallidotomy, including cortical areas of the hemisphere that did not undergo surgical treatment. These network-related metabolic changes may be due to enhanced cortical afferent synaptic activity from the ventral thalamus following surgical reduction in pallidothalamic inhibitory output.[46,52,67]

PET activation studies using [^{15}O]H_2O lend credence to the notion of pallidotomy-induced modulation of the cortico-striato-pallido-thalamo-cortical (CSPTC) motor circuit. Subtraction of resting state from task-specific data allows isolation of changes in rCBF relating to various motor tasks.[30,31] Grafton et al[35] reported movement-related increases in rCBF in the ipsilateral premotor and supplementary motor areas after pallidal ablation. In another study employing network analysis of motor system connectivity, Grafton and colleagues[34] found significant reductions in the strength of interactions between the globus pallidus and the thalamus, and between the thalamus and the mesial frontal motor area. These findings are in accordance with what is known about the CSPTC motor loop, and demonstrate the importance of this motor network in regulating volitional movements.[13,15]

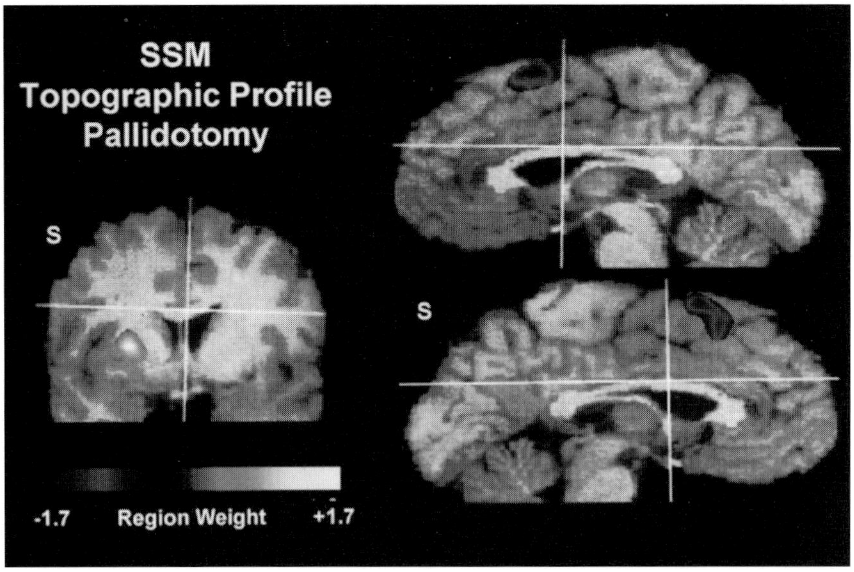

Figure 4: Display of the regional covariance pattern associated with postsurgical changes in glucose metabolism following pallidotomy, identified using the Scaled Subprofile Model (SSM). Regional weights have been overlaid on standardized Talairach transformed magnetic resonance imaging sections *(Left:* coronal, y = –8 mm; *Right:* sagittal, x = ±1 mm). This pattern was characterized by operative declines in lentiform metabolism covarying with bilateral metabolic increases in the supplementary motor area. S = surgical side. (Reproduced from Eidelberg et al[28] with permission.)

Pallidotomy

Functional Predictors of Clinical Outcome

In addition to adding to our understanding of the network modulations occurring with pallidotomy, FDG-PET may be useful in selecting optimal candidates for pallidotomy. Indeed, the authors observed that preoperative lentiform glucose metabolism positively correlates with postoperative clinical improvement in two independent patient populations studied on different tomographs[24,47] (Figure 5). This supports the contention that optimal pallidotomy candidates have functionally overactive lentiform nuclei. The only two patients who had no postoperative improvement in CAPIT ratings had the lowest rates of lentiform glucose metabolism in the entire cohort (Figure 5A). Additionally, a preoperative L-DOPA responsiveness index correlated significantly with percent clinical improvement. In a linear regression analysis, the authors found that preoperative lentiform glucose metabolism was the best predictor for surgical outcome, accounting for nearly 50% of outcome variance, whereas the preoperative L-DOPA responsiveness index accounted for 36.5% of variance. However, combining both these measures accounted for 71% of variance in outcome. The authors believe that L-DOPA responsiveness reflects an individual's capacity for operative modulation of the CSPTC motor circuit. A prior PET study demonstrated reduction in pallidal hypermetabolism with L-DOPA infusion.[11] The authors' findings indicate that optimal candidates for pallidotomy should have a functionally suppressible pallidum. Combining preoperative FDG-PET measurements of lentiform metabolism with clinicopharmacological estimates of the patient's individual capacity for network modulation can provide useful and complementary criteria for patient selection for pallidotomy.

FDG-PET is also a powerful tool in the differential diagnosis of parkinsonism.[20,22,26] Atypical parkinsonian syndromes are akinetic-rigid syndromes clinically characterized by progressive

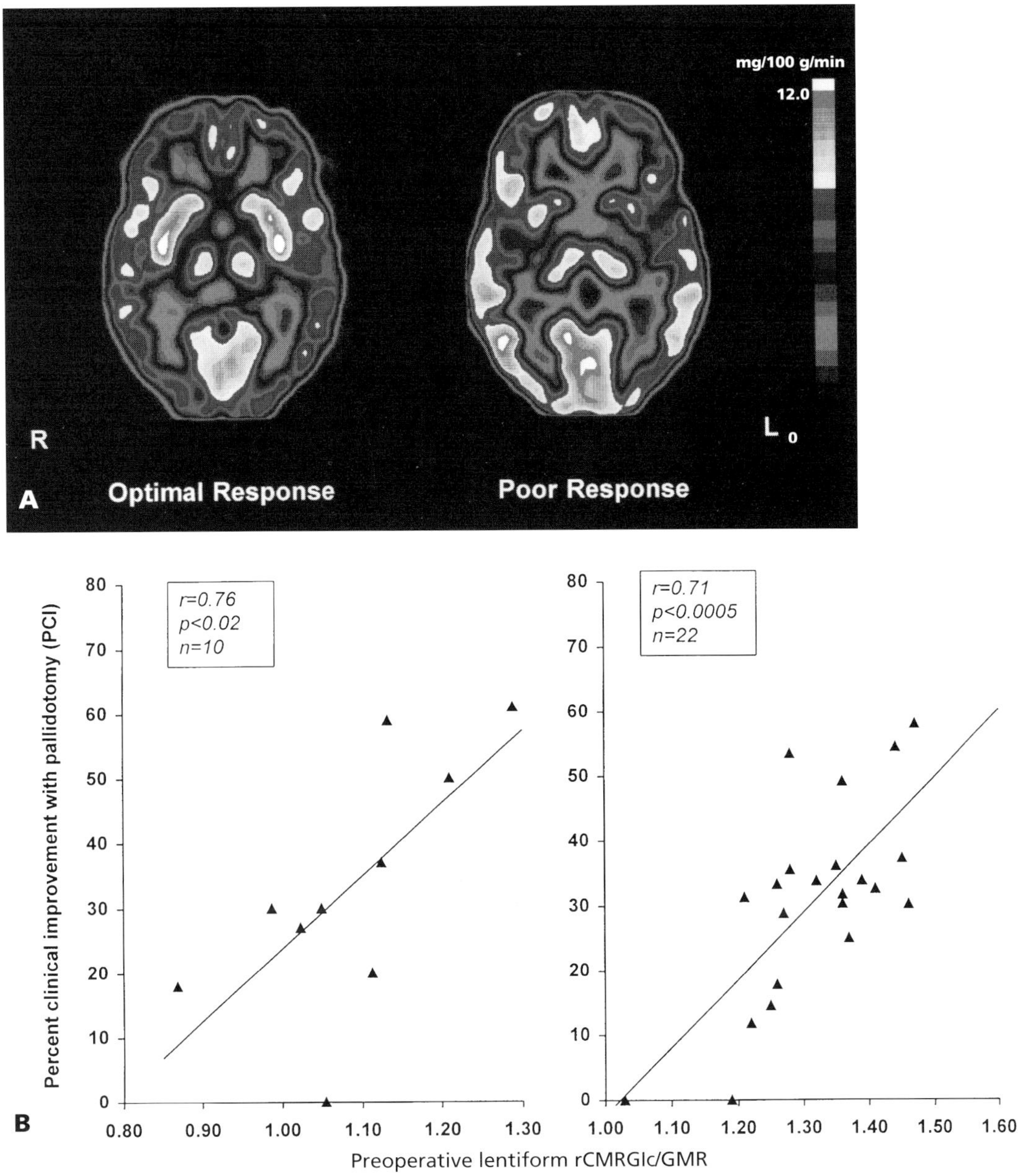

Figure 5: A) Preoperative [^{18}F]FDG-PET images from two patients with idiopathic Parkinson's disease who underwent right unilateral pallidotomy. *Left:* A patient with preoperative lentiform glucose hypermetabolism had an optimum surgical outcome. *Right:* A patient with a lower rate of metabolism in the lentiform nucleus had no therapeutic response to surgery. Both pallidotomy lesions were comparable in size and location. The color stripe represents regional rates of glucose metabolism in mg/100 g/min. **B)** Correlation between preoperative lentiform glucose metabolism normalized by the global mean (rCMRG/GMR) and percent clinical improvement (PCI) in contralateral limb CAPIT scores measured 3 months following pallidotomy. Preoperative lentiform metabolism correlated significantly with PCI in two independent patient cohorts scanned on different tomography devices (*Left:* SuperPET 3000, Scanditronix, Essex, Massachusetts, full width at half maximum (FWHM) = 7.5 mm; *Right:* GE Advance, General Electric, Milwaukee, Wisconsin, FWHM = 4.3 mm).

rigidity, usually without tremor, and minimal or absent response to dopaminergic therapy.[74] Although these conditions are pathologically heterogeneous, they are often clinically indistinguishable from each other as well as from Parkinson's disease. Because patients with atypical Parkinson's disease show little improvement with pallidotomy, it is important to identify them when selecting candidates for surgery. Although lack of response to dopaminergic therapy is highly predictive of atypical parkinsonism, differential diagnosis cannot be made solely on the basis of this clinical feature. A retrospective study of 23 pathologically confirmed cases of multiple system atrophy revealed that 15 responded to L-DOPA initially, while the remaining 8 patients remained partially responsive up to the time of death.[41] The authors recently performed FDG-PET imaging on a cohort of 43 patients diagnosed with atypical Parkinson's disease and 56 patients with classical idiopathic Parkinson's disease. The FDG-PET data from the atypical group was characterized by reductions in caudate and lentiform nuclei and in the thalamus relative to the classical group. A linear combination of caudate, lentiform, and thalamic metabolic values accurately differentiated the two clinical groups studied on different tomographs.[48]

Anatomical Correlates

Preoperative FDG-PET measures can be construed as meaningful indicators of outcome only if the pallidum itself is anatomically normal before surgery and if the pallidotomy lesion is placed accurately. Indeed, patients with coexisting vascular lesions of the basal ganglia may not be appropriate surgical candidates. Similarly, this procedure may not be beneficial for patients with parkinsonism secondary to other forms of pallidal pathology, such as manganese intoxication.[71]

The issues of optimal lesion localization and volume are unresolved. The use of microelectrode recording allows tailoring of the pallidal target for individual patients.[62,79] The authors have recently explored the relationship between lesion site and surgical outcome using postoperative magnetic resonance imaging measurements.[47] In this series of 22 patients, lesions were fine-tuned by microelectrode recording to be localized to the middle of the GPi as far posteriorly and ventrally as possible, to allow for at least 6 mm of depth with a 45°-50° angle to the anterior commissure (AC)-posterior commissure (PC) plane. In this patient group, pallidal lesions were comparable in location across subjects and agreed well with the proposed target. (The coordinates of the ventral end of the lesion were $x = 19.6 \pm 1.4$ mm, $y = 0.7 \pm 1.6$ mm, and $z = -4.4 \pm 1.2$ mm, scaled to the AC-PC line length of 23 mm. The volume of the lesion was 262 ± 76 mm^3.) In accordance with earlier studies, the authors found no evidence of a relationship between operative outcome and the position and size of the surgical lesion.[24,37,39] Given the limited variability in target location, it is not surprising that no association between lesion coordinates and clinical outcome could be discerned in the data. Instead, the authors found that lesions of comparable position in the posteroventral pallidum were associated with striking individual differences in postoperative motor improvement. It was also noted that with the average 6-mm diameter of the pallidal lesions, there was apt to be considerable overlap in lesion position across patients. Therefore, given the limited variability in target location, it is not surprising that no association between lesion coordinates and clinical outcome could be discerned in the authors' data.

SUMMARY

To assess surgical outcome, reliable in vivo markers of neuronal activity are needed. Currently available clinical scales are relatively insensitive and inherently variable, and may not accurately reflect the extent of neuropathological change. Alternatively, quantitative functional brain imaging markers may be suitable as outcome measures for the surgical treatment of Parkinson's disease. The authors have found that PET serves as a useful tool in predicting optimal candidates for certain surgical interventions.

Considerable attention has been dedicated to the development of novel data analysis methods for the characterization and quantification of neural networks in functional brain imaging data. Moreover, new radiotracer techniques have been developed to quantify neurochemical deficits associated with neurodegenerative processes. A major contribution of this research has been a combined approach utilizing both network analysis strategies and in vivo neurochemical measurements to investigate the relationships between localized neuronal attrition and the expression of widely distributed functional brain networks. These complementary PET techniques may greatly advance the understanding of the pathophysiology of Parkinson's disease and the functional changes that occur with surgical treatment.

REFERENCES

1. Abi-Dargham A, Gandelman MS, DeErausquin G: SPECT imaging of dopamine transporters in human brain with iodine-123 fluoroalkyl analogs of ßCIT. **J Nucl Med 37:**1129-1133, 1996
2. Alexander GE, Crutcher MD, DeLong MR: Basal ganglia-thalamocortical circuits: parallel substrates for motor, oculomotor, "prefrontal" and "limbic" functions. **Prog Brain Res 85:**119-146, 1990
3. Alexander GE, Moeller JR: Application of the scaled subprofile model to functional imaging in neuropsychiatric disorders: a principal component approach to modeling brain function in disease. **Hum Brain Mapp 2:**1-16, 1994
4. Antonini A, Vontobel P, Psylla M, et al: Complementary positron emission tomographic studies of the striatal dopaminergic system in Parkinson's disease. **Arch Neurol 52:**1183-1190, 1995
5. Asenbaum S, Brücke T, Pirker W, et al: Imaging of dopamine transporters with iodine-123-ßCIT and SPECT in Parkinson's disease. **J Nucl Med 38:**1-6, 1997
6. Baños G, Daniel PM, Pratt OE: The effect of age upon the entry of some amino acids into the brain, and their incorporation into cerebral protein. **Dev Med Child Neurol 20:**335-346, 1978
7. Baron JC, Levasseur, Mazoyer B, et al: Thalamocortical diaschesis: positron emission tomography in humans. **J Neurol Neurosurg Psychiatry 55:**935-942, 1992
8. Baron MS, Vitek JL, Bakay RAE, et al: Treatment of advanced Parkinson's disease by GPi pallidotomy: 1-year results of a pilot study. **Ann Neurol 40:** 355-366, 1996
9. Bergman H, Wichmann T, Karmon B, et al: The primate subthalamic nucleus. II. Neuronal activity in the MPTP model of Parkinsonism. **J Neurophysiol 72:**507-520, 1994
10. Björklund A, Stenevi U: Reconstruction of nigrostriatal dopamine pathway by intracerebral nigral transplant. **Brain Res 177:**555-560, 1979
11. Blesa R, Blin J, Miletich R, et al: Levodopa-reduced glucose metabolism in striatopallidothalamo-cortical circuit in Parkinson's disease. **Neurology 41 (Suppl 1):**359,1991 (Abstract)
12. Brooks DJ, Salmon EP, Mathias CJ, et al: The relationship between locomotor disability, autonomic dysfunction, and the integrity of the striatal dopaminergic system in patients with multiple system atrophy, pure autonomic failure, and Parkinson's disease, studied with PET. **Brain 113:**1539-1552, 1990
13. Ceballos-Baumann AO, Obeso JA, Vitek JL, et al: Restoration of thalamocortical activity after posteroventral pallidotomy in Parkinson's disease. **Lancet 344:**814, 1994 (letter)
14. Chaly T, Dhawan V, Kazumata K, et al: Radiosynthesis of [^{18}F]N-3-fluoropropyl-2-ß-carbomethoxy-3-ß-(4-iodophenyl)nortropane and the first human study with positron emission tomography. **Nucl Med Biol 23:**999-1004, 1996
15. DeLong MR: Primate models of movement disorders of basal ganglia origin. **Trends Neurosci 13:** 281-285, 1990
16. Dhawan V, Ishikawa T, Patlak C, et al: Combined F-DOPA and 3OMFD PET studies in Parkinson's disease. **J Nucl Med 37:**209-216, 1996
17. Dogali M, Fazzini E, Kolodny E, et al: Stereotactic ventral pallidotomy for Parkinson's disease. **Neurology 45:**753-761, 1995
18. Dusart I, Nothias F, Roudier F, et al: Visualization of fetal cell suspension grafts in the excitotoxically lesioned adult rat thalamus. **Brain Res Dev Brain Res 48:**215-228, 1989
19. Eidelberg D, Moeller JR, Dhawan V, et al: The metabolic anatomy of Parkinson's disease: complementary [^{18}F]-fluorodeoxyglucose and [^{18}F]-fluorodopa positron emission tomographic studies. **Mov Disord 5:** 203-213, 1990
20. Eidelberg D, Moeller JR, Dhawan V, et al: The metabolic topography of parkinsonism. **J Cereb Blood Flow Metab 14:**783-801, 1994
21. Eidelberg D, Moeller JR, Ishikawa T, et al: Assessment of disease severity in parkinsonism with fluorine-18-fluorodeoxyglucose and PET. **J Nucl Med 36:**378-383, 1995
22. Eidelberg D, Moeller JR, Ishikawa T, et al: Early differential diagnosis of Parkinson's disease with ^{18}F-fluorodeoxyglucose and positron emission tomography. **Neurology 45:**1995-2004, 1995
23. Eidelberg D, Moeller JR, Ishikawa T, et al: The metabolic topography of idiopathic torsion dystonia. **Brain 118:**1473-1484, 1995
24. Eidelberg D, Moeller JR, Ishikawa T, et al: Regional metabolic correlates of surgical outcome following unilateral pallidotomy for Parkinson's disease. **Ann Neurol 39:**450-459, 1996
25. Eidelberg D, Moeller JR, Kazumata K, et al: Metabolic correlates of pallidal neuronal activity in Parkinson's disease. **Brain 120:**1315-1324, 1997
26. Eidelberg D, Takikawa S, Dhawan V, et al: Striatal ^{18}F-DOPA uptake: absence of an aging effect. **J Cereb Blood Flow Metab 13:**881-888, 1993
27. Fahn S: Fetal-tissue transplants in Parkinson's disease. **N Engl J Med 327:**1589-1590, 1992 (Editorial)
28. Folkerth RD, Durso RD: Survival and proliferation of nonneural tissues, with obstruction of cerebral ventricles, in a parkinsonian patient treated with fetal allografts. **Neurology 46:**1219-1225, 1996
29. Freed CR, Breeze RE, Rosenberg NL, et al: Survival of implanted fetal dopamine cells and neurologic improvement 12 to 46 months after transplantation for Parkinson's disease. **N Engl J Med 327:**1549-1555, 1992

30. Friston KJ, Frith CD, Liddle PF, et al: The relationship between global and local changes in PET scans. **J Cereb Blood Flow Metab 10:**458-466, 1990
31. Friston KJ, Holmes KJ, Worsely KJ: Statistical parametric maps in functional imaging: a general linear approach. **Hum Brain Mapp 2:**189-210, 1995
32. Frost JJ, Rosier AJ, Reich SG, et al: Positron emission tomographic imaging of the dopamine transporter with ^{11}C-WIN 35,428 reveals marked declines in mild Parkinson's disease. **Ann Neurol 34:**423-431, 1993
33. Geny C, Naimi-Sadaoui S, Jeny R, et al: Long-term delayed vascularization of human neural transplants to the rat brain. **J Neurosci 14:**7553-7562, 1994
34. Grafton ST, Sutton J, Couldwell W, et al: Network analysis of motor system connectivity in Parkinson's disease: modulation of thalamocortical interactions after pallidotomy. **Hum Brain Mapp 2:**45-55, 1994
35. Grafton ST, Waters C, Sutton J, et al: Pallidotomy increases activity of motor association cortex in Parkinson's disease: a positron emission tomographic study. **Ann Neurol 37:**776-783, 1995
36. Guttman M, Burns RS, Martin WRW, et al: PET studies of parkinsonian patients treated with autologous adrenal implants. **Can J Neurol Sci 16:**305-309, 1989
37. Hanieh A, Maloney AFJ: Localization of stereotaxic lesions in the treatment of parkinsonism: a clinicopathological comparison. **J Neurosurg 31:**393-399, 1969
38. Hardebo JE, Falck B, Owman CH: A comparative study on the uptake and subsequent decarboxylation of monoamine precursors in cerebral microvessels. **Acta Physiol Scand 107:**161-167, 1979
39. Hariz MI: Correlation between clinical outcome and size and site of the lesion in computed tomography guided thalamotomy and pallidotomy. **Stereotact Funct Neurosurg 54/55:**172-185, 1990
40. Huang SC, Yu DC, Barrio JR, et al: Kinetics and modeling of L-6-[^{18}F]fluoro-DOPA in human positron emission tomographic studies. **J Cereb Blood Flow Metab 11:**898-913, 1991
41. Hughes AJ, Colosimo C, Kleedorfer B, et al: The dopaminergic response in multiple system atrophy. **J Neurol Neurosurg Psychiatry 55:**1009-1013, 1992
42. Innis RB, Seibyl JP, Scanley BE, et al: Single photon emission computed tomographic imaging demonstrates loss of striatal dopamine transporters in Parkinson's disease. **Proc Natl Acad Sci USA 90:** 11965-11969, 1993
43. Ishikawa T, Dhawan V, Chaly T, et al: Clinical significance of striatal DOPA decarboxylase activity in Parkinson's disease. **J Nucl Med 37:**216-222, 1996
44. Ishikawa T, Dhawan V, Chaly T, et al: Fluorodopa positron emission tomography with an inhibitor of catechol-O-methyltransferase: effect of the plasma 3-O-methyldopa fraction on data analysis. **J Cereb Blood Flow Metab 16:**854-863, 1996
45. Ishikawa T, Dhawan V, Kazumata K, et al: Comparative nigrostriatal dopaminergic imaging with iodine-123-ßCIT-FP/SPECT and fluorine-18-FDOPA/PET. **J Nucl Med 37:**1760-1765, 1996
46. Kadekaro M, Crane AM, Sokoloff L: Differential effects of electrical stimulation of sciatic nerve on metabolic activity in spinal cord and dorsal root ganglion in the rat. **Proc Natl Acad Sci USA 82:** 6010-6013, 1985
47. Kazumata K, Antonini A, Dhawan V, et al: Preoperative indicators of clinical outcome following stereotaxic pallidotomy. **Neurology 49:**1083-1089, 1997
48. Kazumata K, Ishikawa T, Dhawan V, et al: Differential diagnosis of parkinsonism with [^{18}F]fluorodeoxyglucose and PET. **Neurology 46 (Suppl 2):**A454, 1996 (Abstract)
49. Kish SJ, Zhong XH, Hornykiewicz O, et al: Striatal 3, 4-dihydroxyphenylalanine decarboxylase in aging: disparity between postmortem and positron emission computed tomography studies. **Ann Neurol 38:** 260-264, 1995
50. Kordower JH, Freeman TB, Snow BJ, et al: Neuropathological evidence of graft survival and striatal reinnervation after the transplantation of fetal mesencephalic tissue in a patient with Parkinson's disease. **New Engl J Med 332:**1118-1124, 1995
51. Kozlowski MR, Marshall JF: Plasticity of [^{14}C]2-deoxy-D-glucose incorporation into neostriatum and related structures in response to dopamine neuron damage and apomorphine replacement. **Brain Res 197:**167-183, 1980
52. Kuwabara H, Cumming P, Reith J, et al: Human striatal L-dopa decarboxylase activity estimated *in vivo* using 6-[^{18}F]fluoro-dopa and positron emission tomography: error analysis and application to normal subjects. **J Cereb Blood Flow Metab 13:**43-56, 1993
53. Laihinen AO, Rinne JO, Någren KÅ, et al: PET studies on brain monoamine transporters with carbon-11-ßCIT in Parkinson's disease. **J Nucl Med 36:** 1263-1267, 1996
54. Laitinen LV, Bergenheim AT, Hariz MI: Leksell's posteroventral pallidotomy in the treatment of Parkinson's disease. **J Neurosurg 76:**53-61, 1992
55. Langston JW, Widner H, Goetz CG, et al: Core assessment program for intracerebral transplantations (CAPIT). **Mov Disord 7:**2-13, 1992
56. Leenders KL, Salmon EP, Tyrrell P, et al:The nigrostriatal dopaminergic system assessed *in vivo* by positron emission tomography in healthy volunteer subjects and patients with Parkinson's disease. **Arch Neurol 47:**1290-1298, 1990
57. Lindvall O, Brundin P, Widner H, et al: Grafts of fetal dopamine neurons survive and improve motor function in Parkinson's disease. **Science 247:**574-577, 1990
58. Lindvall O, Sawle G, Widner H, et al: Evidence for long-term survival and function of dopaminergic grafts in progressive Parkinson's disease. **Ann Neurol 35:**172-180, 1994
59. Lindvall O, Widner H, Rehncrona S, et al: Transplantation of fetal dopamine neurons in Parkinson's disease: one-year clinical and neurophysiological observations in two patients with putaminal implants. **Ann Neurol 31:**155-165, 1992
60. Logan J, Fowler JS, Volkow ND, et al: Graphical analysis of reversible radioligand binding from time activity measurements applied to N-^{11}C-methyl-(-)-cocaine PET studies in human subjects. **J Cereb Blood Flow Metab 10:**740-747, 1989
61. Loizou LA: Uptake of monoamines into central neurones and the blood-brain barrier in the infant rat. **Br J Pharmacol 40:**800-813, 1970
62. Lozano A, Hutchison W, Kiss Z, et al: Methods for microelectrode-guided posteroventral pallidotomy.

J Neurosurg 84:194-202, 1996

63. Lozano AM, Lang AE, Galvez-Jimenez N, et al: Effect of GPi pallidotomy on motor function in Parkinson's disease. **Lancet 346:**1383-1387, 1995
64. Marek KL, Seibyl JP, Zoghbi SS, et al: [^{123}I]ß-CIT/SPECT imaging demonstrates bilateral loss of dopamine transporters in hemi-Parkinson's disease. **Neurology 46:**231-237, 1996
65. Martin WRW, Perlmutter JS: Assessment of fetal tissue transplantation in Parkinson's disease: does PET play a role? **Neurology 44:**1777-1780, 1994
66. Mata M, Fink DJ, Gainer H: Activity-dependent energy metabolism in rat posterior pituitary primarily reflects sodium pump activity. **J Neurochem 34:** 213-215, 1980
67. Mitchell IJ, Boyce S, Sambrook MA, et al: A 2-deoxyglucose study of the effects of dopamine agonists on the parkinsonian primate brain. **Brain 115:**809-824, 1994
68. Moeller JR, Strother SC: A regional covariance approach to the analysis of functional patterns in positron emission tomographic dopamine transportera. **J Cereb Blood Flow Metab 11:**A121-A135, 1991
69. Moeller JR, Strother SC, Sidtis JJ, et al: Scaled subprofile model: a statistical approach to the analysis of functional patterns in positron emission tomographic data. **J Cereb Blood Flow Metab 7:**649-658, 1987
70. Neumeyer JL, Wang S, Gao Y, et al: *N*-W-fluoroalkyl analogs of (1R)-2ß-carbomethoxy-3ß-(4-iodophenyl)tropane (ß-CIT): radiotracers for positron emission tomography and single photon emission computed tomography imaging of dopamine transporters. **J Med Chem 37:**1558-1561, 1994
71. Olanow CW, Good PF, Shinotoh H, et al: Manganese intoxication in the rhesus monkey: a clinical, imaging, pathologic, and biochemical study. **Neurology 46:**492-498, 1996
72. Pate BD, Kawamata T, Yamada T, et al: Correlation of striatal fluorodopa uptake in the MPTP monkey with dopaminergic indices. **Ann Neurol 34:**331-338, 1993
73. Patlak CS, Blasberg RG: Graphical evaluation of blood-to-brain transfer constants from multiple-time uptake data. Generalizations. **J Cereb Blood Flow Metab 5:**584-590, 1985
74. Quinn N: Multiple system atrophy—the nature of the beast. **J Neurol Neurosurg Psychiatry 52 (Suppl):** 78-89, 1989
75. Remy P, Samson Y, Hantraye P, et al: Clinical correlates of [^{18}F]fluorodopa uptake in five grafted parkinsonian patients. **Ann Neurol 38:**580-588, 1995
76. Sanberg PR, Nash DR, Calderon SF, et al: Neural transplants disrupt the blood-brain barrier and allow peripherally acting drugs to exert a centrally mediated behavioral effect. **Exp Neurol 102:**149-152, 1988
77. Sawle GV, Bloomfield PM, Björklund A, et al: Transplantation of fetal dopamine neurons in Parkinson's disease: PET[^{18}F]6-L-fluorodopa studies in two patients with putaminal implants. **Ann Neurol 31:** 166-173, 1992
78. Sawle GV, Myers R: The role of positron emission tomography in the assessment of human neurotransplantation. **Trends Neurosci 16:**172-176, 1993
79. Schaltenbrand G, Wahren W: **Atlas for Stereotaxy of the Human Brain.** Stuttgart: Thieme, 1977
80. Schwartz WJ, Smith CB, Davidsen L, et al: Metabolic mapping of functional activity in the hypothalamo-neurohypophysial system of the rat. **Science 205:** 723-725, 1979
81. Seibyl JP, Marek KL, Quilan D, et al: Decreased single-photon emission computed tomographic [^{123}I]ß-CIT striatal uptake correlates with symptom severity in Parkinson's disease. **Ann Neurol 38:**589-598, 1995
82. Snow BJ, Tooyama I, McGeer EG, et al: Human positron emission tomographic [^{18}F]fluorodopa studies correlate with dopamine cell counts and levels. **Ann Neurol 34:**324-330, 1993
83. Sokoloff L: Relationship between functional activity and energy metabolism in the nervous system: whether, where and why?, in Lassen NA, Ingvar DH, Raichle ME, et al (eds): **Brain Work and Mental Activity.** Copenhagen: Munksgaard, 1991, pp 52-64
84. Sterio D, Beriĉ A, Dogali M, et al: Neurophysiological properties of pallidal neurons in Parkinson's disease. **Ann Neurol 35:**586-591, 1994
85. Takikawa S, Dhawan V, Chaly T, et al: Input functions for 6-[Fluorine-18]Fluorodopa quantitation in Parkinsonism: comparative studies and clinical correlations. **J Nucl Med 35:**955-963, 1994
86. van Dyck CH, Seibyl JP, Malison RT, et al: Age-related decline in striatal dopamine transporter binding with iodine-123-ß-CIT SPECT. **J Nucl Med 36:**1175-1181, 1995
87. Volkow ND, Ding YS, Fowler JS, et al: A new PET ligand for the dopamine transporter. Studies in the human brain. **J Nucl Med 36:**2162-2168, 1995
88. Widner H, Tetrud J, Rehncrona S, et al: Bilateral fetal mesencephalic grafting in two patients with parkinsonism induced by 1-methyl-4-phenyl-1,2,3,6-tetrahydropyridine (MPTP). **N Engl J Med 327:** 1556-1563, 1992
89. Wilson JM, Levey AI, Rajput A, et al: Differential changes in neurochemical markers of striatal dopamine nerve terminals in idiopathic Parkinson's disease. **Neurology 47:**718-726, 1996
90. Wooten GF, Collins RC: Metabolic effects of unilateral lesion of the substantia nigra. **J Neurosci 1:** 285-291, 1981

CHAPTER 7

Pharmacological Treatment of Movement Disorders

Mitchell F. Brin, MD

Pharmacological Treatment of Parkinson's Disease

Parkinsonism is a neurological syndrome with the following cardinal features: 1) bradykinesia; 2) postural instability; 3) rigidity; 4) rest tremor; and 5) freezing (motor blocks).[86,88] Tremor or rigidity, plus at least one other cardinal feature, should be present before the diagnosis of parkinsonism is made. The parkinsonian syndromes can be classified into three categories: 1) idiopathic (Parkinson's disease); 2) symptomatic, those with a known and identifiable cause; and 3) parkinsonism plus syndromes, in which symptoms of parkinsonism are associated with other neurological abnormalities (see Chapter 1, "Classification of Movement Disorders"). The specific diagnosis depends on details of the clinical history, the neurological examination, and laboratory tests.

Idiopathic parkinsonism, also known as Parkinson's disease, is the most common type of parkinsonism. While the underlying defect that initiates Parkinson's disease is not established, the pathological source of many of the motor symptoms is attributed to nigral cell degeneration and consequent loss of dopamine production. However, many of the motor and neurocognitive symptoms of this progressive neurodegenerative disorder are not explained by dopamine deficiency and remain poorly understood. Because of extensive research into and advances in treatment, the physician beginning pharmacological treatment of Parkinson's disease has a wide range of drugs and protocols available; these can be tailored to each patient. In this chapter, specific therapeutic agents are reviewed and then treatment considerations are discussed.

Levodopa

The pathways of metabolism for levodopa (L-DOPA) and dopamine provide the framework for current L-DOPA-related therapy (Figure 1). The small intestine absorbs L-DOPA via the large neutral amino acid transporter, competing with other amino acids for transport.[118] L-DOPA is rapidly distributed throughout the tissues and

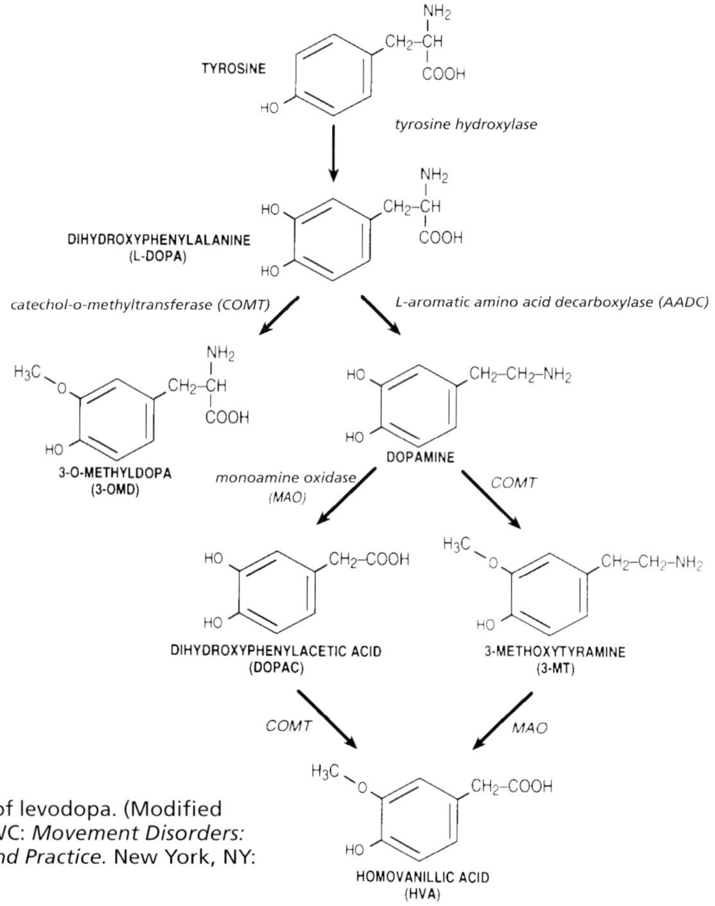

Figure 1: Metabolism of levodopa. (Modified from Watts RL, Koller WC: *Movement Disorders: Neurologic Principles and Practice.* New York, NY: McGraw-Hill, 1997)

absorbed into the central nervous system (CNS) via the same transporter;[207] dietary protein may therefore influence eventual L-DOPA response at either the gut or CNS level.[144]

Peripherally, L-DOPA is rapidly metabolized by aromatic amino acid decarboxylase (AADC) and catechol-O-methyltransferase (COMT), reducing the availability of L-DOPA to the CNS. AADC and COMT are, therefore, targets of inhibitors that potentiate L-DOPA and prolong the therapeutic effect of a single dose.

The current hypothesis of L-DOPA action is that nigral cells take up L-DOPA, convert it to dopamine, and release it to bind with postsynaptic D_1 and D_2 receptors. This hypothesis predicts a loss of L-DOPA efficacy with nigral cell death, a correlation that is not borne out in at least some Parkinson's disease patients. These inconsistencies may be accounted for by up-regulation of receptors or extranigral conversion of L-DOPA,[125] although neither of these phenomena are established as clinically relevant at this time.

Fundamental experiments in the 1950s and early 1960s pointed to dopamine deficiency as the pathophysiological basis of Parkinson's disease.[55,78] In 1961, L-DOPA therapy was shown to be an effective treatment for Parkinson's disease.[16,26] Experiments over the next decade confirmed its efficacy and showed the value of combining decarboxylase inhibitors with L-DOPA to prolong the effect and reduce the required dosage.[63,220] By 1969, the side effects of chronic L-DOPA treatment were described,[62] signaling the end of levodopa's promise as the single magic bullet for Parkinson's disease. These side effects are motor fluctuations or a lack of consistent response to oral dosing of the drug. Patients experience end-of-dose "wearing off" characterized by a marked worsening of Parkinson's disease symptoms at the end of a dose. Many patients also experience "peak-dose dyskinesias," hyperkinetic involuntary movements that characteristically appear after the drug is maximally absorbed and transported into the brain. Nonetheless, L-DOPA remains the most effective single drug treatment for Parkinson's disease, and its extraordinary effect on the early parkinsonian patient remains the standard by which other treatments are judged.

L-DOPA is typically administered as a combination formulation with an AADC inhibitor. The addition of an AADC inhibitor, either carbidopa or benserazide, decreases peripheral L-DOPA metabolism, thereby reducing the amount of L-DOPA needed for clinical efficacy and increasing the transport of L-DOPA into the brain. Co-administration of L-DOPA with an AADC inhibitor has become standard therapy.

Sustained-release formulations, which delay the onset of peak L-DOPA levels and prolong its plasma clearance, are available. By smoothing out fluctuations in drug levels, response oscillations may be lessened.[29] COMT inhibitors may further increase the effectiveness of orally administered L-DOPA, probably by decreasing peripheral 3-O-methyldopa production, which competes with transport of L-DOPA into the brain.

L-DOPA (with an AADC inhibitor) is usually started at 100 mg once daily, gradually increasing to 100 mg three times a day, with further adjustments as needed. Dosage increases are made following evaluation of benefit and side effects, and are usually spaced 3-14 days apart, unless there is some urgency in dose titration. The dosage for carbidopa (or benserazide equivalents) ranges from 10 to 25 mg per 100 mg L-DOPA, with the goal of administering 100-200 mg/day.

Long-term L-DOPA therapy often leads to late complications, including response oscillations, dyskinesias, and drug-induced psychiatric effects. Early in therapy, most patients have continuous benefit from three or four doses per day; subsequent response oscillations typically develop within 5 years of treatment.[84,127] Even more troubling, some patients develop unpredictable oscillations with no apparent relation to their dosing regimen. Response oscillations may be accompanied by dyskinesias; chorea, with or without dystonia, is common, especially at the time of peak levels. While dose reduction may be effective for peak-dose dyskinesias, many patients have a very narrow therapeutic window, and titrating an effective dose versus reduction of the dyskinesia may be difficult. Strategies include co-administration of dopamine agonists, liquid preparations, or subcutaneous apomorphine (see below). Delayed gastric emptying may be responsible in some cases. Prokinetic drugs, such as cisapride, may be of use in selected patients.[72]

Psychiatric effects of chronic L-DOPA therapy include vivid dreams, hallucinations, and an exacerbation of memory loss, confusion, and anxiety. While some of these effects may be treated symptomatically with other medications, a reduction in L-DOPA may be necessary.

Dopamine Agonists

Dopamine agonists directly stimulate D_1 and D_2 receptors and, unlike L-DOPA, do not require neuronal transformation for their efficacy. They offer the benefit of dopaminergic action without requiring viable dopamine-releasing cells. By substituting dopamine agonists for endogenous or exogenous dopamine sources, the generation of free radicals that may be associated with dopamine turnover may be reduced; thus, dopamine agonists may exert a neuroprotective effect.[193] In spite of these putative advantages, the current dopamine agonists have not proven as clinically effective as L-DOPA and have not replaced L-DOPA as the cornerstone of Parkinson's disease therapy. Side effects, similar for all agonists, include dose-related confusion and hallucinations and orthostatic hypotension. Orthostasis may be ameliorated in many patients by decreasing the speed of drug initiation. Long-term use of ergot-derived dopamine agonists may cause erythromelalgia.[80,233]

Bromocriptine and pergolide are ergot preparations that are currently available in the United States, and a third—lisuride—is available in Europe and elsewhere. A fourth non-ergot agonist, apomorphine, is also available in Europe; it is presently the most potent dopamine agonist available for treatment of Parkinson's disease. Three non-ergot agonists were recently introduced: ropinirole, pramipexole, and cabergoline.

Bromocriptine has been shown to be effective monotherapy in early Parkinson's disease,[167] but as with all dopamine agonists, it is less effective than L-DOPA against parkinsonian symptoms. As a result, only about 30% of patients can be treated with bromocriptine monotherapy for more than 3 years.[167] As monotherapy, bromocriptine is usually administered at a dose of 20-40 mg/day; slightly smaller doses are given as an adjunct to L-DOPA therapy. Effects last from 1 to 6 hours.

Lisuride improves parkinsonian symptoms and reduces motor fluctuations when used as an adjunct to L-DOPA in late-stage Parkinson's disease.[242] Unlike the other dopamine agonists, lisuride is water-soluble and may be administered parenterally or even continuously infused via a minipump, although this approach may cause a higher degree of psychosis.[268] As an oral medication, its duration of action is relatively short (1-3 hours).

Pergolide has been shown to reduce motor fluctuations by 30% or more and to reduce the amount of L-DOPA required for disease management by 25%.[160,178] In a single-blind crossover comparison of pergolide and bromocriptine, pergolide was slightly more effective and better tolerated than bromocriptine.[229] Its duration of effect is 2-8 hours. Pergolide may reduce dopamine turnover and have important effects on free radical scavenging enzymes, giving a theoretical basis for early management with this agent.[91,103]

Apomorphine was first described as an antiparkinsonian drug in 1951,[251] although it has yet to be approved for this indication in more than a few European countries. Its efficacy against late-stage "off period" dyskinesias has been shown in several clinical trials.[95,260,269] Subcutaneous injection may be the most effective and practical delivery method, although rectal and sublingual administration have been used as well. Continuous infusion via a minipump is also possible. Co-administration with the anti-emetic domperidone is often necessary.

The three new dopamine agonists that have been marketed recently, cabergoline, ropinirole, and pramipexole, are non-ergot agents that have no D_1 receptor activity, but have D_2 and, with the exception of cabergoline, D_3 (a subtype of the D_2 receptor) receptor activity. These agents have established antiparkinsonian effects and the side effect profile for hypotension and gastrointestinal discomfort is similar to that of the ergoline dopamine agonists.[235] Experience with these agents is limited, and therefore it cannot be said whether the non-ergot agonists offer any clinical advantage over the established ergot agents.

Monoamine Oxidase B Inhibitors

Dopamine is metabolized to 3,4-dihydroxyphenylacetic acid by monoamine oxidase B (MAO-B). MAO-B inhibitors, therefore, can potentiate dopamine (and L-DOPA) by blocking its degradation. The principal MAO-B inhibitor used in the treatment of Parkinson's disease is selegiline, also known as deprenyl.

Selegiline is commonly used as early monotherapy or in combination therapy with L-DOPA. Its mild efficacy as monotherapy was demonstrated in a large, multicenter study known as DATATOP (Deprenyl and Tocopherol Antioxidative Therapy of Parkinsonism).[223] This and other studies have demonstrated the ability of selegiline to postpone L-DOPA therapy for perhaps 9 months or more.[5,200] However, there remains controversy regarding the mechanism of this effect. Selegiline was hypothesized by early researchers to exert a neuroprotective effect by blocking degradation and subsequent free radical formation, thus prolonging the life of the degenerating nigral cells and postponing the onset of parkinsonian symptoms. Selegiline also has mild, clear symptomatic effects, possibly because of its ability to block dopamine degradation and re-uptake,[81,284] or through its metabolism to methamphetamine.[238] Some authors interpret the results of the DATATOP and later studies as indicating symptomatic improvement rather than neuroprotection,[250] a conclusion supported by follow-up studies showing no statistical difference in therapy needs 3 years after treatment with selegiline versus placebo.[223] However, one noncontrolled, retrospective postmortem study has shown a greater preservation of dopaminergic neurons with selegiline.[241] As an L-DOPA adjunct in late-stage Parkinson's disease, selegiline has been shown to improve motor fluctuations in one half to two thirds of patients,[27,105,243] and to allow a decreased L-DOPA dosage of 15%-30%.[213]

Side effects from selegiline are uncommon and include nausea and dizziness. The absence of serious side effects from selegiline therapy, combined with its as yet unproven potential as a neuroprotective agent leads many clinicians to prescribe selegiline at the time of diagnosis.[201,202]

The standard dose of selegiline is 10 mg/day. L-DOPA side effects may be enhanced by selegiline and often require a decrease in L-DOPA dosage in patients experiencing peak-dose dyskinesias.

Anticholinergics

Anticholinergics are used primarily in *de novo* patients for whom tremor is the predominant complaint. Anticholinergic therapy may have a mild effect on rigidity and tremor, but has little effect on akinesia.[232] Because of their propensity to induce confusion,[76] anticholinergics are not recommended for use in elderly patients, and their use is contraindicated in patients with dementia. Their use is also limited by side effects, including constipation, blurred vision, dizziness, and nausea. Another side effect, dry mouth, may actually be welcomed by the patient in whom sialorrhea may be an unpleasant symptom of the disease. Dosing for trihexyphenidyl, the most widely used anticholinergic, is begun at 0.5-1.0 mg twice daily and gradually increased to 2-3 mg three times daily.

Amantadine

Amantadine is effective against akinesia, rigidity, and, to some extent, tremor.[146,177,221,222] Its mechanism of action is unknown, although it has been shown to have N-methyl-D-aspartate (NMDA)-antagonist properties and anticholinergic properties, and to promote release of stored dopamine in nerve terminals.[150] Because of their NMDA antagonism, amantadine and similar compounds are being explored for their potential neuroprotective effect.[28,194] Amantadine may be started as monotherapy in Parkinson's disease patients with mild impairment. Dosage is 100-300 mg daily for younger patients; lower doses, in the form of an elixir, are administered to older patients.

Clozapine

Clozapine is an "atypical" neuroleptic that has become an important adjunctive therapy for Parkinson's disease.[83] Whereas the classical neuroleptics (phenothiazines and butyrophenones) aggravate Parkinson's disease, those that do not block D_1 and D_2 receptors do not appear to have an adverse effect on Parkinson's disease patients. Clozapine can be effective against tremor that proves resistant to other drugs.[83,98,138,219] In late-stage Parkinson's disease, it can reduce or suppress L-DOPA-induced dyskinesias[13,17] and nocturnal restlessness.[170] It is useful against drug-induced psychosis from L-DOPA and dopamine agonists.[82,281] Effective doses range widely, from 6.25 mg every other day to 200 mg/day.[17,82] The author typically does not administer more than 25 mg/day in Parkinson's disease patients. Side effects include hypotension, sialorrhea, sedation, and seizures. Agranulocytosis occurs in about 1% of patients[8] and requires weekly blood counts in patients taking the drug. If leukopenia is recognized and the drug is promptly discontinued, fatal agranulocytosis is rare.

Approach to Therapy

The single most controversial question is whether medical intervention should be initiated at the time of diagnosis or be postponed until functional impairment becomes limiting. Despite the relative abundance of proven treatments, the management of mid-disease and advanced symptoms remains complex, for four major reasons. First, the most effective treatment for Parkinson's disease, L-DOPA, diminishes in effectiveness in the majority of patients and response fluctuations become common. Second, alternative or adjunct therapies vary in their effectiveness among patients, and so their titration into the treatment regimen may require several attempts to find the most effective combination of drugs and dosage. Third, most of the medications used have the potential for side effects, further complicating dosing decisions and requiring individualization of treatment. Finally, Parkinson's disease is a progressive disease and one whose symptoms vary in their initial distribution, severity, and rate of progression. As a result, treatment must change consonant with a patient's changing status and responsiveness to therapeutics. Therefore, while there is some clinical consensus on the broad outlines of effective Parkinson's disease therapy, there is considerable diversity of opinion over the details.

TABLE 1

Management of Early Parkinson's Disease

Prior to symptomatic disability
Selegiline
Amantadine
Anticholinergics
When symptoms begin to impair function
Begin a dopamine agonist and titrate to maximum benefit
Add levodopa/carbidopa sustained release when additional symptomatic relief is required
If there is urgency for symptomatic relief
Initiate levodopa/carbidopa sustained release for initial relief
Add an agonist after levodopa/carbidopa has provided initial symptomatic relief

Once Parkinson's disease has been diagnosed, the decision to begin pharmacological treatment is influenced by both medical and social aspects. Important factors include work status, initial symptoms, age at onset, and cognitive impairment. The potential benefit of therapy must be weighed against the potential for drug-related adverse effects. The goals of treatment are most often functional improvement (e.g., lessening tremor or increasing speed of movement) and safety (e.g., increasing stability of gait).

Patients may first seek treatment because of tremor, gait impairment, or slowness of movement.[124] The patient's work status may be the single most important factor in treatment choice and timing; maintaining the ability to work is both financially and psychologically paramount for most patients. Symptoms that impair the ability to work (bradykinesia in a factory worker, for example) argue for earlier intervention, while those that do not (mild tremor in a home or office worker, for instance) may not be treated upon initial presentation. Because symptom onset is often unilateral (and ultimately asymmetric), the degree of functional impairment may depend on whether the dominant or nondominant hand is affected first.

Patients recently diagnosed with Parkinson's disease need to be educated about their disease and what they may expect. In addition to the educational efforts provided by the clinical team, patients may be referred to one of the several national Parkinson's disease organizations (for a listing, visit http://www.wemove.org on the World Wide Web). These organizations also sponsor regional support groups, an important source of information and support for patients with Parkinson's disease. Parkinsonian patients may begin to exercise less often because of motor impairments. Education and health promotion programs have been shown to be effective in increasing exercise frequency and health confidence, and decreasing office visits.[195]

Most patients ultimately require a polypharmaceutical approach to maximize therapeutic responsiveness. Drugs are chosen to meet specific goals. Each drug is regulated to optimize the clinical response, balancing therapeutic benefit and adverse effects. When an anti-parkinsonian medication is discontinued, the dose is reduced gradually to minimize the risk of withdrawal syndrome.[285]

Drug choice and timing of the onset of therapy are influenced by the limitations of the drugs themselves. L-DOPA therapy leads to motor fluctuations and dyskinesias after 5 years in about 50% of all Parkinson's disease patients, rising to 80% after 10 years.[84,127] For this reason, alternative treatments are often used early in the younger patient, saving L-DOPA therapy until absolutely required.

Younger patients are most often started on one of the alternatives mentioned above (Table 1), with L-DOPA therapy replacing or joining the other agent as the disease progresses and symptoms become more disabling. Early use of selegiline in all diagnosed Parkinson's disease patients has been advocated by some, based on its potential role as a neuroprotective agent.[147] It is often instituted early as monotherapy and frequently provides at least some symptomatic relief. Anticholinergics or amantadine may be tolerated by younger patients with predominant tremor.

Dopamine agonists are currently used as early monotherapy, especially in young patients, or as an adjunct to L-DOPA either early or late in the illness. As an early adjunct, they have been promoted for their "L-DOPA sparing effect," with the expected benefit of prolonged L-DOPA effectiveness. However, to date this has not been unanimously supported in double-blind trials.[277] In general, the effectiveness of dopamine agonists is less than that of L-DOPA against parkinsonian symptoms. But while many physicians advocate early combination therapy (L-DOPA plus a dopamine agonist), it is also common to add dopamine agonists once L-DOPA monotherapy becomes problematic.

While postponing L-DOPA therapy may be desirable, especially for younger patients, L-DOPA is indicated in patients of any age with severe disability or interference with work performance, for whom other drugs fail to provide adequate treatment. When L-DOPA therapy is initiated, nearly all patients are begun on L-DOPA combined with an AADC inhibitor. Controlled-release preparations may be used from the start, although their more even release may result in less dramatic symptomatic relief. If the diagnosis of idiopathic parkinsonism is in any doubt, the controlled-release formula may not provide the evidence needed to confirm L-DOPA responsiveness. A dopamine agonist may be added within 3-6 months to keep the L-DOPA requirement low.

Motor Fluctuations

After 4-6 years of symptoms, most patients begin to experience a weakening of levodopa's efficacy, probably related to continued loss of storage capacity for dopamine.[197] Suboptimal peak response, rapid wearing off of peak effect, and unpredictable off states indicate a change in L-DOPA responsiveness and require a modification in therapeutic strategy.

Suboptimal peak response may be treated initially by an increased dose of L-DOPA or an agonist. Higher L-DOPA doses may be avoided by an increase in the dopamine agonist dose or by introduction of an agonist or selegiline if not already present. Patients experiencing a rapid wearing off of L-DOPA effects may respond well to a switch to a controlled-release preparation. Liquid L-DOPA/carbidopa preparations may also be helpful;[155] in the author's experience, however, this strategy is not always practical.

Dietary protein may interfere with L-DOPA absorption and metabolism and can contribute to unpredictable off states. Shifting the majority of the protein intake to one meal, usually supper, may offer some relief during the rest of the day.[163,270] Occasionally, apomorphine (if available), usually administered with domperidone, is effective in treating prolonged off states and may be especially useful for "rescuing" patients trapped by unpredictable freezing. The author has found pergolide particularly useful in the management of "off dystonia." In addition, early morning dystonia often responds to an added dose of pergolide at bedtime.

Neuropsychiatric Problems

Neuropsychiatric problems, including cognitive impairment, behavioral impairment, and psychosis, are common in late-stage Parkinson's disease, either as a manifestation of the disease, a side effect of the drugs used to treat it, or a combination of the two. Changes in mental state often accompany Parkinson's disease and may affect treatment choice. Dementia occurs in 15%-25% of patients with Parkinson's disease,[24,145,184,187,224] although the degree of causality in this correlation is debated, with co-occurrence of Parkinson's disease and Alzheimer's disease a likely explanation for at least some of these cases. Depression and anxiety are also common. Cognitive impairment can influence the patient's willingness to undergo therapy and the response to treatment.

Confusion or memory deficit is most common in older Parkinson's disease patients and has been estimated to occur in up to 65% of patients by the age of 85 years.[184] Treatment begins with an attempt to distinguish drug effects from disease effects. Hallucinations and nightmares are often drug-induced, while depression and off-period anxiety are more likely to be related to Parkinson's disease or another, concomitant illness. Drug-related symptoms may be treated by medication reduction, although titrating the reduction of psychiatric symptoms with the concurrent reduction in drug efficacy is difficult because an aggravation of parkinsonian symptoms emerges.

Anticholinergics, amantadine, selegiline, and the dopamine agonists may aggravate cognitive impairment, and their reduction may be indicated as well, usually in the order stated. As a last resort, the dose of L-DOPA/carbidopa may be adjusted downward, although an unacceptable increase in motor symptoms may prevent adequate reduction in dosage.

Estimates of the prevalence of depression range from 10%-90%, with an average of 30%-40%.[75,185] In some patients, mood changes coincide with motor fluctuations, and the depressed state occurs only during the off state.[54] In these patients, managing the response oscillations may be sufficient to treat the depression. In others, the depression is independent of motor fluctuations. Counseling may be an important adjunct to therapy, although medical management of the depression is often required. Low-dose tricyclic antidepressants (amitriptyline, nortriptyline) are often helpful and usually well tolerated, but the anticholinergic effect may aggravate confusion. Selective serotonin re-uptake inhibitors (SSRIs; sertraline, paroxetine) may interact with selegiline,[261] although there is evidence to the contrary,[276] so they may be used together with caution.

Agitation is a possible effect of selegiline, as well as of amantadine, dopamine agonists, and anticholinergics. It is also a common symptom when a patient experiences wearing off. The patient may be asked to keep a diary to ascertain if there is a relationship between motor fluctuations and agitation. Anxiety and panic disorder may be more frequent during motor fluctuations; agitation may occur as an end-of-dose phenomenon when the patient is "turning off." These symptoms may require re-regulation of anti-parkinsonian medications. An increase in the dose of the dopamine agonist is often useful in managing agitation that occurs during wearing-off. Primary agitation unrelated to therapy may also occur and may be treated with anxiolytics, such as short-acting benzodiazepines.

Vivid dreams, progressing to nightmares, hallucinations, and paranoia, may occur in as many as 20% of Parkinson's disease patients[246] and may or may not be a consequence of medical therapy. Hallucinations are most commonly visual, nonthreatening, and involve family members or pets. Symptoms may be caused by any of the medication classes, and treatment begins with reduction or elimination of the suspected drug. Unsatisfactory control may require the introduction of a neuroleptic. Because classical neuroleptics tend to worsen motor symptoms, the atypical neuroleptic clozapine may be the drug of choice, as it rarely aggravates parkinsonian symptoms.[82,83] As noted above, agranulocytosis is a significant adverse effect and weekly blood monitoring is required.

Pharmacological Treatment of Dystonia

Dystonia is one of the most challenging conditions to treat because the underlying pathophysiology is unknown. The term "dystonia" does not represent a homogeneous disorder and there are numerous etiologies. Dystonia is a neurological syndrome dominated by involuntary muscle contractions that may be sustained (tonic), spasmodic (rapid or clonic), patterned, or repetitive. The muscle movements frequently cause abnormal postures, including twisting (e.g., torticollis), flexion or extension (e.g., anterocollis, retrocollis, writer's cramp), or adduction or abduction (e.g., blepharospasm, spasmodic dysphonia). Dystonia can involve any voluntary muscle. Because the movements and resulting postures are often unusual and the condition is rare, it is one of the most frequently misdiagnosed neurological conditions.[89] The prevalence of the condition is unknown, but at least 150,000 cases of idiopathic dystonia are estimated in the U.S.[206,259] About 1 in 3000 people is diagnosed with dystonia, but the true prevalence is probably much higher. Cervical dystonia is probably the most commonly diagnosed form of focal dystonia, but graphospasm (writer's cramp) may be the most prevalent form of dystonia in the general population.

Because dystonia is a clinical syndrome, patients may be classified according to clinical distribution and symptomatology, age at onset, and etiology. Classification may be important, as it can give clues about prognosis and also an approach to management. According to the etiological classification, patients with idiopathic disease have no evidence by history, examination, or laboratory studies of any identifiable cause for the dystonic symptoms. However, patients may have in their history factors that precipitate the onset of dystonic symptoms.[131] Therefore, there must be a normal perinatal and early developmental history and no prior history of neurological illness or exposure to drugs known to cause acquired dystonia (e.g., phenothiazines). There must also be normal intellectual, pyramidal, cerebellar, and sensory examinations, as well as normal diagnostic studies.[47,180] Patients who have the abnormalities noted above are classified as having symptomatic dystonia.

The clinical phenomenology will often be a clue to etiology. Primary dystonia is typically action-induced; symptoms are enhanced with use of the affected body part and the region may appear normal at rest. Secondary dystonia frequently results in fixed dystonic postures. The presence of extensive dystonia limited to one side of the body (hemidystonia) suggests a secondary etiology.

When classified by distribution, patients are categorized as having focal, segmental, or generalized symptoms. Focal dystonic symptoms involve one small group of muscles in one body part, segmental disease involves a contiguous group of muscles, and generalized dystonia is widespread. Common examples of focal dystonia include blepharospasm (forced, involuntary eye closure), oromandibular dystonia (face, jaw, or tongue), torticollis or cervical dystonia (neck), writer's cramp (action-induced dystonic contraction of hand muscles), and spasmodic dysphonia (vocal cords).

In families with dystonia, various members may have generalized, segmental, or focal dystonia, suggesting that those with milder manifestations are related to the more generalized cases. This gives rise to the concept that the less involved individuals represent formes frustes or more limited manifestations of generalized dystonia. The presence of dystonic symptoms in other family members supports the concept that the focal involvement is dystonic and genetic in these cases.

There is clinical and genetic heterogeneity among patients with idiopathic dystonic symptomatology; family and linkage studies indicate that several of these subtypes have different genetic bases. These subtypes include autosomal dominant dopa-responsive dystonia,[156,210,211] X-linked Filipino torsion dystonia,[153,154,165,262,278] and autosomal dominant (non-dopa-responsive) idiopathic torsion dystonia due to the DYT1 gene mapped to chromosome 9q34.[152,217,244] Ozelius et al[218] recently described the protein associated with the DYT1 mutation, named Torsin A. Both dopa-responsive dystonia and X-linked torsion dystonia are rare, "variant" forms of idiopathic torsion dystonia in which parkinsonism as well as dystonia are common expressions of the disease gene. In contrast, studies of families in which dystonia is due to the DYT1 gene describe dystonia as the only clinical abnormality.

Leube et al[168] recently described a German family with autosomal dominant, primarily segmental cranial dystonia and a gene localized to chromosome 18p. Almasy et al[6,7] described childhood-onset dystonia in the Amish-Mennonite population, with linkage to chromosome 8 (for additional information, visit http://www3.ncbi.nlm.nih.gov/Omim/ on the World Wide Web).

Despite advances in our understanding of the genetics of many forms of dystonia, no gene-directed therapy is available at this time. Genetic studies have supported the assertion that something is wrong in the basal ganglia and its connections,[218,234] but neurochemical,[67,126,137] biochemical,[40] anatomical,[212,286,287] and neuroimaging[42,57,79,230] studies have not revealed a common neurochemical substrate. Although presumed for many years to be primarily a motor disorder, the motor signs of dystonia may be, in part, a reflection of aberrant sensory input.[116,117,140]

Specific pharmacotherapy is not available for most cases of dystonia; for most patients, intervention is supportive and symptomatic. However, there are several common treatment themes and principles that apply to patients with dystonic symptoms. During the neurological evaluation, the physician evaluates the patient in an attempt to diagnose an underlying cause or contributing factors. If an underlying biochemical basis is identified, then specific therapy is instituted. Therapeutic options are first reviewed and then guidelines are offered on an approach to therapy.

Supportive and Physical Therapy

The most extensive support system is the network of concerned patients who participate in support groups and international foundations that promote education and research on dystonia (for a listing, visit http://www.wemove.org on the World Wide Web). Reactive or primary depression may aggravate disability,[129,130,151,161,198,264] and patients may benefit from supportive psychotherapy.

Physical measures include braces that mimic the simple "geste antagonistique," a sensory trick that many patients report. The author does not recommend rigid braces because they often result in patient discomfort. Biofeedback[44,45,59,60,96,135,139,148,149,172] or physical therapy may provide limited benefit for some. Manipulation-based therapists (physical therapists, chiropractors) should not use force in therapy, but should use modalities to assist patients in using their own resources to compensate for postural abnormalities. None of these therapies have yet been subjected to double-blind evaluation.

Pharmacological Therapies

Agents from nearly every neuropharmacological class have been tried in primary dystonia, and no single agent representing a specific neurotransmitter system has emerged as efficacious. With the exception of dopa-responsive dystonia, there is no consistent beneficial response observed among family members expressing the same genetic defect, or among otherwise phenotypically similar individuals. A small percentage of patients (up to 15%[110]) respond to a variety of agents, possibly representing a therapeutic effect. Alternatively, this may be a placebo response or recall bias reflected in retrospective chart reviews. Early results with many therapies (such as carbamazepine and mexiletine) have been promising, only to be tempered by subsequent reports[99,100,128,214,215,272] or symptoms of dystonia due to the drug.[64,164,258]

Disorders With Specific Pharmacotherapy

Specific pharmacotherapy directed at an underlying, identified biochemical defect is available only for a limited number of patients,[36] such as those with Wilson's disease, which is treated with drugs that deplete copper and/or interfere with copper absorption. The best treatment for tardive dystonia is prophylaxis: avoidance of offending medications when possible. Acute drug-induced dystonia can be caused by dopamine-receptor blocking agents (DRBAs), including antipsychotic[1,114,141,143,176,181] and antiemetic agents,[245] anticonvulsants,[58,65,258] and quinine-related drugs.[2,119,267] Acute DRBA-induced dystonia may be relieved by intravenous administration of 50 mg diphenhydramine (Benadryl). Intravenous anticholinergics, benzodiazepines, or methylphenidate can also be used.[56] It is not known whether an acute drug-induced dystonic reaction predisposes one to persistent tardive dystonia;[50,101] many patients resume DRBA therapy without further acute reactions. Dystonic reactions associated with anticonvulsant therapy may be treated by decreasing the dose or discontinuing the offending agent.[143]

Dopa-responsive dystonia usually starts in childhood with gait disturbance and is often familial.[92,211] Most patients respond dramatically to <500 mg/day of L-DOPA with carbidopa.[208,209] For this reason, treatment with L-DOPA is often the first-line pharmaceutical approach to patients with limb-onset dystonia.

Paroxysmal dystonias are preferentially treated with the anticonvulsants carbamazepine or phenytoin if kinesigenic,[108,173,179] carbamazepine if nocturnal,[30,122,175,192] or with the addition of acetazolamide when nonkinesigenic.[23,186,204,252]

Anticholinergics

Open-label[33,85,102,159,182] and double-blind[48] studies have substantiated the benefit of anticholinergics in approximately 50% of children and 40% of adults with focal, segmental, or generalized dystonia. Children will tolerate high doses, often in excess of 40 mg/day.[85] The biochemical basis for this benefit in dystonia is unknown; it is relatively uncommon for patients to derive substantial benefit from an anticholinergic agent. Centrally acting cholinergic therapy may aggravate dystonia.[263]

Central and peripheral adverse effects of anticholinergic agents limit the dosage for most patients. The side effects include dry mouth, blurred vision (due to paralysis of accommodation), and urinary retention, which can be treated acutely by a dose reduction or symptomatically with peripheral anticholinesterase agents, such as pyridostigmine tablets or pilocarpine (a muscarinic agonist) eye drops. Central adverse effects may be insidious and dose-limiting and include confusion, drowsiness, hallucinations, personality change, and forgetfulness. No anticholinergic has been found to be more efficacious than another. The author's unconfirmed clinical impression is that ethopropazine is better tolerated compared to trihexyphenidyl in the adult population.

Benzodiazepines

Benzodiazepines directly bind to the gamma-aminobutyric acid $(GABA)_A$ receptor/ion channel complex and allosterically modulate receptor activity[123] by displacing an endogenous inhibitor of this receptor.[62] Side effects include sedation, depression, personality change, and psychosis; these are controlled by modifying the dose. Dystonia patients may tolerate exceedingly high doses (e.g., 120 mg/day diazepam) if the dosage is increased slowly.

Several open-label studies in adults and children have found diazepam to be useful.[106,110] There are no data on whether any particular benzodiazepine is superior. Prior to 1980, diazepam was prescribed primarily; subsequently, clonazepam and lorazepam began to be used. This switch was, in part, due to adverse publicity about diazepam, as encountered for example in the 1967 bestseller *Valley of the Dolls* by Jacqueline Susann.

Baclofen

Oral baclofen is a GABA agonist that stimulates the $GABA_B$ autoreceptor, which, when stimulated, confers an inhibitory function.[61] In experimental systems,[271] baclofen inhibits the release of noradrenaline,[31] acetylcholine[43] from peripheral nerve endings, and acetylcholine,[68] noradrenaline,[32] dopamine,[32,237] serotonin,[32,109,249] and glutamate[231] from CNS neurons. It is used orally to treat spasticity,[90,142,240,248,283] primary dystonia,[35,106,110,111,247] and myoclonus,[157,191] and has occasionally been reported to be of value in managing the off-state dystonia associated with Parkinson's disease.[166] The mechanism of benefit in dystonia is not known. Adverse effects include sedation, nausea, and, rarely, hepatitis.

Dopaminergics: Stimulation, Blocking, and Depletion

Levodopa therapy is tried in all patients with limb-onset dystonia. With the exception of dopa-responsive dystonia, a minority of patients with primary dystonia respond to L-DOPA or dopamine agonist therapy.[110, 158] An increased proportion of patients (up to 78%) respond to dopamine blocking and depleting agents. Although dopamine blocking agents may be efficacious, persistent tardive symptoms may occur,[46,49] effectively aggravating the underlying primary disease. The atypical neuroleptic agent clozapine has shown promise in selected patients with primary or symptomatic dystonia;[253,279] however, an acute dystonic reaction has been associated with this drug.[141] Experience with olanzapine is limited.

Tetrabenazine is a presynaptic catecholamine depleting agent with some blocking activity.[236] Although there are rare reports of acute dystonic reactions[52] or neuroleptic malignant syndrome,[51, 183,216] there has not been a report of tardive symptoms from this drug. Double-blind[132] and open-treatment[133,136] studies document efficacy in treating primary and secondary dystonia. The author's clinical experience has demonstrated that the addition of lithium may ameliorate the parkinsonian and depressive effects of tetrabenazine while enhancing the beneficial treatment effect on dystonia. When used alone, lithium does not have a significant beneficial effect in patients with dystonia.

Other pharmacotherapeutic agents, either alone or in combination, are used as well in dystonia when traditional therapies fail. These include most classes of CNS active agents, often with limited benefit.

Intrathecal Therapy

Chronic intrathecal baclofen (CITB) infusion via an implantable pump has been effective in relieving spasticity of the limbs and bladder associated with demyelinating disease, cerebral or spinal cord trauma, cerebral palsy, transverse myelitis, postencephalitic spasticity, and hereditary spasticity, in addition to stiff-person syndrome.[4,162,190,227,228] Subsequent to the report of Narayan et al,[203] the author and others have reported on the benefit of CITB in managing patients with primary and symptomatic childhood and adult dystonia in whom other therapies failed.[3,41,94,203,226] Prior to implantation of a CITB pump, the patient has usually been evaluated on a course of oral baclofen and traditional dystonia therapy, including an anticholinergic and a benzodiazepine, and either failed or had unacceptable adverse effects. Patients are screened with pre-implantation boluses of intrathecal baclofen. The benefit appears to be greatest in children with symptomatic dystonia, although adults with symptomatic and primary dystonia may derive benefit. It is difficult to predict which patients will benefit with chronic therapy. Approximately 60% of the author's patients who benefit from screening and then undergo pump implantation have persistent benefit.

Local Therapies

Phenol

Phenol is the major oxidized metabolite of benzene, which, like alcohol, causes tissue necrosis. Phenol is utilized extensively in the management of spasticity[189,282] and occasionally in the management of dystonia. Complications include severe pain in the region injected, chronic dysesthesia, excessive motor weakness, peripheral edema, sensory loss, wound infection, and systemic side effects in the case of overdose, including tremor, seizures, and cardiovascular collapse.

Botulinum Toxin Type A

Botulinum toxin type A has proven to be dramatically effective therapy for many focal dystonias. It is currently considered the treatment of choice and is offered as primary therapy for most cases of blepharospasm, cervical dystonia, spasmodic dysphonia, jaw dystonia, and many cases of limb dystonia both with and without tremor.[9-12,37,134,196,205] The list of areas treated has expanded to include dystonic and nondystonic involuntary movements, including those spasms associated with numerous etiologies and anatomical regions (Table 2).

TABLE 2

BOTULINUM TOXIN THERAPY FOR CONDITIONS CHARACTERIZED BY EXCESSIVE MUSCLE CONTRACTION*

Dystonic spasms
Blepharospasm
Cervical dystonia
Laryngeal dystonia
Oromandibular dystonia
Occupational cramps
Limb dystonia
Dystonic tremor
Nondystonic excessive muscle contraction
Back spasm
Bladder: detrusor sphincter dyssynergia
Bruxism
Cosmetic (hyperfunctional facial lines): brow furrows, frown lines, crows' feet, platysma lines
Gastrointestinal: achalasia, anismus (constipation), cricopharyngeal spasm, lower esophageal sphincter spasms, rectal spasms, rectal fissures
Eyelid spasms: hemifacial spasm and synkinesis, benign eyelid fasciculation
Headache (muscle contraction, migraine)
Hyperhydrosis
Myokymia
Oscillopsia
Presurgical stabilization
Spasticity: stroke, cerebral palsy, head injury, paraplegia, multiple sclerosis
Sports medicine injuries
Stuttering
Tics
Temporomandibular joint associated muscle spasm
Tremor: Parkinson's disease, essential tremor, hereditary chin tremor
Vaginismus

*Modified from Brin.[38]

The bacteria *Clostridium botulinum* produce seven serologically distinct toxins, designated A, B, C, D, E, F, and G;[256] type A is used in routine treatment. Botulinum toxin exerts its effect at the neuromuscular junction by inhibiting the release of acetylcholine and, when injected in graded amounts, causes a controlled weakness. Botulinum toxin type A does not affect the synthesis or storage of acetylcholine.[115,257]

The preparations of botulinum toxin are distinct and are not generic.[39,171] Although each of the products is measured in units of biological activity, BOTOX units are distinct from Dysport units and NeuroBloc (type B toxin) units. Therefore, it is critical that treating physicians note which product is being utilized, particularly when treating patients in a setting in which multiple products and/or serotypes are available.

The results of botulinum toxin type A therapy for each treatment location are summarized in various treatises on the subject.[9,134,196] In general, a satisfactory result from local injections of botulinum toxin type A occurs in >90% of treated cases of blepharospasm, hemifacial spasm, and laryngeal dystonia. Over 75% of patients with cervical dystonia and jaw-closing oromandibular dystonia derive significant benefit. Patients with upper limb dystonia are more challenging to treat because of the variety of postures present and the potential for hand weakness. Nevertheless, many patients obtain relief from this therapy. The onset of effect is usually within 72 hours and often peaks at 1 week. Most patients experience meaningful relief of symptoms for 3-4 months, although selected patients derive a longer duration of benefit. Toxin-related side effects are typically reversible and related to excessive weakness in the injected or adjacent muscles. An occasional patient may develop a rash or flu-like syndrome; with rare exceptions, these are self-limited.

Antibodies to botulinum toxin type A have been detected rarely in patients exposed either by food poisoning[225] or by therapeutic indications.[25,70,71,73,74,107,120,255,265] Some of the patients who developed botulinum toxin type A antibodies have benefited from injections of immunologically distinct preparations. The benefits of botulinum toxin type F appear to last only about 1 month.[112,113,174,239,254] Botulinum toxin type B is currently in clinical trial.[169,266]

Botulinum toxin type A injections have several advantages over primary pharmacological or surgical therapy in the management of intractable disease. Systemic pharmacological effects are rare; permanent destruction of tissue does not occur. Graded degrees of weakening can be achieved by varying the dose injected. Most adverse effects are transient. If the patient has a strong response to therapy and too much weakness occurs, strength gradually returns. The patient's acceptance is high, and in most cases, botulinum toxin type A therapy is preferred to alternative pharmacotherapies, which can be added as needed.

Peripheral Surgery

With the development of botulinum toxin therapy, only rarely are patients referred for peripheral surgery.[18,22,66,77,121] Prior to the availability of botulinum toxin, patients with blepharospasm underwent selective myectomy[188] and differential section of the facial nerve;[53] results of these treatments were usually inconsistent. Dedo[69] described dramatic relief of spasmodic dysphonia symptoms by sectioning the recurrent laryngeal nerve. The initial favorable reports were temporized by Aronson and DeSanto,[14,15] who reviewed 33 patients treated with surgery. After 3 years, only 36% of patients had persistent improvement and only one patient achieved a persistent normal voice; adverse effects included breathiness, hoarseness, diplophonia, and falsetto. Of the 64% with failed voices at 3 years, 48% were worse than before surgery.

Currently, the most common indication for surgery is resistance to botulinum toxin type A therapy in patients with cervical dystonia. Selective denervation procedures[19,21] are best performed by surgeons who specialize in such procedures. Surgery may be successful in managing patients with primary rotatory torticollis, laterocollis, or retrocollis. However, the surgery carries the risk of permanent excessive weakness and dysphagia. The author has obtained excellent results in properly selected patients referred for surgery; the pessimistic view of this procedure[93] is not shared by other authors,[20,34,77,97] including this one. Cervical stimulation has been championed by some,[273-275] but was shown to be of no sustained benefit.[87,104]

An Approach to Managing Patients With Dystonia

The treatment of primary and most cases of secondary dystonia is similar. At the time of the

TABLE 3

THERAPEUTIC OPTIONS IN DYSTONIA

Supportive and social treatment
Physical therapies
Oral and intrathecal pharmacotherapy
Injection therapy
Surgical therapy
Peripheral surgery
CNS surgery

initial consultation, the patient is introduced to the five basic treatment options, acknowledging that in most cases the choice is the patient's (Table 3). Although a patient may be an obvious candidate for a specific intervention, he or she needs to be aware of the options, including those that may not be chosen.

Pharmacotherapy may be dramatically useful in patients with known biochemical or enzymatic defects. In all patients, the benefits of pharmacotherapy must be weighed against the limitations of systemic adverse effects. In an effort to avoid tardive complications,[280] classical neuroleptics that block D_1 and D_2 dopamine receptors are avoided unless absolutely mandatory.

The choice of drug to initiate treatment usually depends on the patient's age, prior exposure to medications, other concurrent medications or medical problems, and the biases of the physician and patient. Drug dosage is initially low, gradually increased as tolerated, and adjusted to identify the most efficacious dose with a minimum of adverse effects ("regulation of dose"). If a medication is of no benefit at a dose that causes adverse effects, it is gradually tapered and discontinued. If a medication is helpful, it can be continued at the regulated dose, and the next medication added. When a medication is removed from a treatment program, the dose is tapered and only rarely abruptly discontinued.

Botulinum toxin injection therapy has the overall benefit of treating focal and regional dystonic postures and spasms, typically without systemic adverse effects. For most patients with focal dystonia or symptoms limited to one region, local injections of botulinum toxin are the core treatment. For those who cannot be treated effectively with botulinum toxin or for botulinum toxin type A therapy failures, pharmacotherapy is instituted. Physical therapies are recommended as complementary treatment for most botulinum toxin type A patients in an attempt to extend the toxin's benefit. Botulinum toxin type A may substantially change motor patterns, requiring physical therapy to help the patient relearn normal postures and functional control. Although it has not been proven in a formal study, physical therapy may extend the benefit of botulinum toxin type A treatment for cervical dystonia. The benefit from botulinum toxin for spasmodic dysphonia can be augmented with speech therapy.[199]

When relief from more generalized symptoms is required, systemic pharmacotherapy is introduced; botulinum toxin type A can also be used for focal or regional control. Until a direct, genetics-based diagnosis for dopa-responsive dystonia is available, levodopa therapy should always be tried. L-DOPA is tried in all patients with young onset (age <30 years) and in those with onset in a limb. The combination of L-DOPA and decarboxylase inhibitor is begun with small doses of L-DOPA (100 mg), which are gradually increased as tolerated. Most dopa-responsive dystonia patients respond to doses of <1000 mg/day. If there is no response, then the drug is tapered and discontinued.

Next, either an anticholinergic or a benzodiazepine may be introduced. Young patients tolerate both medications well. As discussed above, early assessment of an anticholinergic is appropriate in children. After the dose of anticholinergic agent is regulated, a benzodiazepine is introduced. In adults, a benzodiazepine is usually introduced early in the disease because the cognitive side effects from anticholinergics are poorly tolerated. In both children and adults, after anticholinergics and benzodiazepines are tested, oral baclofen is introduced and the dose regulated.

If this initial approach fails, then one needs to consider introducing tetrabenazine or screening with CITB. As noted above, other oral pharmacotherapeutic agents have been tried, with limited but definite success. Tricyclic antidepressants are often tried early because of the combined anticholinergic and antidepressant effects.

Destructive surgical procedures (thalamotomy, pallidotomy, cervical rhizotomy) are usually reserved for patients in whom more conservative therapies fail. It is hoped that better understanding of dystonia will permit more specific therapies in the near future.

Therapies can be utilized alone or, in most situations, in combination. Many patients receiving botulinum toxin type A continue on low-dose benzodiazepines to aid in prolonging the interval between treatments.

In refractory cases, when all other measures have failed, peripheral or brain surgery is considered. Deep brain stimulation may become an alternative to destructive neurosurgical procedures. With the advancing understanding of the genetics of dystonia, it is hoped that specific therapy to either halt the progression of or bring relief from dystonic spasms, will be available shortly.

References

1. Aguilar EJ, Keshavan MS, Martínez-Quiles MD, et al: Predictors of acute dystonia in first-episode psychotic patients. **Am J Psychiatry 151:**1819-1821, 1994
2. Akindele MO, Odejide AO: Amodiaquine-induced involuntary movements. **Br Med J 2:**214-215, 1976
3. Albright AL, Barry MJ, Fasick P, et al: Continuous intrathecal baclofen infusion for symptomatic generalized dystonia. **Neurosurgery 38:**934-939, 1996
4. Albright AL, Cervi A, Singletary J: Intrathecal baclofen for spasticity in cerebral palsy. **JAMA 265:** 1418-1422, 1991
5. Allain H, Pollak P, Neukirch HC: Symptomatic effect of selegiline in *de novo* parkinsonian patients. The French Selegiline Multicenter Trial. **Mov Disord 8 (Suppl 1):**S36-S40, 1993
6. Almasy L, Bressman SB, de Leon D, et al: Idiopathic torsion dystonia linked to chromosome 8 markers in a family of German Mennonite origin. **Neurology 48 (Suppl 2):**A395, 1997 (Abstract)
7. Almasy L, Bressman SB, Raymond D, et al: Idiopathic torsion dystonia linked to chromosome 8 in two Mennonite families. **Ann Neurol 42:**670-673, 1997
8. Alvir JMJ, Lieberman JA, Safferman AZ, et al: Clozapine-induced agranulocytosis. Incidence and risk factors in the United States. **N Engl J Med 329:** 162-167, 1993
9. American Academy of Neurology: Assessment: The clinical usefulness of botulinum toxin-A in treating neurologic disorders. Report of the Therapeutics and Technology Assessment Subcommittee of the American Academy of Neurology. **Neurology 40:** 1332-1336, 1990
10. American Academy of Ophthalmology: Botulinum-A toxin for ocular muscle disorders. **Lancet 1:**76-77, 1986
11. American Academy of Ophthalmology: Botulinum toxin therapy of eye muscle disorders. Safety and effectiveness. **Ophthalmology 96 (Suppl):**37-41, 1989
12. American Academy of Otolaryngology, Section of Head and Neck Surgery: Policy Statement: BOTOX for spasmodic dysphonia. **AAO-HNS Bull 9 (December):**8, 1990
13. Arevalo GJG, Gershanik OS: Modulatory effect of clozapine on levodopa response in Parkinson's disease: a preliminary study. **Mov Disord 8:**349-354, 1993
14. Aronson AE, DeSanto LW: Adductor spastic dysphonia: 1½ years after recurrent laryngeal nerve resection. **Ann Otol Rhinol Laryngol 90:**2-6, 1981
15. Aronson AE, DeSanto LW: Adductor spastic dysphonia: three years after recurrent laryngeal nerve resection. **Laryngoscope 93:**1-8, 1983
16. Barbeau A, Sourkes TL, Murphy CF: Les catecholamines dans la maladie de Parkinson, in de Ajuriaguerra J (ed): **Monoamines et Système Nerveaux Central.** Geneva: Georg, 1962, pp 247-262
17. Bennett JP Jr, Landow ER, Dietrich S, et al: Suppression of dyskinesias in advanced Parkinson's disease: moderate daily clozapine doses provide long-term dyskinesia reduction. **Mov Disord 9:**409-414, 1994
18. Bertrand C, Molina-Negro P, Bouvier G, et al: Observations and analysis of results in 131 cases of spasmodic torticollis after selective denervation. **Appl Neurophysiol 50:**319-323, 1987
19. Bertrand C, Molina Negro P, Martinez SN: Technical aspects of selective peripheral denervation for spasmodic torticollis. **Appl Neurophysiol 45:**326-330, 1982
20. Bertrand CM: Selective peripheral denervation for spasmodic torticollis: surgical technique, results, and observations in 260 cases. **Surg Neurol 40:**96-103, 1993
21. Bertrand CM, Lenz FA: Surgical treatment of dystonias, in Tsui JKC, Calne DB (eds): **Handbook of Dystonia.** New York, NY: Marcel Dekker, 1995, pp 329-346
22. Bertrand CM, Molina-Negro P: Selective peripheral denervation in 111 cases of spasmodic torticollis: rationale and results. **Adv Neurol 50:**637-643, 1988
23. Biary N, Singh B, Bahou Y, et al: Posttraumatic paroxysmal nocturnal hemidystonia. **Mov Disord 9:** 98-99, 1994
24. Biggins CA, Boyd JL, Harrop FM, et al: A controlled, longitudinal study of dementia in Parkinson's disease. **J Neurol Neurosurg Psychiatry 55:**566-571, 1992
25. Biglan AW, Gonnering R, Lockhart LB, et al: Absence of antibody production in patients treated with botulinum A toxin. **Am J Ophthalmol 101:** 232-235, 1986
26. Birkmayer W, Hornykiewicz O: [The L-3,4-dioxyphenylalanin (Dopa)-effect in Parkinson-akinesia.] **Wien Klin Wochenschr 73:**787-788, 1961 (Ger)
27. Birkmayer W, Riederer P, Youdim MB, et al: The potentiation of the anti akinetic effect after L-dopa treatment by an inhibitor of MAO-B, Deprenil. **J Neural Transm 36:**303-326, 1975
28. Blanchet PJ, Papa SM, Metman LV, et al: Modulation of levodopa-induced motor response complications

by NMDA antagonists in Parkinson's disease. **Neurosci Biobehav Rev 21**:447-453, 1997

29. Block G, Liss C, Reines S, et al: Comparison of immediate-release and controlled-release carbidopa/levodopa in Parkinson's disease. A multicenter 5-year study. The CR First Study Group. **Eur Neurol 37**:23-27, 1997
30. Borrow S, Tattersall ML, Hartman D, et al: Sleep disorders. Consider nocturnal paroxysmal dystonia. **Br Med J 306**:1476-1477, 1993 (Letter)
31. Bowery NG, Doble A, Hill DR, et al: Bicuculline-insensitive GABA receptors on peripheral autonomic nerve terminals. **Eur J Pharmacol 71**:53-70, 1981
32. Bowery NG, Hill DR, Hudson AL, et al: Baclofen decreases neurotransmitter release in the mammalian CNS by an action at a novel GABA receptor. **Nature 283**:92-94, 1980
33. Brans JWM, Lindeboom R, Snoek JW, et al: Botulinum toxin versus trihexyphenidyl in cervical dystonia: a prospective, randomized, double-blind controlled trial. **Neurology 46**:1066-1072, 1996
34. Braun V, Richter HP: Selective peripheral denervation for the treatment of spasmodic torticollis. **Neurosurgery 35**:58-63, 1994
35. Brennan MJ, Ruff P, Sandyk R: Efficacy of a combination of sodium valproate and baclofen in Meige's disease (idiopathic orofacial dystonia). **Br Med J 285**:853, 1982
36. Bressman SB, Greene PE: Treatment of hyperkinetic movement disorders. **Neurol Clin 8**:51-75, 1990
37. Brin MF (ed): Spasticity: etiology, evaluation, management, and the role of botulinum toxin type A: a training syllabus developed by the Spasticity Study Group. **Muscle Nerve 20**:S1-S231, 1997
38. Brin MF: Treatment of dystonia, in Jankovic J, Tolosa E (eds): **Parkinson's Disease and Movement Disorders**. Baltimore, Md: Williams & Wilkins (In press)
39. Brin MF, Blitzer A: Botulinum toxin: dangerous terminology errors. **J R Soc Med 86**:493-494, 1993 (Letter)
40. Brin MF, Moskowitz C, Fahn S: Dystonia clinical research center tissue resource facility: investigations on collected tissue. **Adv Neurol 50**:215-222, 1988
41. Brin MF, Sadiq S, Goodman R, et al: Intrathecal baclofen (IT-B) for dystonia. **Neurology 44 (Suppl 1)**:A338, 1994 (Abstract)
42. Brooks D: PET studies on dystonia. **Focus Dystonia** 14-15, 1994 (Abstract)
43. Brown DA, Higgins AJ: Presynaptic effects of γ-aminobutyric acid in isolated rat superior cervical ganglia. **Br J Pharmacol 66**:108p-109p, 1979
44. Brudny J, Grynbaum BB, Korein J: Spasmodic torticollis: treatment by feedback display of the EMG. **Arch Phys Med Rehabil 55**:403-408, 1974
45. Brudny J, Korein J, Grynbaum BB, et al: EMG feedback therapy: review of treatment of 114 patients. **Arch Phys Med Rehabil 57**:55-61, 1976
46. Burke RE: Neuroleptic-induced tardive dyskinesia variants, in Lang AE, Weiner WJ (eds): **Drug-Induced Movement Disorders**. Mt. Kisco, NY: Futura, 1992, pp 167-198
47. Burke RE, Brin MF, Fahn S, et al: Analysis of the clinical course of non-Jewish, autosomal dominant torsion dystonia. **Mov Disord 1**:163-178, 1986
48. Burke RE, Fahn S: Double-blind evaluation of trihexyphenidyl in dystonia. **Adv Neurol 37**:189-192, 1983
49. Burke RE, Fahn S, Jankovic J, et al: Tardive dystonia and inappropriate use of neuroleptic drugs. **Lancet 1**:1299, 1982 (Letter)
50. Burke RE, Fahn S, Jankovic J, et al: Tardive dystonia: late-onset and persistent dystonia caused by antipsychotic drugs. **Neurology 32**:1335-1346, 1982
51. Burke RE, Fahn S, Mayeux R, et al: Neuroleptic malignant syndrome caused by dopamine-depleting drugs in a patient with Huntington disease. **Neurology 31**:1022-1026, 1981
52. Burke RE, Reches A, Traub MM, et al: Tetrabenazine induces acute dystonic reactions. **Ann Neurol 17**:200-202, 1985
53. Callahan A: Blepharospasm with resection of part of orbicularis nerve supply. Correction of intractable cases. **Arch Ophthalmol 70**:508-511, 1963
54. Cantello R, Gilli M, Riccio A, et al: Mood changes associated with "end-of-dose deterioration" in Parkinson's disease: a controlled study. **J Neurol Neurosurg Psychiatry 49**:1182-1190, 1986
55. Carlsson A, Lindqvist M, Magnusson T: 3,4,dihydroxyphenylalanine and 5-hydroxytryptophan as reserpine antagonists. **Nature 180**:1200, 1957
56. Casey DE: Neuroleptic-induced acute dystonia, in Lang AE, Weiner WJ (eds): **Drug-Induced Movement Disorders**. Mt. Kisco, NY: Futura, 1992, pp 21-40
57. Ceballos-Baumann AO, Passingham RE, Warner T, et al: Overactive prefrontal and underactive motor cortical areas in idiopathic dystonia. **Ann Neurol 37**:363-372, 1995
58. Chadwick D, Reynolds EH, Marsden CD: Anticonvulsant-induced dyskinesias: a comparison with dyskinesias induced by neuroleptics. **J Neurol Neurosurg Psychiatry 39**:1210-1218, 1976
59. Chan J, Brin M, Fahn S: Idiopathic cervical dystonia: clinical characteristics. **Mov Disord 6**:119-126, 1991
60. Christensen JEJ: New treatment of spasmodic torticollis. **Lancet 338**:573, 1991 (Letter)
61. Cooper JR, Bloom FE, Roth RH: **The Biochemical Basis of Neuropharmacology**. New York, NY: Oxford University Press, 1991
62. Cotzias GC, Papavasiliou PS, Gellene R: Modification of parkinsonism—chronic treatment with L-dopa. **N Engl J Med 280**:337-345, 1969
63. Cotzias GC, Van Woert MH, Schiffer LM: Aromatic amino acids and modification of parkinsonism. **N Engl J Med 276**:374-379, 1967
64. Critchley EMR, Phillips M: Unusual idiosyncratic reactions to carbamazepine. **J Neurol Neurosurg Psychiatry 51**:1238, 1988 (Letter)
65. Crosley CJ, Swender PT: Dystonia associated with carbamazepine administration: experience in brain-damaged children. **Pediatrics 63**:612-615, 1979
66. Davis DH, Ahlskog JE, Litchy WJ, et al: Selective peripheral denervation for torticollis: preliminary results. **Mayo Clin Proc 66**:365-371, 1991
67. de Yebenes JG, Brin MF, Mena MA, et al: Neurochemical findings in neuroacanthocytosis. **Mov Disord 3**:300-312, 1988
68. DeBoer P, Westerink BHC: GABAergic modulation of striatal cholinergic interneurons: an *in vivo* microdialysis study. **J Neurochem 62**:70-75, 1994

69. Dedo HH: Recurrent laryngeal nerve section for spastic dysphonia. **Ann Otol Rhinol Laryngol 85:** 451-459, 1976
70. Dezfulian M, Bitar RA, Bartlett JG: Kinetics study of immunological response to *Clostridium botulinum* toxin. **J Clin Microbiol 25:**1336-1337, 1987
71. Dezfulian M, Hatheway CL, Yolken RH, et al: Enzyme-linked immunosorbent assay for detection of *Clostridium botulinum* type A and type B toxins in stool samples of infants with botulism. **J Clin Microbiol 20:**379-383, 1984
72. Djaldetti R, Koren M, Ziv I, et al: Effect of cisapride on response fluctuations in Parkinson's disease. **Mov Disord 10:**81-84, 1995
73. Doellgast GJ, Beard GA, Bottoms JD, et al: Enzyme-linked immunosorbent assay and enzyme-linked coagulation assay for detection of *Clostridium botulinum* neurotoxins A, B, and E and solution-phase complexes with dual-label antibodies. **J Clin Microbiol 32:**105-111, 1994
74. Doellgast GJ, Triscott MX, Beard GA, et al: Sensitive enzyme-linked immunosorbent assay for detection of *Clostridium botulinum* neurotoxins A, B, and E using signal amplification via enzyme-linked coagulation assay. **J Clin Microbiol 31:**2402-2409, 1993
75. Dooneief G, Mirabello E, Bell K, et al: An estimate of the incidence of depression in idiopathic Parkinson's disease. **Arch Neurol 49:**305-307, 1992
76. Dubois B, Danzé F, Pillon B, et al: Cholinergic-dependent cognitive deficits in Parkinson's disease. **Ann Neurol 22:**26-30, 1987
77. Duvoisin RC: Spasmodic torticollis: the role of surgical denervation. **Mayo Clin Proc 66:**433-435, 1991
78. Ehringer H, Hornykiewicz O: [Distribution of noradrenaline and dopamine (3-hydroxytyramine) in the human brain and their behavior in diseases of the extrapyramidal system.] **Klin Wochenschr 38:** 1236-1239, 1960 (Ger)
79. Eidelberg D, Moeller JR, Ishikawa T, et al: The metabolic topography of idiopathic torsion dystonia. **Brain 118:**1473-1484, 1995
80. Eisler T, Hall RP, Kalavar KAR, et al: Erythromelalgia-like eruption in parkinsonian patients treated with bromocriptine. **Neurology 31:**1368-1370, 1981
81. Engberg G, Elebring T, Nissbrandt H: Deprenyl (selegiline), a selective MAO-B inhibitor with active metabolites; effects on locomotor activity, dopaminergic neurotransmission and firing rate of nigral dopamine neurons. **J Pharmacol Exp Ther 259:** 841-847, 1991
82. Factor SA, Brown D, Molho ES, et al: Clozapine: a 2-year open trial in Parkinson's disease patients with psychosis. **Neurology 44:**544-546, 1994
83. Factor SA, Friedman JH: The emerging role of clozapine in the treatment of movement disorders. **Mov Disord 12:**483-496, 1997
84. Fahn S: Adverse effects of levodopa, in Olanow CW, Lieberman AN (eds): **The Scientific Basis for the Treatment of Parkinson's Disease**. Lancashire, England: Parthenon, 1992, pp 89-112
85. Fahn S: High dosage anticholinergic therapy in dystonia. **Neurology 33:**1255-1261, 1983
86. Fahn S: The history of parkinsonism. **Mov Disord 4 (Suppl 1):**S2-S10, 1989
87. Fahn S: Lack of benefit from cervical cord stimulation for dystonia. **N Engl J Med 313:**1229, 1985 (Letter)
88. Fahn S: Parkinson's disease and other basal ganglion disorders, in Asbury AK, McKhann GM, McDonald WI (eds): **Diseases of the Nervous System: Clinical Neurobiology**. Philadelphia, Pa: Ardmore, 1986, pp 1217-1228
89. Fahn S: The varied clinical expressions of dystonia. **Neurol Clin 2:**541-554, 1984
90. Feldman RG, Kelly-Hayes M, Conomy JP, et al: Baclofen for spasticity in multiple sclerosis. Double-blind crossover and three-year study. **Neurology 28:**1094-1098, 1978
91. Felten DL, Felten SY, Steece-Collier K, et al: Age-related decline in the dopaminergic nigrostriatal system: the oxidative hypothesis and protective strategies. **Ann Neurol 32 (Suppl):**S133-S136, 1992
92. Fletcher NA, Holt IJ, Harding AE, et al: Tyrosine hydroxylase and levodopa responsive dystonia. **J Neurol Neurosurg Psychiatry 52:**112-114, 1989
93. Ford B, Greene P, Fahn S: Outcome of cervical ramisectomy for intractable torticollis. **Neurology 46 (Suppl 2):**A273, 1996 (Abstract)
94. Ford B, Greene P, Louis ED, et al: Use of intrathecal baclofen in the treatment of patients with dystonia. **Arch Neurol 53:**1241-1246, 1996
95. Frankel JP, Lees AJ, Kempster PA, et al: Subcutaneous apomorphine in the treatment of Parkinson's disease. **J Neurol Neurosurg Psychiatry 53:**96-101, 1990
96. Friedman A, Fahn S: Spontaneous remissions in spasmodic torticollis. **Neurology 36:**398-400, 1986
97. Friedman AH, Nashold BS Jr, Sharp R, et al: Treatment of spasmodic torticollis with intradural selective rhizotomies. **J Neurosurg 78:**46-53, 1993
98. Friedman JH, Lannon MC: Clozapine-responsive tremor in Parkinson's disease. **Mov Disord 5:** 225-229, 1990
99. Garg BP: Dystonia musculorum deformans. Implications of therapeutic response to levodopa and carbamazepine. **Arch Neurol 39:**376-377, 1982
100. Geller M, Kaplan B, Christoff N: Treatment of dystonic symptoms with carbamazepine. **Adv Neurol 14:**403-410, 1976
101. Giménez-Roldán S, Mateo D, Bartolomé P: Tardive dystonia and severe tardive dyskinesia. A comparison of risk factors and prognosis. **Acta Psychiatr Scand 71:**488-494, 1985
102. Giménez-Roldán S, Mateo D, Martín M: Life-threatening cranial dystonia following trihexyphenidyl withdrawal. **Mov Disord 4:**349-353, 1989
103. Glover V, Clow A, Sandler M: Effects of dopaminergic drugs on superoxide dismutase: implications for senescence. **J Neural Transm Suppl 40:**37-45, 1993
104. Goetz CG, Penn RD, Tanner CM: Efficacy of cervical cord stimulation in dystonia. **Adv Neurol 50:** 645-649, 1988
105. Golbe LI, Lieberman AN, Muenter MD, et al: Deprenyl in the treatment of symptom fluctuations in advanced Parkinson's disease. **Clin Neuropharmacol 11:**45-55, 1988
106. Gollomp SM, Fahn S, Burke RE, et al: Therapeutic trials in Meige syndrome. **Adv Neurol 37:**207-213, 1983
107. Gonnering RS: Negative antibody response to long-term treatment of facial spasm with botulinum toxin. **Am J Ophthalmol 105:**313-315, 1988

108. Goodenough DJ, Fariello RG, Annis BL, et al: Familial and acquired paroxysmal dyskinesias. A proposed classification with delineation of clinical features. **Arch Neurol 35:**827-831, 1978
109. Gray JA, Green AR: $GABA_B$-receptor-mediated inhibition of potassium-evoked release of endogenous 5-hydroxytryptamine from mouse frontal cortex. **Br J Pharmacol 91:**517-522, 1987
110. Greene P, Shale H, Fahn S: Analysis of open-label trials in torsion dystonia using high dosages of anticholinergics and other drugs. **Mov Disord 3:**46-60, 1988
111. Greene PE, Fahn S: Baclofen in the treatment of idiopathic dystonia in children. **Mov Disord 7:** 48-52, 1992
112. Greene PE, Fahn S: Response to botulinum toxin F in seronegative botulinum toxin A—resistant patients. **Mov Disord 11:**181-184, 1996
113. Greene PE, Fahn S: Use of botulinum toxin type F injections to treat torticollis in patients with immunity to botulinum toxin type A. **Mov Disord 8:** 479-483, 1993
114. Grohmann R, Koch R, Schmidt LG: Extrapyramidal symptoms in neuroleptic recipients. **Agents Actions (Suppl) 29:**71-82, 1990
115. Gundersen CB: The effects of botulinum toxin on the synthesis, storage and release of acetylcholine. **Prog Neurobiol 14:**99-119, 1980
116. Hallett M: Is dystonia a sensory disorder? **Ann Neurol 38:**139-140, 1995
117. Hallett M, Toro C: Dystonia and the supplementary sensorimotor area. **Adv Neurol 70:**471-476, 1996
118. Hardie RJ, Malcolm SL, Lees AJ, et al: The pharmacokinetics of intravenous and oral levodopa in patients with Parkinson's disease who exhibit on-off fluctuations. **Br J Clin Pharmacol 22:**429-436, 1986
119. Hassin GB: Quinine and dystonia musculorum deformans. **JAMA 113:**12-14, 1939
120. Hatheway CH, Snyder JD, Seals JE, et al: Antitoxin levels in botulism patients treated with trivalent equine botulism antitoxin to toxin types A, B, and E. **J Infect Dis 150:**407-412, 1984
121. Hernesniemi J, Keränen T: Long-term outcome after surgery for spasmodic torticollis. **Acta Neurochir 103:**128-130, 1990
122. Hirsch E, Sellal F, Maton B, et al: Nocturnal paroxysmal dystonia: a clinical form of focal epilepsy. **Neurophysiol Clin 24:**207-217, 1994
123. Hobbs WR, Rall TW, Verdoorn TA: Hypnotics and sedatives; ethanol, in Hardman JG, Limbird LE, Molinoff PB, et al (eds): **The Pharmacological Basis of Therapeutics**. New York, NY: McGraw-Hill, 1996, pp 361-396
124. Hoehn MM: The natural history of Parkinson's disease in the pre-levodopa and post-levodopa eras. **Neurol Clin 10:**331-339, 1992
125. Hornykiewicz O: Parkinson's disease and the adaptive capacity of the nigrostriatal dopamine system: possible neurochemical mechanisms. **Adv Neurol 60:**140-147, 1993
126. Hornykiewicz O, Kish SJ, Becker LE, et al: Brain neurotransmitters in dystonia musculorum deformans. **N Engl J Med 315:**347-353, 1986
127. Hurtig HI: Problems with current pharmacologic treatment of Parkinson's disease. **Exp Neurol 144:** 10-16, 1997
128. Isgreen WP, Fahn S, Barrett RE, et al: Carbamazepine in torsion in dystonia. **Adv Neurol 14:** 411-416, 1976
129. Jahanshahi M, Marsden CD: Depression in torticollis: a controlled study. **Psychol Med 18:**925-933, 1988
130. Jahanshahi M, Marsden CD: A longitudinal follow-up study of depression, disability, and body concept in torticollis. **Behav Neurol 3:**233-246, 1990
131. Jankovic J: Post-traumatic movement disorders: central and peripheral mechanisms. **Neurology 44:** 2006-2014, 1994
132. Jankovic J: Treatment of hyperkinetic movement disorders with tetrabenazine: a double-blind crossover study. **Ann Neurol 11:**41-47, 1982
133. Jankovic J, Beach J: Long-term effects of tetrabenazine in hyperkinetic movement disorders. **Neurology 48:**358-362, 1997
134. Jankovic J, Hallett M: **Therapy with Botulinum Toxin**. New York, NY: Marcel Dekker, 1994
135. Jankovic J, Leder S, Warner D, et al: Cervical dystonia: clinical findings and associated movement disorders. **Neurology 41:**1088-1091, 1991
136. Jankovic J, Orman J: Tetrabenazine therapy of dystonia, chorea, tics, and other dyskinesias. **Neurology 38:**391-394, 1988
137. Jankovic J, Svendsen CN, Bird ED: Brain neurotransmitters in dystonia. **N Engl J Med 316:**278-279, 1987
138. Jansen ENH: Clozapine in the treatment of tremor in Parkinson's disease. **Acta Neurol Scand 89:** 262-265, 1994
139. Jayne D, Lees AJ, Stern GM: Remission in spasmodic torticollis. **J Neurol Neurosurg Psychiatry 47:** 1236-1237, 1984
140. Kaji R, Rothwell JC, Katayama M, et al: Tonic vibration reflex and muscle afferent block in writer's cramp. **Ann Neurol 38:**155-162, 1995
141. Kastrup O, Gastpar M, Schwarz M: Acute dystonia due to clozapine. **J Neurol Neurosurg Psychiatry 57:** 119, 1994 (Letter)
142. Katz RT: Management of spasticity. **Am J Phys Med Rehabil 67:**108-116, 1988
143. Keepers GA, Casey DE: Clinical management of acute neuroleptic-induced extrapyramidal syndromes. **Curr Psychiatr Ther 23:**139-157, 1986
144. Kempster PA, Wahlqvist ML: Dietary factors in the management of Parkinson's disease. **Nutr Rev 52:** 51-58, 1994
145. Koller WC: How accurately can Parkinson's disease be diagnosed? **Neurology 42 (Suppl 1):**6-16, 1992
146. Koller WC: Pharmacologic treatment of parkinsonian tremor. **Arch Neurol 43:**126-127, 1986
147. Koller WC, Silver DE, Lieberman A: An algorithm for the management of Parkinson's disease. **Neurology 44 (Suppl 10):**S1-S52, 1994
148. Korein J, Brudny J: Integrated EMG feedback in the management of spasmodic torticollis and focal dystonia: a prospective study of 80 patients. **Res Publ Assoc Res Nerv Ment Dis 55:**385-426, 1976
149. Korein J, Brudny J, Grynbaum B, et al: Sensory feedback therapy of spasmodic torticollis and dystonia: results in treatment of 55 patients. **Adv Neurol 14:** 375-402, 1976
150. Kornhuber J, Weller M: Amantadine and the glutamate hypothesis of schizophrenia. Experiences in the treatment of neuroleptic malignant syndrome.

J Neural Transm Gen Sect **92:**57-65, 1993

151. Kraft IA: A psychiatric study of two patients with dystonia musculorum deformans. **South Med J 59:** 284-288, 1966
152. Kramer PL, de Leon D, Ozelius L, et al: Dystonia gene in Ashkenazi Jewish population is located on chromosome 9q32-34. **Ann Neurol 27:**114-120, 1990
153. Kupke KG, Lee LV, Müller U: Assignment of the X-linked torsion dystonia gene to Xq21 by linkage analysis. **Neurology 40:**1438-1442, 1990
154. Kupke KG, Lee LV, Viterbo GH, et al: X-linked recessive torsion dystonia in the Philippines. **Am J Med Genet 36:**237-242, 1990
155. Kurth MC: Using liquid levodopa in the treatment of Parkinson's disease. A practical guide. **Drugs Aging 10:**332-340, 1997
156. Kwiatkowski DJ, Nygaard TG, Schuback DE, et al: Identification of a highly polymorphic microsatellite VNTR within the argininosuccinate synthetase locus: exclusion of the dystonia gene on 9q32-34 as the cause of dopa-responsive dystonia in a large kindred. **Am J Hum Genet 48:**121-128, 1991
157. Lance JW, Bassil GT: Familial intractable hiccup relieved by baclofen. **Lancet 2:**276-277, 1989 (Letter)
158. Lang AE: Dopamine agonists and antagonists in the treatment of idiopathic dystonia. **Adv Neurol 50:** 561-570, 1988
159. Lang AE: High dose anticholinergic therapy in adult dystonia. **Can J Neurol Sci 13:**42-46, 1986
160. Langtry HD, Clissold SP: Pergolide. A review of its pharmacological properties and therapeutic potential in Parkinson's disease. **Drugs 39:**491-506, 1990
161. Lauterbach EC, Price ST, Spears TE, et al: Serotonin responsive and nonresponsive diurnal depressive mood disorders and pathological affect in thalamic infarct associated with myoclonus and blepharospasm. **Biol Psychiatry 35:**488-490, 1994
162. Lazorthes Y, Sallerin-Caute B, Verdie JC, et al: Chronic intrathecal baclofen administration for control of severe spasticity. **J Neurosurg 72:**393-402, 1990
163. Leathwood PD: Neurotransmitter precursors and brain function. **Bibl Nutr Dieta 38:**54-71, 1986
164. Lee JW: Persistent dystonia associated with carbamazepine therapy: a case report. **N Z Med J 107:** 360-361, 1994
165. Lee LV, Kupke KG, Caballar-Gonzaga F, et al: The phenotype of the X-linked dystonia-parkinsonism syndrome. An assessment of 42 cases in the Philippines. **Medicine 70:**179-187, 1991
166. Lees AJ, Shaw KM, Stern GM: Baclofen in Parkinson's disease. **J Neurol Neurosurg Psychiatry 41:** 707-708, 1978
167. Lees AJ, Stern GM: Sustained bromocriptine therapy in previously untreated patients with Parkinson's disease. **J Neurol Neurosurg Psychiatry 44:** 1020-1023, 1981
168. Leube B, Rudnicki D, Ratzlaff T, et al: Idiopathic torsion dystonia: assignment of a gene to chromosome 18p in a German family with adult onset, autosomal dominant inheritance and purely focal distribution. **Hum Mol Genet 5:**1673-1677, 1996
169. Lew MF, Adornato BT, Duane DD, et al: Botulinum toxin type B: a double-blind, placebo-controlled, safety and efficacy study in cervical dystonia. **Neurology 49:**701-707, 1997
170. Linazasoro G, Martí Massó JF, Suárez JA: Nocturnal akathisia in Parkinson's disease: treatment with clozapine. **Mov Disord 8:**171-174, 1993
171. Lorentz IT: Botulinum toxin: dangerous terminology errors. **J R Soc Med 87:**572, 1994 (Letter)
172. Lowenstein DH, Aminoff MJ: The clinical course of spasmodic torticollis. **Neurology 38:**530-532, 1988
173. Luders HO: Paroxysmal choreoathetosis. **Eur Neurol 36 (Suppl 1):**20-23, 1996
174. Ludlow CL, Hallett M, Rhew K, et al: Therapeutic use of type F botulinum toxin. **N Engl J Med 326:** 349-350, 1992 (Letter)
175. Lugaresi E, Cirignotta F, Montagna P: Nocturnal paroxysmal dystonia. **J Neurol Neurosurg Psychiatry 49:**375-380, 1986
176. Malhotra AK, Litman RE, Pickar D: Adverse effects of antipsychotic drugs. **Drug Saf 9:**429-436, 1993
177. Mann DC, Pearce LA, Waterbury L-DOPA: Amantadine for Parkinson's disease. **Neurology 21:**958-962, 1971
178. Markham A, Benfield P: Pergolide: a review of its pharmacology and therapeutic use in Parkinson's disease. **Cns Drugs 7:**328-340, 1997 (Abstract)
179. Marsden CD: Paroxysmal choreoathetosis. **Adv Neurol 70:**467-470, 1996
180. Marsden CD, Harrison MJG: Idiopathic torsion dystonia (dystonia musculorum deformans). A review of forty-two patients. **Brain 97:**793-810, 1974
181. Marsden CD, Jenner P: The pathophysiology of extrapyramidal side-effects of neuroleptic drugs. **Psychol Med 10:**55-72, 1980
182. Marsden CD, Marion MH, Quinn N: The treatment of severe dystonia in children and adults. **J Neurol Neurosurg Psychiatry 47:**1166-1173, 1984
183. Mateo D, Muñoz-Blanco JL, Giménez-Roldán S: Neuroleptic malignant syndrome related to tetrabenazine introduction and haloperidol discontinuation in Huntington's disease. **Clin Neuropharmacol 15:**63-68, 1992
184. Mayeux R, Chen J, Mirabello E, et al: An estimate of the incidence of dementia in idiopathic Parkinson's disease. **Neurology 40:**1513-1517, 1990
185. Mayeux R, Denaro J, Hemenegildo N, et al: A population-based investigation of Parkinson's disease with and without dementia. Relationship to age and gender. **Arch Neurol 49:**492-497, 1992
186. Mayeux R, Fahn S: Paroxysmal dystonic choreoathetosis in a patient with familial ataxia. **Neurology 32:** 1184-1186, 1982
187. Mayeux R, Stern Y, Rosenstein R, et al: An estimate of the prevalence of dementia in idiopathic Parkinson's disease. **Arch Neurol 45:**260-262, 1988
188. McCord CD Jr, Shore J, Putnam JR: Treatment of essential blepharospasm. II. A modification of exposure for the muscle stripping technique. **Arch Ophthalmol 102:**269-273, 1984
189. McDowell FH: Treatment of spasticity. **Drugs 22:** 401-408, 1981
190. McLean BN: Intrathecal baclofen in severe spasticity. **Br J Hosp Med 49:**262-267, 1993
191. Menon MK: Possible value of baclofen in myoclonus. **JAMA 244:**239-240, 1980 (Letter)
192. Montagna P: Nocturnal paroxysmal dystonia and nocturnal wandering. **Neurology 42 (Suppl 6):** 61-67, 1992

193. Montastruc JL, Rascol O, Senard JM: Current status of dopamine agonists in Parkinson's disease management. **Drugs 46**:384-393, 1993
194. Montastruc JL, Rascol O, Senard JM: Glutamate antagonists and Parkinson's disease: a review of clinical data. **Neurosci Biobehav Rev 21**:477-480, 1997 (Abstract)
195. Montgomery EB Jr, Lieberman A, Singh G, et al: Patient education and health promotion can be effective in Parkinson's disease: a randomized controlled trial. **Am J Med 97**:429-435, 1994
196. Moore AP: **Handbook of Botulinum Toxin Treatment**. Oxford: Blackwell Scientific, 1993
197. Mouradian MM, Chase TN: Central mechanisms and levodopa response fluctuations in Parkinson's disease. **Clin Neuropharmacol 11**:378-385, 1988
198. Murry T, Cannito MP, Woodson GE: Spasmodic dysphonia. Emotional status and botulinum toxin treatment. **Arch Otolaryngol Head Neck Surg 120**: 310-316, 1994
199. Murry T, Woodson GE: Combined-modality treatment of adductor spasmodic dysphonia with botulinum toxin and voice therapy. **J Voice 9**:460-465, 1995
200. Myllylä VV, Sotaniemi KA, Vuorinen JA, et al: Selegiline in *de novo* parkinsonian patients: the Finnish study. **Mov Disord 8 (Suppl 1)**:S41-S44, 1993
201. Mytilineou C, Leonardi EK, Radcliffe PM, et al: Deprenyl and desmethylselegiline protect mesencephalic neurons from toxicity induced by glutathione depletion. **J Pharmacol Exp Ther** (In press)
202. Mytilineou C, Radcliffe PM, Olanow CW: L-(-)-desmethylselegiline, a metabolite of selegiline [L-(-)-deprenyl], protects mesencephalic dopamine neurons from excitotoxicity *in vitro*. **J Neurochem 68**:434-436, 1997
203. Narayan RK, Loubser PG, Jankovic J, et al: Intrathecal baclofen for intractable axial dystonia. **Neurology 41**:1141-1142, 1991
204. Nardocci N, Zorzi G, Savoldelli M, et al: Paroxysmal dystonia and paroxysmal tremor in a young patient with multiple sclerosis. **Ital J Neurol Sci 16**:315-319, 1995
205. National Institutes of Health Consensus Development Committee: Clinical use of botulinum toxin. National Institutes of Health Consensus Development Statement, November 12-14, 1990. **Arch Neurol 48**:1294-1298, 1991
206. Nutt JG, Muenter MD, Aronson A, et al: Epidemiology of focal and generalized dystonia in Rochester, Minnesota. **Mov Disord 3**:188-194, 1988
207. Nutt JG, Woodward WR, Hammerstad JP, et al: The "on-off" phenomenon in Parkinson's disease. Relation to levodopa absorption and transport. **N Engl J Med 310**:483-488, 1984
208. Nygaard TG: Dopa-responsive dystonia. **Curr Opin Neurol 8**:310-313, 1995
209. Nygaard TG: Dopa-responsive dystonia, in Tsui JKC, Calne DB (eds): **Handbook of Dystonia**. New York, NY: Marcel Dekker, 1995, pp 213-227
210. Nygaard TG, Marsden CD, Fahn S: Dopa-responsive dystonia: long-term treatment response and prognosis. **Neurology 41**:174-181, 1991
211. Nygaard TG, Trugman JM, de Yebenes JG, et al: Dopa-responsive dystonia: the spectrum of clinical manifestations in a large North American family. **Neurology 40**:66-69, 1990
212. Obeso JA, Giménez-Roldán S: Clinicopathological correlation in symptomatic dystonia. **Adv Neurol 50**:113-122, 1988
213. Oertel WH, Quinn NP: Parkinsonism, in Brandt T, Caplan LR, Dichgans J, et al (eds): **Neurological Disorders: Course and Treatment**. San Diego, Calif: Academic Press, 1996
214. Ohara S, Hayashi H, Miki J, et al: Mexiletine in the treatment of spasmodic torticollis and blepharospasms. **Neurology 48 (Suppl 2)**:A398-A399, 1997 (Abstract)
215. Ohara S, Miki J, Momoi H, et al: Treatment of spasmodic torticollis with mexiletine: a case report. **Mov Disord 12**:466-469, 1997 (Abstract)
216. Ossemann M, Sindic CJ, Laterre C: Tetrabenazine as a cause of neuroleptic malignant syndrome. **Mov Disord 11**:95, 1996 (Letter)
217. Ozelius L, Kramer PL, Moskowitz CB, et al: Human gene for torsion dystonia located on chromosome 9q32-q34. **Neuron 2**:1427-1434, 1989
218. Ozelius LJ, Hewett JW, Page CE, et al: The early-onset torsion dystonia gene (DYT1) encodes an ATP-binding protein. **Nat Genet 17**:40-48, 1997
219. Pakkenberg H, Pakkenberg B: Clozapine in the treatment of tremor. **Acta Neurol Scand 73**:295-297, 1986
220. Papavasiliou PS, Cotzias GC, Düby SE, et al: Levodopa in parkinsonism: potentiation of central effects with a peripheral inhibitor. **N Engl J Med 286**:8-14, 1972
221. Parkes JD, Baxter RCH, Curzon G, et al: Treatment of Parkinson's disease with amantadine and levodopa. A one-year study. **Lancet 1**:1083-1086, 1971
222. Parkes JD, Baxter RCH, Marsden CD, et al: Comparative trial of benzhexol, amantadine, and levodopa in the treatment of Parkinson's disease. **J Neurol Neurosurg Psychiatry 37**:422-426, 1974
223. Parkinson Study Group: DATATOP: a multicenter controlled clinical trial in early Parkinson's disease. **Arch Neurol 46**:1052-1060, 1989
224. Pate DS, Margolin DI: Cognitive slowing in Parkinson's and Alzheimer's patients distinguishing bradyphrenia from dementia. **Neurology 44**: 669-674, 1994
225. Paton JC, Lawrence AJ, Manson JI: Quantitation of *Clostridium botulinum* organisms and toxin in the feces of an infant with botulism. **J Clin Microbiol 15**:1-4, 1982
226. Penn RD, Gianino JM, York MM: Intrathecal baclofen for motor disorders. **Mov Disord 10**: 675-677, 1995
227. Penn RD, Kroin JS: Long-term intrathecal baclofen infusion for treatment of spasticity. **J Neurosurg 66**: 181-185, 1987
228. Penn RD, Mangieri EA: Stiff-man syndrome treated with intrathecal baclofen. **Neurology 43**:2412, 1993
229. Pezzoli G, Martignoni E, Pacchetti C, et al: A crossover, controlled study comparing pergolide with bromocriptine as an adjunct to levodopa for the treatment of Parkinson's disease. **Neurology 45 (Suppl 3)**:S22-S27, 1995
230. Playford ED, Fletcher NA, Sawle GV, et al: Striatal ^{18}[F]dopa uptake in familial idiopathic dystonia. **Brain 116**:1191-1199, 1993
231. Potashner SJ: Baclofen: effects on amino acid release

and metabolism in slices of guinea pig cerebral cortex. **J Neurochem 32**:103-109, 1979
232. Quinn NP: Anti-parkinsonian drugs today. **Drugs 28**:236-262, 1984
233. Rajput AH: Adverse effects of ergot-derivative dopamine agonists, in Olanow CW, Obeso JA (eds): **Dopamine Agonists in Early Parkinson's Disease**. Kent: Wells Medical Limited, 1997, pp 209-216
234. Rajput AH, Gibb WRG, Zhong XH, et al: Dopa-responsive dystonia: pathological and biochemical observations in a case. **Ann Neurol 35**:396-402, 1994
235. Rascol A: Ropinirole: clinical profile, in Olanow CW, Obeso JA (eds): **Dopamine Agonists in Early Parkinson's Disease.** Kent, Wells Medical Limited, 1997, pp 163-175
236. Reches A, Burke RE, Kuhn CM, et al: Tetrabenazine, an amine-depleting drug, also blocks dopamine receptors in rat brain. **J Pharmacol Exp Ther 225**: 515-521, 1983
237. Reimann W, Zumstein A, Starke K: γ-aminobutyric acid can both inhibit and facilitate dopamine release in the caudate nucleus of the rabbit. **J Neurochem 39**:961-969, 1982
238. Reynolds GP, Elsworth JD, Blau K, et al: Deprenyl is metabolized to methamphetamine and amphetamine in man. **Br J Clin Pharmacol 6**:542-544, 1978
239. Rhew K, Ludlow CL, Karp BI, et al: Clinical experience with botulinum toxin F, in Jankovic J, Hallett M (eds): **Therapy With Botulinum Toxin.** New York, NY: Marcel Dekker, 1994, pp 323-328
240. Rice GPA: Pharmacotherapy of spasticity: some theoretical and practical considerations. **Can J Neurol Sci 14**:510-512, 1987
241. Rinne JO: Nigral degeneration in Parkinson's disease in relation to clinical features. **Acta Neurol Scand Suppl 136**:87-90, 1991
242. Rinne UK: Lisuride, a dopamine agonist in the treatment of early Parkinson's disease. **Neurology 39**:336-339, 1989
243. Rinne UK, Siirtola T, Sonninen V: L-deprenyl treatment of on-off phenomena in Parkinson's disease. **J Neural Transm 43**:253-262, 1978
244. Risch NJ, Bressman SB, deLeon D, et al: Segregation analysis of idiopathic torsion dystonia in Ashkenazi Jews suggests autosomal dominant inheritance. **Am J Hum Genet 46**:533-538, 1990
245. Rupniak NM, Jenner P, Marsden CD: Acute dystonia induced by neuroleptic drugs. **Psychopharmacology 88**:403-419, 1986
246. Saint-Cyr JA, Taylor AE, Lang AE: Neuropsychological and psychiatric side effects in the treatment of Parkinson's disease. **Neurology 43 (Suppl 6)**: S47-S52, 1993
247. Sandyk R: Blepharospasm—successful treatment with baclofen and sodium valproate. A case report. **S Afr Med J 64**:955-956, 1983
248. Sawa GM, Paty DW: The use of baclofen in treatment of spasticity in multiple sclerosis. **Can J Neurol Sci 6**:351-354, 1979
249. Schlicker E, Classen K, Göthert M: GABAB receptor-mediated inhibition of serotonin release in the rat brain. **Naunyn Schmiedebergs Arch Pharmacol 326**:99-105, 1984
250. Schulzer M, Mak E, Calne DB: The antiparkinson efficacy of deprenyl derives from transient improvement that is likely to be symptomatic. **Ann Neurol 32**:795-798, 1992
251. Schwab RS, Amador LV, Lettvin JY: Apomorphine in Parkinson's disease. **Trans Am Neurol Assoc 76**: 251-253, 1951
252. Sethi KD, Hess DC, Huffnagle VH, et al: Acetazolamide treatment of paroxysmal dystonia in central demyelinating disease. **Neurology 42**:919-921, 1992
253. Shapleske J, Mickay AP, McKenna PJ: Successful treatment of tardive dystonia with clozapine and clonazepam. **Br J Psychiatry 168**:516-518, 1996
254. Sheean GL, Lees AJ: Botulinum toxin F in the treatment of torticollis clinically resistant to botulinum toxin A. **J Neurol Neurosurg Psychiatry 59**:601-607, 1995
255. Siatkowski RM, Tyutyunikov A, Biglan AW, et al: Serum antibody production to botulinum A toxin. **Ophthalmology 100**:1861-1866, 1993
256. Simpson LL: The origin, structure, and pharmacological activity of botulinum toxin. **Pharmacol Rev 33**:155-188, 1981
257. Simpson LL: Peripheral actions of the botulinum toxins, in Simpson LL (ed): **Botulinum Neurotoxin and Tetanus Toxin.** New York, NY: Academic Press: 1989, pp 153-178
258. Soman P, Jain S, Rajsekhar V, et al: Dystonia—a rare manifestation of carbamazepine toxicity. **Postgrad Med J 70**:54-55, 1994 (Letter)
259. Spinella GM, Sheridan PH: Research opportunities in dystonia: National Institute of Neurological Disorders and Stroke workshop summary. **Neurology 44**:1177-1179, 1994
260. Stibe CM, Lees AJ, Kempster PA, et al: Subcutaneous apomorphine in parkinsonian on-off oscillations. **Lancet 1**:403-406, 1988
261. Suchowersky O, deVries JD: Interaction of fluoxetine and selegiline. **Can J Psychiatry 35**:571-572, 1990 (Letter)
262. Takahashi H, Snow B, Waters C, et al: Evidence for nigrostriatal lesions in Lubag (X-linked dystonia-parkinsonism in the Philippines). **Neurology 42 (Suppl 3)**:441, 1992 (Abstract)
263. Tanner CM, Glantz RH, Klawans HL: Meige disease: acute and chronic cholinergic effects. **Neurology 32**:783-785, 1982
264. Tolosa ES: Clinical features of Meige's disease (idiopathic orofacial dystonia). A report of 17 cases. **Arch Neurol 38**:147-151, 1981
265. Tsui JK, Wong NLM, Wong E, et al: Production of circulating antibodies to botulinum-A toxin in patients receiving repeated injections for dystonia. **Ann Neurol 24**:181, 1988 (Abstract)
266. Tsui JKC, Hayward M, Mak EKM, et al: Botulinum toxin type B in the treatment of cervical dystonia: a pilot study. **Neurology 45**:2109-2110, 1995
267. Umez-Eronini EM, Eronini EA: Chloroquine induced involuntary movements. **Br Med J 1**:945-946, 1977
268. Vaamonde J, Luquin MR, Obeso JA: Subcutaneous lisuride infusion in Parkinson's disease. Response to chronic administration in 34 patients. **Brain 114**: 601-617, 1991
269. van Laar T, Jansen ENH, Essink AWG, et al: Rectal apomorphine: a new treatment modality in Parkinson's disease. **J Neurol Neurosurg Psychiatry 55**: 737-738, 1992 (Letter)
270. Vilming ST: Diettbehandling ved Parkinsons syk-

dom. **Tidsskr Nor Laegeforen 115:**1244-1247, 1995

271. Waldmeier PC, Baumann PA: Presynaptic GABA receptors. **Ann N Y Acad Sci 604:**136-151, 1990
272. Walker RH: Mexiletine in the treatment of dystonia. **Neurology** (In press)
273. Waltz JM, Andreesen WH, Hunt DP: Spinal cord stimulation and motor disorders. **PACE 10:**180-204, 1987
274. Waltz JM, Davis JA: Cervical cord stimulation in the treatment of athetosis and dystonia. **Adv Neurol 37:** 225-237, 1983
275. Waltz JM, Scozzari CA, Hunt DP: Spinal cord stimulation in the treatment of spasmodic torticollis. **Appl Neurophysiol 48:**324-338, 1985
276. Waters CH: Fluoxetine and selegiline—lack of significant interaction. **Can J Neurol Sci 21:**259-261, 1994
277. Weiner WJ, Factor SA, Sanchez-Ramos JR, et al: Early combination therapy (bromocriptine and levodopa) does not prevent motor fluctuations in Parkinson's disease. **Neurology 43:**21-27, 1993
278. Wilhelmsen KC, Weeks DE, Nygaard TG, et al: Genetic mapping of the "Lubag" (X-linked dystonia-parkinsonism) in a Filipino kindred to the pericentromeric region of the X chromosome. **Ann Neurol 29:**124-131, 1991
279. Wolf ME, Mosnaim AD: Improvement of axial dystonia with the administration of clozapine. **Int J Clin Pharmacol Ther 32:**282-283, 1994
280. Wolf ME, Mosnaim AD: **Tardive Dyskinesia: Biological Mechanisms and Clinical Aspects.** Washington, DC: American Psychiatric Press, 1988
281. Wolters EC, Hurwitz TA, Mak E, et al: Clozapine in the treatment of parkinsonian patients with dopaminomimetic psychosis. **Neurology 40:** 832-834, 1990
282. Wood KM: The use of phenol as a neurolytic agent: a review. **Pain 5:**205-229, 1978
283. Wuis EW: Spasticity and drug therapy. **Pharm Weekbl 9:**249-260, 1987
284. Yang HY, Neff NH: The monoamine oxidases of brain: selective inhibition with drugs and the consequences for the metabolism of the biogenic amines. **J Pharmacol Exp Ther 189:**733-740, 1974
285. Young BK, Camicioli R, Ganzini L: Neuropsychiatric adverse effects of antiparkinsonian drugs: characteristics, evaluation and treatment. **Drugs Aging 10:** 367-383, 1997 (Abstract)
286. Zweig RM, Hedreen JC: Brain stem pathology in cranial dystonia. **Adv Neurol 49:**395-407, 1988
287. Zweig RM, Hedreen JC, Jankel WR, et al: Pathology in brainstem regions of individuals with primary dystonia. **Neurology 38:**702-706, 1988

PART B

Treatment of Parkinson's Disease: Ablative Surgical Procedures

CHAPTER 8

THALAMOTOMY: INDICATIONS, TECHNIQUES, AND RESULTS

RICHARD K. OSENBACH, MD, AND KIM J. BURCHIEL, MD, FACS

As one reviews the history of the surgical management of movement disorders, it is impossible not to be struck by the rich legacy left by so many great neurosurgeons who have contributed mightily to this field. Prior to the development of stereotactic surgery, movement disorder surgery involved open procedures on the brain or spinal cord. Sir Victor Horsley, in 1890, performed the first successful cortical resection in a patient with hemiathetosis.[34] Several decades later, Bucy and Case[10] and Klemme[43] were still performing subpial resection of the premotor (area 6) and primary motor (area 4) regions in patients with tremor and dyskinesias. These initial procedures were targeted at interruption of corticospinal pathways. Indeed, it was Bucy's opinion that amelioration of tremor was not possible without destruction of some portion of the corticospinal system. In 1939, Meyers[56] pioneered a new approach to the surgical treatment of Parkinson's disease by resecting the head of the caudate nucleus and later moving on to excision of various portions of the basal ganglia. Meyers later discovered that the best results were obtained by transventricular excision of the internal segment of the globus pallidus (GPi) or interruption of the pallidothalamic outflow at the level of the ansa lenticularis. In 1951, Cooper, while attempting to perform a pedunculotomy through a subtemporal approach, inadvertently injured the anterior choroidal artery, which had to be ligated.[13] Cooper terminated the surgery without cutting the peduncle and noted with some surprise that the patient's contralateral tremor and rigidity were relieved. Cooper subsequently performed ligation of the anterior choroidal artery with considerable success in over 50 patients. Knowing that the anterior choroidal artery irrigates, among other structures, the medial segment of the pallidum, coupled with the results of Cooper's operation, indicated that the medial portion of the globus pallidus along with its efferent pathways played an important role in parkinsonian tremor and rigidity.

In the mid 1950s, based on a keen knowledge of the connections between the GPi and the ventral thalamus along with the observation that the efferent outflow from the GPi and the cerebellum converge in the ventral lateral (VL) nucleus of the thalamus, Hassler and Riechert[31] made the bold proposal that destruction of the VL thalamus might alleviate tremor. Therefore, in 1954,

Hassler performed the first thalamotomy in a patient with Parkinson's disease. By the late 1950s, nearly two decades after Meyers first targeted the basal ganglia, stereotactic thalamotomy had become the treatment of choice for a wide variety of movement disorders, including the tremor and rigidity of Parkinson's disease.

Since the early 1960s, the VL nucleus, and more specifically the ventral intermediate (VIM) nucleus, has been recognized as the target for lesions to control tremor.[13,14,19,36] Indeed, during the 1960s, several thousand thalamotomies were performed in patients with Parkinson's disease. Although many of these procedures were performed using the target suggested by Hassler and Riechert, several variations or modifications of the original target were developed, including thalamocapsulotomy (a lesion close to the thalamic border), subthalamotomy (a lesion in the zona incerta just below the ventral oral [VO] nucleus), and campotomy (a lesion in the fields of Forel), as well as lesions in the prelemniscal and prerubral areas.

Following the discovery of levodopa (L-DOPA) in the late 1960s, pharmacological therapy became preferred over thalamotomy for the treatment of the bradykinesia and tremor of parkinsonism. Not surprisingly, the number of stereotactic procedures performed to alleviate movement disorders fell precipitously.[23] This decline occurred despite continued evolution in stereotactic techniques and improvements in electrophysiology, such as the physiological specificity attained with the use of microelectrode recordings,[80] with an attendant improvement in clinical outcome.

Clinical experience over the last 25 years has shown that the effectiveness of L-DOPA wanes within 2-5 years in >50% of patients, and many, if not most, patients return to the point of disability present prior to therapy within 7 years. Due to the short half-life of L-DOPA, dramatic "on"-"off" cycles sometimes dominate the patient's daily life. There are also associated diurnal variations in performance, involuntary movements, and dementia, constituting the "levodopa syndrome."[3,4,15,17,49,52,54,65,69,76] Consequently, the past decade has witnessed a renaissance in the surgical treatment of movement disorders, namely, pallidotomy, thalamotomy, and, most recently, thalamic stimulation. This renewed interest in surgery has been prompted by the growing realization of the limitations of drug therapy for Parkinson's disease and other conditions, the interest in transplantation from both autogenous and fetal tissue sources, improvements in neuroimaging capabilities, enhanced stereotactic surgical techniques, and innovative therapies such as thalamic stimulation for control of abnormal movements. This chapter explores the role of thalamotomy in the treatment of movement disorders, indications for the procedure, patient selection, current methodology, surgical morbidity, and expected postsurgical functional outcome.

Semiology of Movement Disorders

A detailed discussion of the various movement disorders is beyond the scope of this chapter (see Chapter 1, "Classification of Movement Disorders"). However, a brief review of the various movement disorders is germane to the discussion of thalamotomy, because many different conditions can potentially be effectively managed with this procedure. In general, there are seven categories of movement disorders for which surgical management may be a consideration: 1) tremor; 2) dystonia/dyskinesia; 3) spasticity; 4) chorea/ athetosis; 5) hemiballismus; 6) myoclonus; and 7) hemifacial spasm.

Tremor is by far the most common movement disorder. By definition, tremor consists of an "involuntary rhythmic oscillation within one plane around a joint due to alternate contraction and relaxation of antagonist groups of muscles." There are fundamentally three types of tremor: 1) resting (e.g., parkinsonian); 2) postural (essential); and 3) kinetic or intention tremor (e.g., from multiple sclerosis, or post-traumatic). (Many neurologists prefer the term "kinetic" over "intention" tremor because the tremor is involuntary and not intentional.) It is important to realize that many patients may display more than one type of tremor. For example, although parkinsonian tremor is primarily present at rest, some patients display postural and/or kinetic components. Because of the variability in clinical presentation of patients with tremor, it is essential that neurosurgeons involved in performing surgery on these patients work closely with a neurologist who has a special interest and expertise in this field. Interestingly, most types of tremor are benefited by VL thalamotomy, to a greater or lesser extent, despite the obvious differences in etiology and pathophysiology.

Dystonia is a general term that indicates an alteration in motor tone characterized by co-contraction or simultaneous contraction of antagonistic muscle groups. The posture can be long-lasting, and may be superimposed on normal movements. The most common dystonia is torticollis, which involves the neck and shoulders. Another example of dystonia that can occasionally be successfully treated with thalamotomy is dystonia musculorum deformans. Dyskinesia is another general term that indicates impairment of motor control characterized by irregular involuntary movements. There are several types of dyskinesia for which thalamotomy may be beneficial. Parkinson's patients often develop levodopa-induced dyskinesias during on periods, which can be as disabling as rigidity and bradykinesia. Also, tardive dyskinesia associated with the use of psychotropic medications may occasionally respond to thalamotomy. Although dyskinesias have been treated with thalamotomy, pallidotomy is currently the preferred surgical procedure for abolition of these movements.

Hemiballistic movements are "gross, violent, ceaseless (while awake) flinging movements particularly of the proximal musculature of the upper extremities."[67] Choreic movements are characterized by sudden, irregular fast jerks, typically occurring in a restricted region of the body. Athetosis is recognized by slower, more writhing tonic movements, which have a somewhat faster time course than dystonic postures. It is interesting that the involuntary movements of Huntington's chorea may sometimes respond to thalamotomy. In fact, the first patient treated for a movement disorder using stereotactic surgery had Huntington's disease.

Rigidity is an "exaggeration of tonic stretch reflexes." It can be seen in parkinsonism, cerebral palsy, and forms of dystonia. Hypokinesia is a restriction of voluntary movement, and bradykinesia is extreme slowness of voluntary movement, sometimes to the point of virtual immobility or freezing. Bradykinesia and tremor are quantitatively assessed by the Hoehn and Yahr scale (see Table 2 in Chapter 10, "Pallidotomy: Clinical Results"),[33] and tremor can be scored with a similar instrument developed by Fahn et al.[21] This chapter is primarily directed at the use of thalamotomy for the management of medically refractory tremor.

Thalamic Anatomy and Pathophysiology

Because this chapter focuses on the use of thalamotomy, a review of the pertinent thalamic anatomy is in order. Thalamic anatomy is classified using two different terminologies, the Hassler scheme and the Anglo-American terminology (Figure 1). Hassler subdivided the VL nucleus into the more rostral VO and the VIM nuclei. The VO was further divided into anterior (VOA) and posterior (VOP) portions. The VOP, VOA, and VIM nuclei correspond to the VL nucleus in the Anglo-American terminology, while the ventral caudal (VC) or the main somatosensory nucleus corresponds to the ventral posteromedial and ventral posterolateral nuclei. The Hassler terminology will be utilized throughout the remainder of this discussion.

Hassler noted that the VOA received the pallidal outflow, while the cerebellar efferents projected to the VOP. Furthermore, lesions in the VOA appeared to be more effective for rigidity, while destruction of the VOP more effectively treated tremor. The currently preferred target for tremor, namely, the VIM, lies immediately rostral to the VC and caudal to the VOP. Histologically, the VIM is recognizable by its sparsely scattered, large (30-50 μm), dark-staining neurons. The VIM is structurally quite distinct from the VOP and VOA, which contain smaller, more densely-packed neurons. In contrast, the border between the VIM and VC is less distinct. The VIM is approximately 10 mm in lateral and superoinferior dimensions, 3-4 mm in anteroposterior (AP) thickness, and the long axis is inclined 20° anteriorly.[60] This three-dimensional configuration is important to keep in mind when planning a trajectory for VIM thalamotomy, as well as in lesion generation.

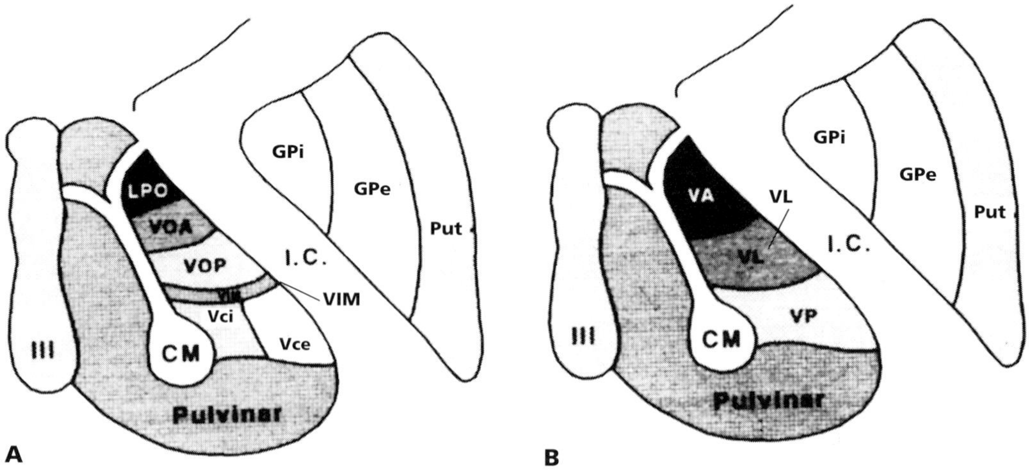

Figure 1: Terminology of the thalamic nuclei. **A)** Hassler classification system. **B)** Anglo-American classification system. LPO = lateral polaris; VOA = ventral oral anterior; VOP = ventral oral posterior; VIM = ventral intermediate; Vci = ventral caudal internal; Vce = ventral caudal external; CM = centrum medianum; VA = ventral anterior; VL = ventral lateral; VP = ventral posterior; GPi = internal segment of the globus pallidus; GPe = external segment of the globus pallidus; Put = putamen; I.C. = intercommissural region; III = third ventricle.

Our understanding of the physiology of motor control continues to evolve; however, a current concept of the functional connectivity with the basal ganglia-thalamocortical "motor loop," as proposed by Bergman and colleagues,[6] is reviewed in Chapter 4, "Pathophysiology of Movement Disorders of Basal Ganglia Origin."

A second pathway that converges on the VL nucleus may explain the rather nonspecific efficacy of lesions in the VL (VIM) nucleus for the alleviation of tremor of many etiologies.[30] Fibers from the contralateral cerebellum traverse the brachium conjunctivum and the thalamic peduncle to reach the posterolateral VL (VOP and VIM) (Figure 2). Cellular activity that is highly correlated with the frequency of parkinsonian tremor ("tremor cells") can be recorded from within the VIM,[47,48] which implies that oscillating excitation from the cerebellar pathway may be responsible for clinical tremor. Lesions placed posteriorly in the VL (VIM) would therefore be expected to abolish tremor, whereas more anterior (VOA) lesions would reduce bradykinesia and rigidity. In fact, this expectation has been borne out in several series.[63,73] Larger lesions in the VL or extension of the lesions into the fields of Forel, which contain fibers from the cerebellum and GPi, would alleviate both tremor and bradykinesia. Ojemann and Ward[63] have discussed the "area of successful lesions" with the locations highly clustered around the VL. The variability of reported outcome after thalamotomy, particularly in those patients for whom hypokinesia is a prominent symptom, may be a reflection of the degree to which these additional, more anterior or subthalamic targets are exploited.

In patients with predominant tremor, a number of groups have reported hyperactive cellular activity in the VL thalamus. In one report by Ohye et al,[61] extracellular recordings were made from the VIM nucleus under local anesthesia in cases with tremor mainly due to Parkinson's disease and essential tremor. The VIM was identified tentatively by characteristic high background activity which contrasted to that found in its more quiescent rostral part and by superimposed large-amplitude, spontaneously active units. In this high-activity zone, approximately one of every five recorded units responded to natural stimulation applied to contralateral body parts. Among them, approximately 90% responded to a passive or active movement of a joint. Several lines of evidence suggested that

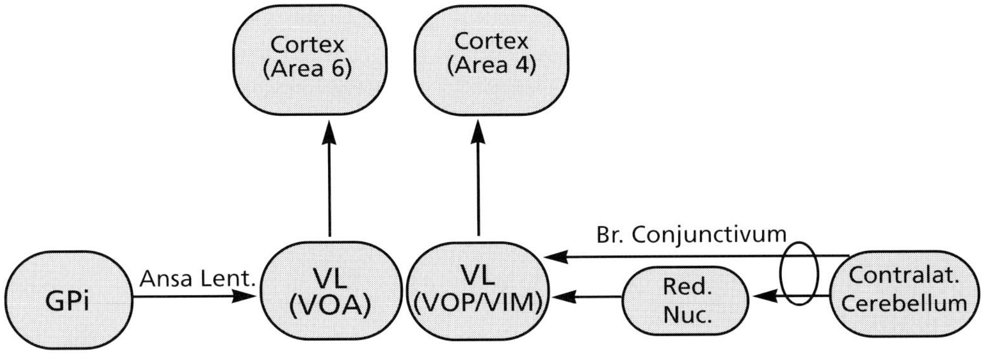

Figure 2: Schematic diagram illustrating cerebellar projections to the VL thalamus. The contralateral cerebellar outflow (primarily from the dentate nucleus) traverses the superior cerebellar peduncle and projects directly as well as indirectly (via the red nucleus) to the VOP and VIM subnuclei of the motor thalamus. These nuclei, in turn, project chiefly to the primary motor cortex (area 4). The more anterior portion of the VL, namely the VOA, receives the pallidofugal output via the ansa lenticularis and projects to the premotor area (area 6). Br. = brachium; Lent. = lenticularis; Nuc. = nucleus.

probably muscle receptors were responsible. The remainder of the units (approximately 10%) responded to light touch applied to the contralateral skin surface. Convergent responses between kinesthetic and tactile units were never encountered. Kinesthetic and tactile neurons were also geographically separated. Neurons with sensory responses were clustered mostly within the confines of the VIM, probably extending caudally to the ventrocaudalis externus anterior of Hassler. Evidence for a somatotopic representation in the VIM nucleus was obtained. Electrical stimulation of the appropriate peripheral nerve produced responses of the same thalamic unit(s) that responded to natural stimulation. These investigators ultimately concluded that the VIM receives kinesthetic afferent input from contralateral body parts (mainly from the muscle receptor) and may be concerned with muscle sensation. This may provide further evidence as to how a small, selective coagulation of the physiologically identified VIM has such a constant effect on several different kinds of tremor.

Investigations into the pathophysiology of other movement disorders have supplemented our understanding of movement disorders. For example, two reported cases with hemichorea and levodopa-induced dyskinesia were successfully treated with VIM-VOP thalamotomy.[41] In patients with hemichorea, hyperactive cellular discharges with irregular bursts of activity were recorded in the VOP and VIM, synchronous with the choreiform movements. Choreic movement was abolished by VIM-VOP thalamotomy, mainly affecting the VOP after physiological identification of the VIM. Thus, phasic hyperactivity in some VIM cell populations may be responsible for abnormal movements in addition to tremor. In patients with hemidystonia, the activity of thalamic single units was correlated with the electromyography (EMG) signal by spectral methods. Results of this analysis indicated that a group of thalamic cells shows a concentration of activity, occurring at the same frequency as the EMG activity during dystonia. The activity of these cells may be involved in the generation of dystonic movements.[48]

Cerebral blood flow (CBF) measurements have been used to quantitate cerebral metabolic activity in patients with parkinsonism and other movement disorders. Positron emission tomography (PET) measurements of CBF and the cerebral metabolic rate of oxygen ($CMRO_2$) may be lower in the parietal lobe contralateral to the tremor preoperatively when compared to the normal side. These same regions can show increased CBF and $CMRO_2$ indices following thalamotomy.[39] In addition, neuropsychological impairment that frequently follows unilateral thalamic lesions may be reflected in a depression of synaptic activity in both the overlying and the contralateral cerebral cortices, as measured by PET oxygen consumption and glucose utilization studies.[5]

Indications for Thalamotomy and Patient Selection

VIM thalamotomy is an effective treatment for medically refractory tremor and levodopa-induced dyskinesias. Palliative effects on rigidity and bradykinesia are much less predictable. The best candidates are those patients with tremor-dominant Parkinson's disease and essential tremor, although patients with hyperkinetic movement disorders following head trauma or stroke (tremor, dystonia, hemiballismus) may benefit, as can those with tremor from multiple sclerosis or choreoathetosis due to cerebral palsy (Table 1). These indications will be presented in some detail using Parkinson's disease as a model.

TABLE 1

Movement Disorders for Which Thalamotomy May Be Effective

Tremor-dominant Parkinson's disease, especially unilateral
Essential or familial tremor
Cerebellar (intention) tremor
Multiple sclerosis
Wilson's disease
Rubral tremor
Posttraumatic tremor
Post-stroke tremor
Hemiballismus
Choreoathetosis and cerebral palsy
Dystonia
Spasmodic torticollis

Parkinson's Disease

In Parkinson's disease, consideration for unilateral VIM thalamotomy should include those patients with one or more of the criteria[59,60] listed in Table 2.

TABLE 2

Patient Selection Criteria for Thalamotomy in the Treatment of Parkinson's Disease

Tremor-dominant cases
Unilateral Parkinson's disease (juvenile, idiopathic, and postencephalitic)
Cases with marked asymmetry in motor symptoms
Levodopa-induced dyskinesias
Refractory to medical therapy
Intolerant of medical therapy (i.e., nausea/vomiting)
Expected improvement in quality of life
Lack of significant cognitive dysfunction

In the past, patients with bilateral tremor who had a good result from the first operation were often selected for a contralateral procedure. However, as a result of the significant morbidity associated with bilateral thalamic lesions, bilateral thalamotomy has largely been abandoned in favor of thalamic stimulation.

Atypical syndromes with parkinsonian features not uncommonly may be confused with Parkinson's disease. This is significant, because the prognosis for improvement with VIM thalamotomy is much poorer in these cases. Parkinson's disease should not be confused with disorders such as striatonigral degeneration, olivopontocerebellar degeneration, Shy-Drager syndrome, progressive supranuclear palsy, parkinsonism-dementia complex, presenile dementia associated with parkinsonism, toxic or drug-induced disorders, Creutzfeldt-Jakob disease, or amyotrophic lateral sclerosis associated with parkinsonism.[55]

Essential Tremor

Next to Parkinson's disease, essential or familial tremor is the diagnosis most tractable to surgical therapy using VIM thalamotomy. Procedures are most often performed unilaterally, targeting the thalamus contralateral to the most severely affected side. Patients who obtain a good result can then be considered for contralateral VIM stimulation 6 months following the initial procedure. With long-term follow-up, the majority of patients enjoy continued significant amelioration of their tremor and disability.[25,26]

Interestingly, voice tremor can be abolished or greatly alleviated in almost three quarters of patients.

Intention Tremor

Intention tremor is volitional (i.e., associated with motion) but may be postural, is usually bilateral, and the etiology is variable. Disorders or lesions that affect the motor control loop from cerebellum to cortex all have the potential to produce tremor. The cause may be postencephalitic syndrome, posttraumatic, or due to abnormalities of the cerebellum or its efferent tracts (dentate nucleus, brachium conjunctivum), multiple sclerosis, or Wilson's disease. Intention tremor responds well to thalamotomy, particularly in the posterior VL (VOP and VIM). Some authors have reported results in this subset of patients to be comparable to those in patients with parkinsonian or essential tremor. Short-term improvement in tremor and disability has been reported in 85%-93% of patients, with sustained improvement reported in about 72%-82%.[13,27,44] Although the authors concur that thalamotomy can be beneficial in this group of patients, the authors' experience would suggest that the results of thalamotomy for patients in this subgroup are somewhat less favorable and that thalamotomy may be associated with a higher morbidity in these patients (see below).

Dystonia

Dystonia is a "disturbance in the attitude or posture of a segment of or of the entire body."[63] The posture is relatively long-lasting, i.e., many minutes, or occasionally days. Common etiologies include dystonia musculorum deformans (DMD), brain injury, degenerative diseases, cerebrovascular disease, encephalitis, meningitis, basal ganglion gliomas, and arteriovenous malformations in the putamen. Stereotactic thalamotomy is particularly useful in contralateral hemidystonia. The risk of adverse effects is less than with bilateral thalamotomy, which may need to be employed when generalized dystonia is severely disabling and not responsive to pharmacotherapy.[20]

DMD is probably the most commonly encountered syndrome with dystonia as its chief symptom. DMD is familial, being transferred as an autosomal dominant trait with variable penetrance. Clinical progression of this disorder usually arrests by age 35 years, so age should be a criterion for patient selection. Between 25% and 70% of patients are improved by the procedure.[2,12,63] In this group with likely more diffuse disease, post-thalamotomy dysphonia occurs in as many as 18%-33% of cases.[63]

Tasker's group[81,95] has reported the results of VL thalamotomy in secondary dystonia and in both typical and atypical DMD. They found that thalamotomy resulted in a 25%-50% long-term improvement in dystonia and limb function in roughly one quarter of the patients, and better than 50% improvement in about one third. Midline features responded poorly, and manual dexterity was little changed in secondary cases because of underlying paralysis, but improved 38% in cases of DMD. Involvement of the neck and trunk or of three to four limbs, or progressive disability predicted a poorer result. Phasic, tonic, familial, and nonfamilial dystonia responded equally well and age at surgery made no difference. Morbidity was significant, with a 27% incidence of complications (including one postoperative death) in the cases with secondary dystonia, and a 21% overall morbidity rate in cases of typical or atypical DMD. The target areas of thalamotomy were the VIM and VOP nuclei.

Spasmodic Torticollis

Spasmodic torticollis is a regional dystonia characterized by an abnormality of posture affecting the head and neck. There is a predominantly dystonic quality to the movement, with occasional superimposed athetotic or myoclonic jerking. The disorder may occur with other disorders, such as DMD, choreoathetosis, Huntington's chorea, and occasionally parkinsonism. Although in the past it has been suggested to be largely a psychiatric condition, prevailing opinion is that it is neurological in origin and that it is part of the spectrum of other dystonias.

VL thalamotomy has been used for the treatment of spasmodic torticollis, but usually bilateral lesions are required. Good results have been reported in 60%-80% of patients.[2,13,57] Intraoperative stimulation at the target site may produce dystonia at a distinctly unusual low threshold from this area. Furthermore, stimulation in the fields of Forel may also provoke torticollis with sternocleidomastoid contraction.[70]

A variety of targets have been tried: the medial VL nucleus by Cooper,[13] the zona incerta by Mundinger et al,[57] and the lateral VL by Bertrand.[7] The target for the latter series was 6/10 intercommissural (IC) line posterior to the anterior commissure (AC)—about 10.5 mm anterior to the posterior commissure (PC), 1/10 the IC distance superior (2.5 mm), and 5/10 lateral (13 mm). Although Bertrand was once a proponent of thalamotomy for this disorder, his group has since concluded that torticollis is a highly localized dystonia and that VL thalamotomy should therefore be superseded by selective peripheral denervation (see Chapter 18, "Surgical Treatment of Spasmodic Torticollis: Selective Peripheral Denervation Revisited").[8] The results of his and other variations on a denervating procedure have been impressive and currently these operations dominate the surgical treatment of torticollis.

Hemiballismus

Hemiballismus is an uncommon movement disorder frequently related to injury in the region of the subthalamic nucleus. VL thalamotomy is probably the surgical procedure of choice in medically intractable cases. Fifty percent of cases can be expected to improve.[13,57] Posttraumatic hemiballismus may also respond to VIM thalamotomy.[50]

Choreoathetosis and Cerebral Palsy

This is probably one of the most controversial indications for thalamotomy, because results have been highly variable. Narabayashi and Kubota[58] have seen improvement in 78% of patients with cerebral palsy. The improvement was mainly in facial grimacing, leg scissoring, foot inversion, thumb abduction, and shoulder and rectus muscle spasm. Lesions to treat cerebral palsy have been placed anteriorly in the VL or in the fields of Forel.[58] In contrast, Spiegel et al[77] noted no improvement in athetosis with lesions in the fields of Forel. Mundinger et al[57] noted 18% marked improvement and 32% modest improvement in choreoathetosis. Other authors have reported little improvement in choreoathetosis but better results in choreic and dystonic movements.[13,45,91]

Postischemic Movement Disorders

Only small numbers of patients have been reported who underwent thalamotomy for movement disorders that occurred as a result of ischemia. Hyperkinetic movement disorders, such as chorea, dystonia, and tremor, which may occur after aneurysm clipping, removal of intracerebral hematoma, or resection of extra-axial tumors, can be successfully treated with VL thalamotomy.[79] Postural tremors after a cerebrovascular accident may also respond to VL thalamotomy.[93]

Posttraumatic Movement Disorders

Posttraumatic movement disorders may be alleviated by thalamotomy. Following severe closed head injury, an infrequently encountered posttraumatic entity of dystonic hemiplegia or hemiparesis, which may be alleviated by thalamotomy, can occur but does not have a specific neuroanatomical basis. Intention tremor following severe head injuries, rarely associated with hydrocephalus and without other significant cerebellar findings, can develop as a dysfunction of the cerebellofugal outflow system (see Figure 2). Bilateral VL thalamotomies staged 4-6 months apart have been successful in alleviating severe and medically intractable intention tremor,[67] with reported success in up to 86% of patients,[53] and in hemiballismus.[50] In general, caution should be exercised in the use of thalamotomy for posttraumatic tremor. When head injury is diffuse, or at least bilateral, the usual redundancy of the motor control system may be compromised. Even unilateral lesions can result in devastating neurological compromise, predominantly hypophonia and dysphagia.

PROCEDURE FOR VIM THALAMOTOMY

The technique of VIM thalamotomy, including neuroimaging, described below is the one that has been developed and refined by the senior author (KJB).

Stereotactic Frame Application

Patients are met in the holding area of the recovery room early on the morning of surgery. An intravenous line is placed in the normal or less severely affected arm and patients are given analgesics (fentanyl) and sedation (midazolam) sparingly, on an as-needed basis, because often age, varying levels of dementia, fatigue, a long procedure, and the cumulative effects of medications can lead to a rapidly deteriorating level of cooperation and/or reliability toward the later and more crucial aspects of the operation. Maintenance of good rapport and verbal contact of both the surgeon and the anesthesiologist with the patient is preferable to escalating doses of medications.

Application of the frame is most easily accomplished by two persons to ensure that it is applied properly. Indeed, proper application of the frame is one of the most, if not the most, critical part of the entire procedure. The authors employ the Leksell G frame (Elekta, Atlanta, Georgia), although the procedure can be performed using any type of frame. Numerous stereotactic frame systems are available, most of which are both computed tomography (CT)- and magnetic resonance imaging (MRI)-compatible. However, the authors have found that a system which can be used for CT, MRI, and radiographic localization for functional stereotactic surgery, and also for the more common tumor biopsies, stereotactic surgical planning, and radiosurgery is the most usable and cost-effective. A review of the currently available stereotactic frames can be found in the recent publication by Gildenberg and Tasker.[24]

Once the patient has been adequately sedated, he or she is placed upright for application of the frame. The key to correct placement is to apply the base of the frame parallel to the orbitomeatal plane. Foam padding is used in the external auditory canal to alleviate the discomfort of placing the earbars during frame alignment and attachment. A local anesthetic mixture consisting of equal parts 0.5% marcaine and 1% lidocaine with epinephrine (1:200,000) is utilized to infiltrate the scalp at the pin insertion sites. Following application of the frame, the patient is transported to radiology for imaging and target selection.

Neuroimaging and Target Selection

Over the past decade, CT and MRI localization for stereotactic surgery has become standard methodology. It is uncommon for ventriculography to be used, and when it is, it is usually to validate the accuracy of a new system in comparison to a "gold standard,"[46] or a redundant method of target localization.[38]

Stereotactic Atlases

The practitioner of functional stereotactic surgery should be very familiar with one or more of the classic stereotactic atlases, such as the Schaltenbrand and Bailey,[74] Schaltenbrand and Wahren,[75] and Van Buren and Borke.[90] A number of these have now been integrated into computer-generated graphical planning systems (see below and Chapter 16, "Interactive Computer-Assisted Image-Guided Technology as an Adjuvant to Neurosurgery for Movement Disorders"), but reference to the original is a desirable redundancy and may be required as a back-up approach, in the event of computer or software failure. Some of the older atlases are out of print, but older editions can be restored and preserved as a tangible link to the beginnings of stereotactic surgery.

Ventriculography

Although ventriculography is now rarely used, it was the forerunner of CT and MRI applications in functional stereotaxy and remains an important method for target localization, if merely from a historical perspective. Intraoperative radiography is required, with precise align-

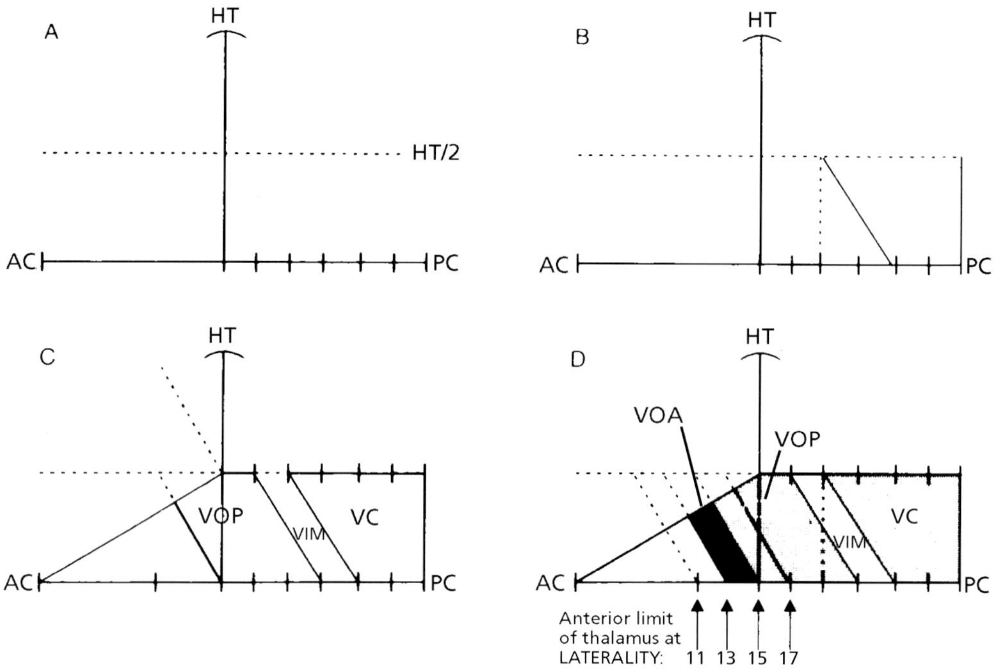

Figure 3: Guiot method for localization of the VIM using ventriculography.[80] See text for explanatory details.

ment of the biplanar x-ray tubes. Dedicated operating rooms with permanent fixed systems with long projection baselines are desirable, but less commonly available than was the case two to three decades ago. Currently, portable x-ray machines often must be used, requiring laborious calibration prior to each case. Still, in operating rooms that can support radiography, ventriculography can offer an independent method of corroborating target localization and following the progress of the electrode trajectory and location.

One advantage of the preoperative CT scan or MRI is that the appropriate frontal horn can be designated as an alternate stereotactic target. A ventriculostomy is then performed stereotactically, simplifying the procedure significantly in patients with small ventricles. Lacking preoperative imaging, a third ventriculostomy is performed with a standard technique. Once the ventricle is cannulated, radiocontrast (and if necessary air) is injected to determine the location of the anterior and posterior commissures.

The VIM nucleus can be localized using ventriculography and the Guiot method (Figure 3).[80] The lateral x-ray is used to identify the AC and PC, and the IC line is then constructed. From the midpoint of the IC line, a perpendicular line is extended to the floor of the lateral ventricle (the "thalamic height" [HT]). The midpoint of this line is marked, and a line paralleling and of equal length to the IC line is drawn (HT/2) (Figure 3A). Both the IC and HT/2 lines are divided into twelfths beginning at the PC, and then a line is drawn from 2/12 IC to 4/12 HT/2 (Figure 3B), and a second line is drawn from 3/12 IC to 5/12 HT/2 (Figure 3C). The quadrilateral space defined by these lines and the IC and HT/2 lines predicts the AP (y axis) and superior-inferior (z axis) dimensions of the VIM (Figure 3D). The lateral location (x axis) is derived from the AP x-rays.

Computed Tomography and Magnetic Resonance Imaging

Axial CT has proven reliable for image-based stereotaxis,[64,70,83] and intraoperative CT has been successful in monitoring the progress of elec-

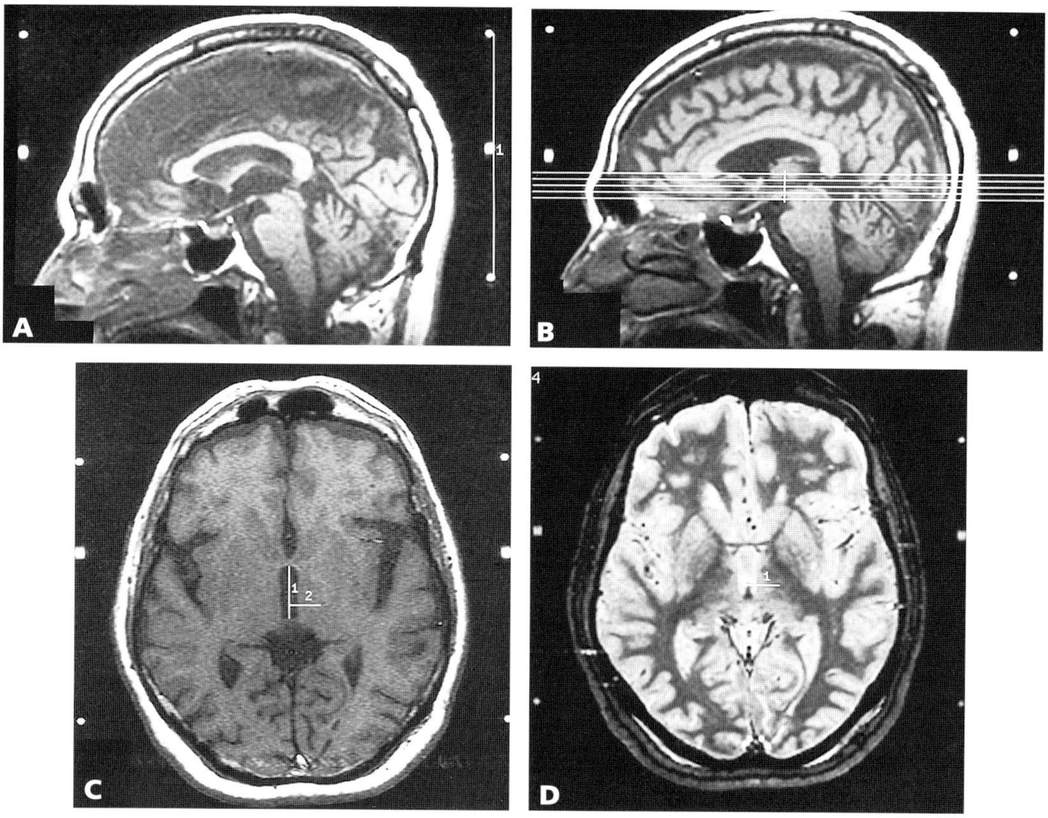

Figure 4: Target localization using MRI. **A)** Sagittal T1-weighted localizer image for determining the AC, PC, and AC-PC line in the sagittal plane. **B)** Sagittal T1-weighted image showing position of the axial slices above and below, as well as parallel to, the AC-PC line. **C)** Axial T-weighted image demonstrating the AC-PC line (labeled 1). The AP target coordinate has been calculated at 25% of the AC-PC line anterior to the PC. From this point, the lateral target coordinate (labeled 2) has been drawn. **D)** T2-weighted, fast spin echo inversion recovery (FSE IR) sequence showing the lateral target coordinate (labeled 1) in relation to the internal capsule.

trode localization.[88] CT localization avoids the potential for magnetic distortion of spatial localization, but lacks the increased spatial resolution of MRI.

Although high-field (1.5-T) MRI localization has been successfully implemented for stereotactic functional procedures,[38,51] questions still remain as to reliability and accuracy.[11,28,73] Essentially all investigators believe that physiological confirmation of the lesion site is imperative. Currently, the authors use MRI as the sole imaging technique in all patients undergoing stereotactic thalamotomy or, for that matter, pallidotomy. For patients in whom MRI is contraindicated (i.e., patients with pacemakers, cochlear implants, aneurysm clips, etc.), CT is used as an alternative imaging modality.

The initial MRI sequence consists of a sagittal T1-weighted image on which the initial identification of the AC and PC is made and the AC-PC line constructed (Figure 4A). Axial slices 3 mm thick are then calculated parallel to and on either side of the AC-PC line (Figure 4B) and then the axial images are obtained. Ideally, if the stereotactic frame has been applied correctly, there will be an axial slice on which both the AC and PC are clearly seen (Figure 4C). This image is then chosen for selecting the target. In the event that the AC and PC cannot be identified on the same image, one should choose the image on which the PC is best visualized, because the target for VIM thalamotomy is much closer to the PC than to the AC. However, if the discrepancy is extremely large, one should think about removing and reapplying the frame.

Once the appropriate axial image has been

selected, the cursor on the MRI console is employed to mark both the AC and PC and construct the AC-PC line and calculate its length. A point is then calculated at a distance of 25% of the AC-PC line anterior to the PC (or posterior to the midcommissural point), which defines the AP target coordinate (Figure 4C). From this point, a second line is constructed 13-15 mm lateral to the midline to obtain the lateral target coordinate (Figure 4D). In patients with significant atrophy in whom the width of the third ventricle exceeds 6 mm, the lateral coordinate is calculated at a distance of 11 mm from the lateral aspect of the third ventricular wall. For VIM thalamotomy, the vertical coordinate is taken to be on the IC plane. While the target is being selected from the T1-weighted axial images, additional T2-weighted axial and coronal images are obtained. The purpose of these images is to better define the relationship of the target to the internal capsule, which is better visualized using T2-weighted sequences (Figure 4D). The imaging protocol developed by the senior author (KJB) is outlined in Table 3.

The MRI coordinates (anterior-posterior, right-left, superior-inferior) are then mathematically transformed into Leksell frame coordinates, adjusting for the center of the frame using simple arithmetic calculations. These coordinates are independently verified using a computer digitizing tablet and the final Leksell coordinates are obtained. Alternatively, the Leksell SurgiPlan computer work station (Elekta) can be used to directly obtain the frame coordinates from the MRI images. Following completion of the MRI, the patient is then transported to the operating room.

The measurements described above are those used by the authors and have provided reliable results. However, other thalamic targets exist and they generally fall into two groups based on whether one is attempting to treat tremor or rigidity. Although rigidity and bradykinesia theoretically can also be controlled by thalamotomy, the current preference is to perform pallidotomy for these symptoms.[63]

There is strong evidence that lesions in the VIM or VOP, concentrated at the 13.5-15.0 sagittal plane, effectively abolish tremor regardless of etiology.[60,85] Based on the somatotopic organization of the VIM, targeting for upper extremity tremor places a lesion in the VIM just rostral to the junction of the "labial commissure" and the thumb area in the VC; lesions for lower extremity tremor are directed more laterally, at the boundary of the VIM and the internal capsule (Figure 5).

Other "tremor targets" have been described that involve more of the VOP than the VIM. Goodman and Rea[28] place their lesions 5-9 mm anterior to the PC, 13-15 mm lateral to the midline, and on the IC plane about at the junction of the VOP and VIM. Taren et al,[80] Kelly et al,[42] and Ohye[60] all place their lesions in a similar location, slightly more anteriorly at the VOA/VOP interface. Coordinates for this target are 2-3 mm posterior to the midpoint of the IC line,

TABLE 3

Magnetic Resonance Imaging Protocol for Stereotactic Thalamotomy*

Sagittal localizer (T1-weighted)
  Select AC-PC plane

Axial oblique images (3 mm) parallel to AC-PC line (T1-weighted)
  Identify AC and PC on same image
  Construct AC-PC line
  AP coordinate: 25% of AC-PC line posterior to midcommissural point
  Lateral coordinate: 13-17 mm from midline
  Vertical coordinate: on IC plane

Axial oblique images (FSE IR, T1-weighted, 200 msec): same plane as previous series

Coronal images (FSE IR, T1-weighted, 200 msec): orthogonal to frame

Details for the FSE IR series
  TI = 200 msec
  TE = min. full msec
  TR = 3000 msec
  COILTYPE = quad head
  AUTOCF = water
  IMAGINGMODE = 2-dimensional
  PULSESEQ = SE
  IMAGEOPT = fast IR
  FOV (field of view) = 28 cm
  SLICETHICKNESS = 3 mm
  INTERSCANSPACE = 0 mm
  ACQMATRIX = 256 × 256
  NEX = 2
  BANDWIDTH = 32 kHz

*Imaging performed on a GE Signa (version 5.3) 1.5-T scanner (General Electric, Milwaukee, Wisconsin).

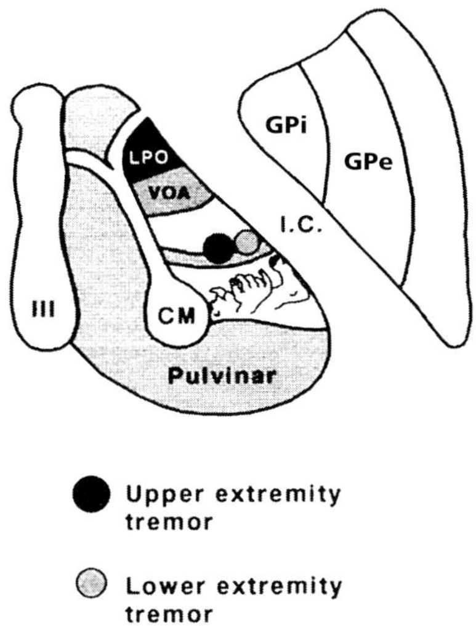

Figure 5: Schematic diagram of the thalamus, internal capsule, and pallidum demonstrating the somatotopic organization of the thalamic nuclei. Lesions to treat upper extremity tremor are ideally placed just rostral to the junction of the "labial commissure" and thumb representation in the VC. Lesions for lower extremity tremor need to be directed more laterally, near the boundary of the VIM with the internal capsule. See Figure 1 legend for abbreviations. (Adapted from Kelly PJ: Principles of stereotactic surgery, in Youmans JR (ed): *Neurological Surgery. A Comprehensive Reference Guide to the Diagnosis and Management of Neurosurgical Problems.* 3rd ed. Philadelphia, Pa: WB Saunders, 1990, pp 4183-4226, with permission.)

1-3 mm above the IC plane, and 12-14.5 mm lateral to the midline. Broggi et al[9] prefer a combination of the VOA, VOP, and zona incerta. These intermediate targets may produce a lesion that involves both the VIM and the VOA/VOP.

The "rigidity target" is more anterior still, well into the VOA. The coordinates are 1.5 mm anterior to the midpoint of the IC line, 12.5 mm lateral to the midline or 10 mm lateral to the wall of the third ventricle (i.e., 13 mm lateral if the third ventricle is 6 mm), and 2.5 mm above the IC plane.[80]

The visualization of the anterior and posterior commissures, and of differentiating separate basal ganglia, thalamus and internal capsule, and other fiber tracts by special sequences, such as proton density imaging, is exciting.[40] In some settings, good correlation has been found between visualization using MRI and the actual thalamic target coordinates determined by ventriculography and semi-microelectrode recording.[38] Others have suggested that each modality has its place in the armamentarium, and that CT and MRI data should be entered into a common data set that is coregistered to stereotactic frame space, for use in planning and performing the procedure.[29,88]

Computer-Assisted Techniques

Microcomputer technology has advanced to the point where it is feasible to bring computer-assisted stereotactic surgical planning into the operating room. A wide variety of systems now employ computer-resident atlases that can be warped and superimposed on the digital anatomical database of the patient's CT or MRI data. Examples include the Schaltenbrand and Bailey atlas, recommended by Hardy et al,[29] Tasker et al,[83] and Yoshida;[97] the Schaltenbrand and Wahren atlas, used by Hardy et al, Kall,[37] and Struppler and Lipinski;[78] and the Andrew and Watkins atlas, preferred by Goodman and Rea.[28]

Application of computer-resident atlases appears to give acceptable results when compared to ventriculography and microelectrode recordings in the same patient.[38,83] Not surprisingly, discrepancies between physiological and computer-generated atlas data are more likely to crop up in cases of stroke, multiple sclerosis, severe head injury, or after craniotomy.[83] Computer-assisted construction of target overlays has been used,[29,37] as have autocad (computer-assisted design) programs to plot electrode trajectories and homunculi.[82] More sophisticated computer graphic techniques can take an MRI, delineate internal landmarks, store the data, and later, by pattern recognition methods, reconstruct these invisible landmarks within the reference frame of plain intraoperative radiography.[66]

Surgical Technique

Thalamotomy is almost always performed under local anesthesia to allow for the necessary patient participation in target localization (microelectrode recordings, stimulation mapping) and to immediately observe the effects of test and final lesions. Blood pressure is carefully monitored before, during, and after the procedure and is held at normotensive levels, even if pharmacological control is necessary. Indeed, failure to strictly control blood pressure following thalamotomy can result in a disastrous thalamic hemorrhage.

The patient is placed on the operating table and the head is secured to the table using an adaptor to the Mayfield head holder. A small area is shaved in the precoronal area and prepared with an antiseptic solution. The Leksell frame coordinates are set and are always verified by a second member of the surgical team. The arc system is then attached to the head frame.

The scalp is anesthetized with local anesthetic and a stab incision is made. The beginning of the electrode trajectory is from a twist drill hole, centered from 25 to about 35 mm lateral to the midline. The authors prefer the more lateral approach, because the VIM is angled slightly laterally as well. A trajectory based on the inclination and configuration of the VIM is chosen, approximately 65°-70° to the sagittal plane and 80° in the coronal plane. Using this trajectory, the electrode should approximately pass into the VIM along the longitudinal axis. Although one can also use a burr hole, there is at least the theoretical possibility of the escape of excessive amounts of cerebrospinal fluid (CSF) during the procedure, especially in elderly patients with significant atrophy. CSF leakage may lead to small degrees of brain shift, which may alter the stereotactic target. Some surgeons get around this problem by "sealing" the subarachnoid space with tissue glue after passing the electrode. Some authors would also argue that the risk of hemorrhage from traversing a cortical vein is substantially less with a burr hole. However, in several hundred stereotactic procedures performed by the senior author (KJB) through a twist drill hole, there has not been a single case of hemorrhage.

After the twist drill hole has been made, the dura is penetrated using a smaller drill bit and a gentle oscillating motion. A cannula is then inserted, again using a gentle rapid oscillating motion, and the obturator removed. The stimulating-lesioning electrode (which has been calibrated to the target) is then placed through the cannula. Physiological corroboration of the target (described in detail below) is then performed.

Physiological Localization

Despite the power of current imaging modalities, individual anatomical variations mandate physiological confirmation of stereotactic targets. There are a number of electrophysiological techniques that can be utilized for target localization during stereotactic functional procedures. These techniques include neural noise recording, impedance monitoring, evoked potentials, macrostimulation, and microelectrode recording. Evoked potential recordings from either macroelectrodes or semi-microelectrodes can be used to localize the VIM.[78] For more discrete localization, microelectrode recordings are preferable.

Neural noise recording, using an audioamplifier and either semi-microelectrodes or true microelectrodes, is capable of detecting spontaneous neuronal activity. Electrical interrogation of various structures in the brain has shown that each possesses its own unique pattern of spontaneous activity. Thus, various structures can be identified as an electrode passes through a given trajectory. Although neural noise recording is quite helpful in locating the various regions of the globus pallidus, it is of limited utility in performing VL thalamotomy.

Electrical impedance recording can theoretically differentiate between various brain structures. Indeed, impedance recording has proven useful in procedures such as percutaneous cordotomy. Impedance recording can differentiate between large white matter tracts, nuclei, and CSF, but not between individual nuclei. Impedance recording has otherwise not proven useful for physiological localization during thalamotomy.

Somatosensory evoked potentials (SSEPs) have been utilized for physiological investigation of the thalamus. Using peripheral nerve stimulation, SSEPs can be recorded from either macro- or microelectrodes from within the VC and VIM nuclei. Alternatively, they can be recorded from scalp electrodes following thalamic stimulation. Using these methods, the origins of various components of the evoked potentials have been elucidated.[1] Although evoked potentials have come to play a critical role in the performance of many neurosurgical procedures, they have not been found to be particularly practical or beneficial during thalamotomy.

The simplest method of physiological investigation of brain structures is the use of electrical stimulation, which can be performed using either a macro- or microelectrode. Macroelectrode stimulation is safe, technically simple, quick, and inexpensive. Macrostimulation requires a minimal amount of equipment and can be performed using the same electrode that is used for lesion-making. Using macrostimulation, one can identify a wide variety of structures, as well as detect somatotopic organization. In general, the use of monophasic versus biphasic impulses and other variations in stimulation parameters have minimal influence on the induced response other than threshold.[84] Also, with some exceptions, the quality of the response is independent of the stimulation parameters. The influence of electrical stimulation on involuntary movement such as tremor is frequency-sensitive, with frequencies between 130 and 180 Hz being most effective. In the normal motor pathways, the difference between inducing a single twitch or tetanization depends on whether low- or high-frequency pulses are used. The effects elicited by sensory stimulation are most pronounced in the 10-500 Hz range. Indeed, stimulation may go undetected at very low and high rates (<5 Hz and ≥1000 Hz, respectively). If a microelectrode or semimicroelectrode is used for stimulation, the induced effects will be essentially identical to those achieved by macrostimulation. The only differences will be threshold levels and effects related to current spread.

Microelectrode recording represents the most elegant and sophisticated method currently available for physiological interrogation and mapping of brain structures. There are two techniques available for microelectrode recording—the use of semi-microelectrodes or true microelectrodes. The semi-microelectrode technique as introduced by Albe-Fessard utilizes a larger, more rugged, low-impedance semi-microelectrode that is relatively easy to handle.[42,60,61,80,96] The impedance of these electrodes measures around 100 kΩ. The typical configuration is a bipolar electrode with a 100-μm central tip and a second concentric ring electrode with an interelectrode distance of around 0.4 mm.[80] Although far simpler compared to microelectrode recording, semi-microelectrodes are limited in their ability to detect "neural noise" from groups of neurons or electroencephalographic-like "field potentials." Individual cellular action potentials cannot typically be discriminated. Its limitations notwithstanding, this is more than adequate for most routine localization applications.

Tasker and others[47,48,62,84,85,87] have championed the use of high-impedance (around 1 MΩ) true microelectrodes with a tip diameter of around 1 μm. This technique has the advantage of being able to differentiate the activity of individual neurons, and may provide more precise localization. The other advantage of microelectrodes is their ability to precisely detect somatotopy. On the other hand, the methodology is more difficult than the use of semi-microelectrodes, particularly in the electrically "hostile" environment of the operating room, and the electrodes are fragile. For investigation into the electrophysiology of movement and sensation, the technique is unsurpassed. Frequency power spectrum analysis of microelectrode or semi-microelectrode data can also yield profiles characteristic for each subcortical structure.[48,96] The relative advantages and disadvantages of the common techniques used for physiological localization during thalamotomy are summarized in Table 4.

There is considerable debate as to the necessity for microelectrode recordings in the performance of thalamotomy and, more recently, thalamic stimulation for tremor control. There are basically two schools of thought regarding physiological localization during thalamotomy. Some neurosurgeons believe that the use of microelectrodes is essential for proper physiological localization and for creating a selective lesion in the thalamus. Others, including the authors, believe that macrostimulation is adequate for physiological corroboration during thalamotomy and that microelectrode recordings, while they may be useful, are not necessary. The authors currently employ only macrostimulation for physiological localization during thalamotomy. Stimulation is performed using the same electrode utilized for making the lesion, which consists of a 2-mm exposed tip that is 1.2 mm in diameter. The power source consists of the RFG-3CF lesion generator (Radionics, Burlington, Massachusetts), which has been modified to accommodate high-frequency stimulation of up to 300 Hz. Frequently, even before performing electrical stimulation, passing the electrode to the target will

TABLE 4

COMPARISION OF VARIOUS METHODS OF ELECTROPHYSIOLOGICAL LOCALIZATION*

	Electrical Stimulation	Microelectrode Recording
Degree of safety	High	High
Cost	Low	High
Technical problems	Very low	Moderate to high
Sophistication of back-up equipment required	Low	High
Speed of exploration	Rapid	Slow
Ability to stimulate and record with same electrode	No	Yes
Durability for repeated use	High	Low to Moderate
Ability to detect somatotopy	Good	Exquisite
Variety of structures identified	High	Low
Ability to identify nearby structures	Good	None

* Modified from Tasker and Kiss.[84]

produce a "microthalamotomy" effect with some reduction of tremor. This provides early evidence that the electrode has reached the proper target. Sensory (50-Hz) and motor (2-Hz) stimulation (1 msec pulse duration, constant voltage) are performed to ensure that the electrode is not too near the VC nucleus or internal capsule, respectively. Knowing the amount of current spread with an electrode of this size and configuration, sensory or motor thresholds exceeding 0.5 V and 1.0 V, respectively, are considered acceptable so as to ensure that the lesion will not extend into either the VC or the internal capsule. If the sensory threshold is <0.5 V, the target is adjusted more anteriorly; motor thresholds of <1.0 V dictate that the target be adjusted more medially. Using this protocol, the authors have had excellent success with minimal morbidity related to inadvertent lesioning of the internal capsule or the VC. In fact, in many patients, only a single electrode trajectory is required (Figure 6). The final step in target localization involves the use of high-frequency (130-200 Hz) stimulation to produce tremor arrest. Cessation of tremor at relatively low thresholds (0.1-0.5 V) is *a priori* evidence that the electrode is situated in the proper area.

Electrophysiological Properties and Localization of the VIM

Many investigators believe that the VIM is the relay nucleus for kinesthetic sensation; the VOA and VOP receive pallidal and cerebellar input, respectively. As noted above, the border between the VIM and VOP is fairly discrete; however, the boundary that separates the VIM from the VC is indistinct. Similar to the VC, it is only within the basal two thirds of the VIM that one can identify and record from specific neurons. Microelectrode recording in the VIM typically reveals noisy, high-voltage spontaneous activity, albeit less than that observed in the VC.[84] The neurons in the VIM respond to passive joint movement or pressure on muscle bellies or other deep structures, such as tendons. The discharges may be phasic or tonic, and may be either rapidly or slowly adapting, but similar to tactile cells, kinesthetic cells do not fatigue with repetitive stimulation.

The "kinesthetic neurons" in the "high-activity" zone at the VIM target (encountered first at the anterior border of the VIM) respond to deep (not superficial) movements of the joints.[60] Kinesthetic (VIM) and tactile (VC) responses do

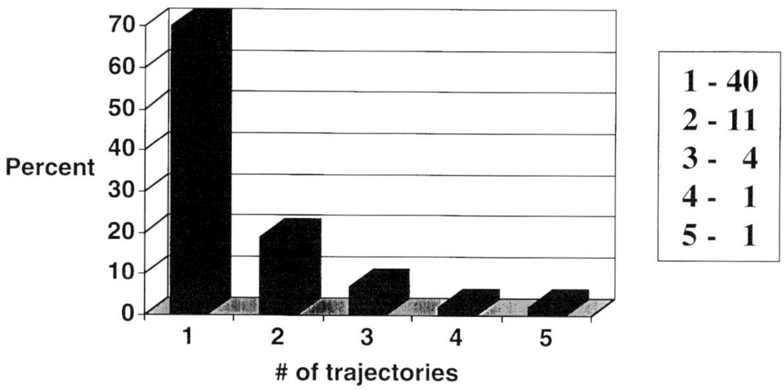

Figure 6: Number of electrode trajectories in 57 thalamotomies for medically refractory tremor.

not overlap, and the area of kinesthetic responses is always anterior to the zone responding to tactile stimuli. There is a distinct topographic orientation, with the lower limb dorsolateral, upper limb ventromedial, and face most medial.[60,80]

Numerous investigators have demonstrated that in patients with tremor, kinesthetic cells in the VIM discharge at tremor frequency and that this firing ceases when tremor is arrested (Figure 7). This suggests that this rhythmic firing simply represents an "evoked potential" in response to movement. Indeed, it does not appear that spontaneous tremor cells are the underlying cause of tremor. Tremor cells can be more readily identified in patients with Parkinson's disease than in those with tremor due to other causes. Although the reason for this is unclear, Tasker and Kiss[84] have suggested that perhaps tremor cells are more numerous in Parkinson's disease because the tremor is continuously present at rest and therefore continually activates kinesthetic cells.

The VIM can also be localized using both macro- and microstimulation. Microstimulation (60-100 Hz, 0.3-1.0 mA) in the kinesthetic area often produces an "electric shock" sensation in the contralateral homotopic region of the body. The responses are similar to those obtained with stimulation in the VC, with a few important differences. First, stimulation in the VC most commonly produces numbness or paresthesias.[60,61] Secondly, with either macro- or microstimulation, the threshold response is considerably higher than that observed with stimulation in the VC. For example, with microelectrode stimulation, thresholds in the VIM are on the order of 10-20 μA compared to as little as 2 μA in the VC.[84] Also, the projected fields are substantially larger with stimulation in the VIM, whereas they are more discreet with stimulation of the VC.

Creation of the Lesion

Once the target has been confirmed using some method of physiological localization, one is ready to create a lesion. The authors initially perform test lesions at lower temperatures (45°C) for short durations (usually 10 sec) to prevent irreversible neurological deficits. The lesion created in this fashion is reversible and any neurological dysfunction detected should prompt a reassessment of the target. Alternatively, microinjections of lidocaine can serve the same purpose.[16] Three lesions are typically made. The first is made at the target, i.e., on the level of the commissural plane. The customary lesion for patients with essential or parkinsonian tremor is made at a temperature of 70°C for 60 seconds, which produces a lesion volume of 40-60 mm^3.[3,55,86] In patients with tremor due to multiple sclerosis or trauma, a larger lesion is usually required to achieve an equivalent effect. After the first lesion is made, the patient is then examined for any evidence of neurological deficit and the effect of the lesion on the tremor. Two more lesions are then made at 2-mm intervals above the first, using identical parameters. If after three lesions have been made there is residual tremor,

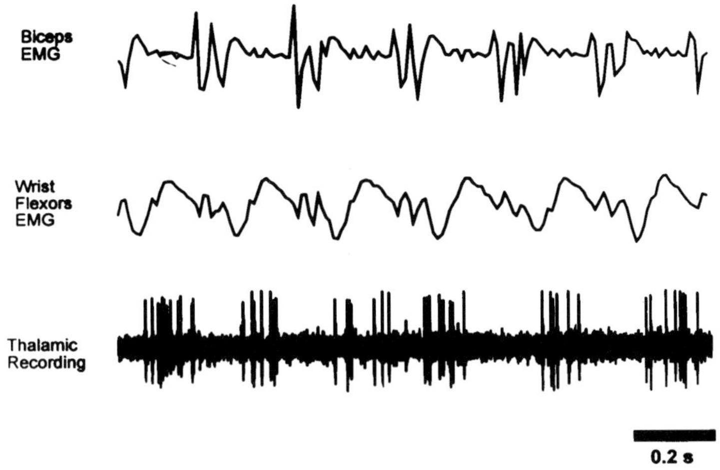

Figure 7: Tremor cells recorded from the VIM *(bottom)*. Note the correlation between the neuronal discharges from the tremor cells and the EMG. These discharges stop when the tremor ceases.

the previous lesions can be enlarged by increasing the lesioning temperature. Another option is to make a fourth lesion 2 mm below the commissural plane, which should incorporate the pallidofugal and cerebellofugal input.

After all lesions have been made, the cannula and electrode assembly are withdrawn as a unit. A single suture is all that is needed to close the stab wound in the scalp. The patient is then transported to the surgical intensive care unit and kept at rest until the following morning, maintaining strict blood pressure control. The majority of patients are discharged the following day.

Thalamotomy for Tremor: Clinical Experience

The authors have reviewed the recent experience with MRI-guided stereotactic thalamotomy for tremor at their institution. Between 1994 and 1997, 57 thalamotomies were performed in 54 patients with medically refractory tremor. There were 35 men and 19 women in this series, with an average age of 67 years (age range 20-83 years). The average duration of tremor in all patients was 16.5 years. Forty-six (81%) of the 57 procedures were performed on the left side. The initial procedure was always carried out to treat the most severely affected side. Unilateral thalamotomy was performed in 52 of the 54 patients (96%); bilateral procedures were performed in only two patients, both early in 1995. Because of the significant risks associated with bilateral lesions (discussed below), the authors no longer perform bilateral thalamotomy. The tremor was related to either Parkinson's disease (30 patients, 55.6%) or essential tremor (21 patients, 39%) in nearly 95% of patients. One patient had post-traumatic tremor and another rubral tremor. The last patient developed tremor following resection of a meningioma.

All patients underwent stereotactic thalamotomy according to the protocol described above. The only significant changes that occurred during this period involved a change in the lesioning electrode. The original electrode had a 4-mm exposed tip with a 2-mm diameter. Consequently, early in the series, because of the larger electrode size, most patients had only two lesions. After switching to the small electrode (2- to 3-mm exposed tip, 1.2-mm diameter), it was necessary to create three lesions to achieve the same result.

Outcome

The outcomes in regard to tremor relief were

excellent overall. Forty-three thalamotomies (79%) resulted in complete relief of tremor with improvements in functional capacity. Twelve (22%) resulted in nearly complete resolution of tremor and, from a functional standpoint, improvement to a significant degree. Therefore, 55 of 57 thalamotomies (97%) resulted in either complete or nearly complete tremor arrest. Two patients (4%) remained with moderate tremor. Tremor recurred at variable intervals in five patients (9%). One of these patients underwent a repeat procedure, which successfully relieved the tremor.

The authors' results, as well as those of others, indicate that thalamotomy is a highly effective procedure in treating tremor regardless of etiology, but especially in patients with parkinsonian or essential tremor.[55,84] Indeed, abolition of the tremor occurs in 94%-100% of patients with either Parkinson's disease or essential tremor.[22,32,42,60] The early prognosis for posttraumatic and post-stroke tremor is less satisfactory.[60] Improvement in contralateral extremity tremor after thalamotomy even occurs in some patients and may occasionally persist over time. It should be noted that thalamotomy is most effective in relieving appendicular tremor. Midline symptoms, such as head tremor and voice tremor, seem to respond less well and may progress relentlessly, and limit function in one quarter of the patients.[68,89,92] Specifically, Van Buren et al[89] found that in general, impairment from the midline symptoms and speech deficits exceeded any gains from the reduced tremor, and their average patient functioned less well post-thalamotomy. Therefore, before proceeding with thalamotomy, patients should be informed as to the reasonable improvements that can be expected in order to avoid disappointment due to unrealistic expectations.

It has been suggested that the effects of thalamotomy tend to wane over time. Indeed, long-term follow-up for as long as 10 years after unilateral thalamotomy indicates that about 48% of patients may return to their preoperative condition and 22%-40% continue to show improvement from their preoperative baseline.[9,55] In patients with Parkinson's disease, it is necessary to continue pharmacological therapy, as surgical treatment does not arrest general disease progression.[9]

Complications of Thalamotomy

The risks of thalamotomy are relatively small. The mortality rate is approximately 0.5%, with intracranial hemorrhage being the major source of mortality. Therefore, all patients should be carefully screened for a personal or family history of bleeding problems or coagulopathy. Aspirin, or aspirin-containing products such as nonprescription cold remedies, should be discontinued for at least 1 week prior to surgery. Patients with hypertension should be maintained under good blood pressure control, as uncontrolled hypertension is the single most important risk factor for hemorrhage following thalamotomy. The presence of significant cerebral atrophy may also place patients at increased risk of subdural hematoma from traction and tearing of bridging veins. In the authors' series of thalamotomy, there was not a single occurrence of intracranial hemorrhage. In fact, in the considerable experience of the senior author (KJB) over a period of more than 15 years, there has never been a clinically significant hemorrhagic complication from thalamotomy, or pallidotomy for that matter.

In the authors' series of 57 thalamotomies (January 1994 to April 1997), there were a total of 11 complications related to the procedure. This number includes all patients, even those with transient minor degrees of neurological dysfunction. Seven patients developed mild transient dysphasia manifested primarily by word-finding difficulty or contralateral weakness. In several patients, the weakness developed 2-3 days following surgery and was believed to be related to encroachment on the internal capsule by edema related to the lesion. Permanent complications occurred in only four patients (7.4%). Three of these complications occurred in patients whose tremor was due to a condition other than Parkinson's disease or essential tremor. The patient with rubral tremor had mild persistent upper extremity weakness following surgery. The patient with posttraumatic tremor developed a mild hemiparesis and mild dysnomia. The patient in whom tremor developed following removal of a meningioma was left with a mild expressive dysphasia and hemiparesis as well as mild dysarthria. The authors believe that these patients probably had underlying subclinical brain dysfunction, making them more susceptible to the complications of thalamotomy.

There has recently been significant debate regarding the performance of bilateral thalamotomy. Some investigators, including the authors, currently are of the opinion that bilateral thalamotomy should not be performed, although there are others who question this tenet.[80] This is especially true now that the contralateral side can be treated by deep brain stimulation. However, it is clear that much of the major morbidity of thalamotomy is related to bilateral lesions, typically from previous contralateral thalamotomy. This caveat usually applies to the "second side," in cases in which bilateral thalamotomy is necessary. However, even unilateral thalamotomy can be hazardous in other conditions that may be associated with bilateral damage, such as head injury or multiple sclerosis. The predominant complication is speech and/or language impairment, characterized by low voice volume (hypophonia), dysarthria, or dysphasia.[22] This complication can be expected in approximately 18% of patients after staged bilateral thalamotomy.[55,60] Significant dysphagia may also occur following bilateral thalamotomy. Transient confusion can be seen in 10% of patients. Other potential complications include transient central facial weakness (8%), numbness of the mouth or fingers (5%), paresthesias (1%-2%), arm dyspraxia, abulia, unilateral auditory neglect, and neglect of the contralateral extremity.[22,32,35,55,94]

Memory and language dysfunctions following thalamotomy are probably more common than traditionally thought or recognized. Significant changes in memory and language function may occur in up to 39% of patients. The risk after bilateral thalamotomy is approximately 60%, whereas only 31% of patients will suffer this complication after unilateral lesions. It appears that patients who show tissue loss on brain imaging or who have evidence of a previous thalamic lesion are most at risk for memory and language dysfunction postoperatively. Preoperative memory and language evaluation and CT appear to be of value in predicting which patients might be at greatest risk for postoperative memory and language dysfunction. About one half of the patients can be expected to recover to baseline within several months.[71]

Radiographic Follow-Up Following Thalamotomy

The location and extent of thalamic lesions following thalamotomy can be identified with postoperative imaging. During the acute stage, CT scans show a relatively large area of low attenuation which, with time, diminishes in size. The lesion demonstrated on contrast-enhanced CT scans at Day 14 gives the best anatomical mapping of the actual histological defect.[18]

Early (≤7 days) and late (8 days to 5 months) MRIs show a progressive shrinkage of the lesion over a period of months after the procedure. The lesion is characterized by edema during the acute phase, followed by coagulative necrosis and hemosiderin deposition. Lesion size stabilizes by around 7 months postoperatively.[86]

Summary

VL thalamotomy remains an excellent choice for the control of tremor in patients with a wide variety of disorders. Parkinson's disease and essential tremor are the best indications, but other disorders also respond. Improvement of bradykinesia and rigidity in Parkinson's disease is achievable, but not as dramatically as hyperkinetic symptoms. Indeed, individuals with significant rigidity or bradykinesia should likely be considered for pallidotomy. Morbidity from thalamotomy is most common with bilateral lesions, and innovative therapies such as thalamic stimulation may have a role when a second contralateral procedure is needed.

Thalamotomy is an effective procedure that has probably been underutilized over the past two decades. With renewed interest in stereotactic neurosurgery, improved imaging modalities, and well-established target localization techniques, the procedure is effective with a high degree of safety. The growing enthusiasm for brain grafting has also stimulated interest in the surgical treatment of movement disorders, and clearly this technique will evolve and progress as well. In the authors' opinion, the results of ablative surgery are certainly equivalent to those of deep brain stimulation (see Chapter 12, "Chronic Deep Brain Stimulation: Clinical Results") and still far exceed those of tissue implantation (see

Chapter 13, "Human Fetal Tissue Transplantation for the Treatment of Movement Disorders"). For a select group of indications, thalamotomy should be considered in the forefront of options for patients with movement disorders.

References

1. Albe-Fessard D, Guiot G, Hardy J: Electrophysiological localization and identification of subcortical structures in man by recording spontaneous and evoked activities. **Electroencephalogr Clin Neurophysiol 15:**1052-1053, 1963 (Abstract)
2. Andrew J, Fowler CJ, Harrison MJG: Stereotaxic thalamotomy in 55 cases of dystonia. **Brain 106:** 981-1000, 1983
3. Barbeau A: Long-term appraisal of levodopa therapy. **Neurology 22 (Suppl):**22-24, 1972
4. Barbeau A: The nonsurgical treatment of "Parkinson's disease": a personal view, in Morley TP (ed): **Current Controversies in Neurosurgery.** Philadelphia, Pa: WB Saunders, 1976, pp 419-428
5. Baron JC, Levasseur M, Mazoyer B, et al: Thalamocortical diaschisis: positron emission tomography in humans. **J Neurol Neurosurg Psychiatry 55:**935-942, 1992
6. Bergman H, Wichmann T, DeLong MR: Reversal of experimental parkinsonism by lesions of the subthalamic nucleus. **Science 249:**1436-1438, 1990
7. Bertrand C: The treatment of spasmodic torticollis with particular reference to thalamotomy, in Morley TP (ed): **Current Controversies in Neurosurgery.** Philadelphia, Pa: WB Saunders, 1976, pp 455-460
8. Bertrand C, Molina Negro P, Martinez SN: Technical aspects of selective peripheral denervation for spasmodic torticollis. **Appl Neurophysiol 45:**326-330, 1982
9. Broggi G, Giorgi C, Servello D: Stereotactic neurosurgery in the treatment of tremor. **Acta Neurochir Suppl 39:**73-76, 1987
10. Bucy PC, Case JT: Tremor: physiologic mechanism and abolition by surgical means. **Arch Neurol Psychiatry 41:**721-746, 1939
11. Burchiel KJ: Image-based functional neurosurgery. **Clin Neurosurg 39:**314-330, 1993
12. Cooper IS: Dystonia: Surgical approaches to treatment and physiologic implications, in Yahr MD (ed): **The Basal Ganglia.** New York, NY: Raven Press, 1976, pp 369-384
13. Cooper IS: **Involuntary Movement Disorders.** New York, NY: Harper & Row, 1969
14. Cooper IS: **Parkinsonism: Its Medical and Surgical Therapy.** Springfield, Ill: Charles C Thomas, 1961
15. Direnfeld LK, Feldman RG, Alexander MP, et al: Is L-dopa drug holiday useful? **Neurology 30:**785-788, 1980
16. Dostrovsky JO, Sher GD, Davis KD, et al: Microinjection of lidocaine into human thalamus: a useful tool in stereotactic surgery. **Stereotact Funct Neurosurg 60:**168-174, 1993
17. Eadie MJ: Problems in the contemporary treatment of parkinsonism. **Med J Aust 142:**113-117, 1985
18. Ebisutani D, Matsumoto K, Murayama Y, et al: CT appearance of experimental thalamic radiofrequency lesion in dog. **Appl Neurophysiol 50:**465-470, 1987
19. Fager CA: Effectiveness of stereoencephalotomy in treatment of Parkinson's disease. **JAMA 179:**703-707, 1962
20. Fahn S: Systemic therapy of dystonia. **Can J Neurol Sci 14:**528-532, 1987
21. Fahn S, Tolosa E, Marin C: Clinical rating scale for tremor, in Jankovic J, Tolosa E (eds): **Parkinson's Disease and Movement Disorders.** Baltimore, Md: Urban & Schwarzenberg, 1987, pp 225-234
22. Fox MW, Ahlskog JE, Kelly PJ: Stereotactic ventrolateralis thalamotomy for medically refractory tremor in post-levodopa era Parkinson's disease patients. **J Neurosurg 75:**723-730, 1991
23. Gildenberg PL: Stereotactic neurosurgery: present and past, in Heilbrun MP (ed): **Stereotactic Neurosurgery.** Baltimore, Md: Williams & Wilkins, 1988, pp 1-15
24. Gildenberg PL, Tasker RR: **Textbook of Stereotactic and Functional Neurosurgery.** New York, NY: McGraw-Hill, 1997
25. Goldman MS, Ahlskog JE, Kelly PJ: The symptomatic and functional outcome of stereotactic thalamotomy for medically intractable essential tremor. **J Neurosurg 76:**924-928, 1992
26. Goldman MS, Kelly PJ: Stereotactic thalamotomy for medically intractable essential tremor. **Stereotact Funct Neurosurg 58:**22-25, 1992
27. Goldman MS, Kelly PJ: Symptomatic and functional outcome of stereotactic ventralis lateralis thalamotomy for intention tremor. **J Neurosurg 77:**223-229, 1992
28. Goodman JH, Rea GL: Microcomputer management of stereotactic atlas data, in Kelly PJ, Kall BA (eds): **Computers in Stereotactic Neurosurgery.** Boston, Mass: Blackwell, 1992, pp 100-108
29. Hardy TL, Brynildson L, Bronson B: Computer rendering of stereotactic atlas data and whole-brain mapping with computed tomography and magnetic resonance imaging, in Kelly PJ, Kall BA (eds): **Computers in Stereotactic Neurosurgery.** Boston, Mass: Blackwell, 1992, pp 109-133
30. Hassler R, Mundinger F, Riechert T: Correlations between clinical and autoptic findings in stereotaxic operations of parkinsonism. **Confin Neurol 26:** 282-290, 1965
31. Hassler R, Riechert T: Indikationen und Lokalisations-methode der gezielten Hirnoperationenen. **Nervenarzt 25:**441-447, 1954
32. Heikkinen ER: Stereotactic neurosurgery: new aspects of an old method. **Ann Clin Res 47 (Suppl 18):**73-83, 1986
33. Hoehn MM, Yahr MD: Parkinsonism: onset, progression and mortality. **Neurology 17:**427-442, 1967
34. Horsley V: The Linacre lecture on the function of the so-called motor area of the brain. **Br Med J 2:** 125-132, 1909
35. Hugdahl K, Wester K, Asbjørnsen A: Auditory neglect after right frontal lobe and right pulvinar thalamic lesions. **Brain Lang 41:**465-473, 1991
36. Jinnai D, Nishimoto A, Matsumoto K, et al: Pallidotomy and thalamocapsulotomy for parkinsonism. **Excerpta Medica 36:**E94-E95, 1961
37. Kall BA: Computer-assisted stereotactic functional neurosurgery, in Kelly PJ, Kall BA (eds): **Computers**

in Stereotactic Neurosurgery. Boston, Mass: Blackwell, 1992, pp 134-142
38. Kall BA, Goerss SJ, Kelly PJ: A new multimodality correlative imaging technique for VOP/VIM (VL) thalamotomy procedures. **Stereotact Funct Neurosurg 58:**45-51, 1992
39. Katayama Y, Tsubokawa T, Tsukiyama T, et al: Changes in regional cerebral blood flow and oxygen metabolism following ventrolateral thalamotomy in Parkinson syndrome as revealed by positron emission tomography. **Appl Neurophysiol 49:**76-85, 1986
40. Kawashima Y, Chen HJ, Takahashi A, et al: Application of magnetic resonance imaging in functional stereotactic thalamotomy for the evaluation of individual variations of the thalamus. **Stereotact Funct Neurosurg 58:**33-38, 1992
41. Kawashima Y, Takahashi A, Hirato M, et al: Stereotactic Vim-Vo-thalamotomy for choreatic movement disorder. **Acta Neurochir Suppl 52:**103-106, 1991
42. Kelly PJ, Ahlskog JE, Goerss SJ, et al: Computer-assisted stereotactic ventralis lateralis thalamotomy with microelectrode recording control in patients with Parkinson's disease. **Mayo Clin Proc 62:** 655-664, 1987
43. Klemme RM: Surgical treatment of dystonia, paralysis agitans, and athetosis. **Arch Neurol Psychiatry 44:** 926, 1940
44. Krayenbühl H, Yasargil M: Relief of intention tremor due to multiple sclerosis by stereotaxic thalamotomy. **Confin Neurol 22:**368-374, 1962
45. Laitinen LV: Short-term results of stereotaxic treatment for infantile cerebral palsy. **Confin Neurol 26:** 258-263, 1965
46. Laitinen LV, Hariz MI: Multi-purpose stereoadapter. **Appl Neurophysiol 50:**68-76, 1987
47. Lenz FA, Martin R, Kwan HC, et al: Thalamic single-unit activity occurring in patients with hemidystonia. **Stereotact Funct Neurosurg 54/55:**159-162, 1990
48. Lenz FA, Tasker RR, Kwan HC, et al: Selection of the optimal lesion site for the relief of parkinsonian tremor on the basis of spectral analysis of neuronal firing patterns. **Appl Neurophysiol 50:**338-343, 1987
49. Lesser RP, Fahn S, Snider SR, et al: Analysis of the clinical problems in parkinsonism and the complications of long-term levodopa therapy. **Neurology 29:** 1253-1260, 1979
50. Levesque MF, Markham CH: Ventral intermediate thalamotomy for posttraumatic hemiballismus. **Stereotact Funct Neurosurg 58:**26-29, 1992
51. Lunsford LD: Magnetic resonance imaging stereotactic thalamotomy: report of a case with comparison to computed tomography. **Neurosurgery 23:**363-367, 1988
52. Markham CH, Diamond SG: Long-term follow-up of early dopa treatment in Parkinson's disease. **Ann Neurol 19:**365-372, 1986
53. Marks PV: Stereotactic surgery for post-traumatic cerebellar syndrome: an analysis of seven cases. **Stereotact Funct Neurosurg 60:**157-167, 1993
54. Marsen CD, Parkes JD: Success and problems of long-term levodopa therapy in Parkinson's disease. **Lancet 1:**345-349, 1977
55. Matsumoto K: Reappraisal of ventrolateral thalamotomy for Parkinson's disease, in Tasker RR (ed): **Neurosurgery: State of the Art Reviews. Stereotactic Surgery.** Philadelphia, Pa: Hanley & Belfus, 1987, pp 209-234
56. Meyers HR: Surgical procedure for postencephalitic tremor with notes on the physiology of premotor fibers. **Arch Neurol Psychiatry 44:**455-459, 1940
57. Mundinger F, Riechert T, Disselhoff J: Long term results of stereotaxic operations on extrapyramidal hyperkinesis (excluding parkinsonism). **Confin Neurol 32:**71-78, 1970
58. Narabayashi H, Kubota K: Reconsideration of ventrolateral thalamotomy for hyperkinesis. **Prog Brain Res 21B:**339-349, 1966
59. Narabayashi H, Maeda T, Yokochi F: Long-term follow-up study of nucleus ventralis intermedius and ventrolateralis thalamotomy using a microelectrode technique in parkinsonism. **Appl Neurophysiol 50:** 330-337, 1987
60. Ohye C: Stereotactic surgery in movement disorders: choice of patient, localization with microelectrodes and long-term results, in Tasker RR (ed): **Neurosurgery: State of the Art Reviews. Stereotactic Surgery.** Philadelphia, Pa: Hanley & Belfus, 1987, pp 193-208
61. Ohye C, Shibazaki T, Hirai T, et al: Microrecording for the study of thalamic organization, for tumor biopsy and removal. **Stereotact Funct Neurosurg 52:**136-144, 1989
62. Ohye C, Shibazaki T, Hirato M, et al: Strategy of selective VIM thalamotomy guided by microrecording. **Stereotact Funct Neurosurg 54/55:**186-191, 1990
63. Ojemann GA, Ward AA Jr: Abnormal movement disorders, in Youmans JR (ed): **Neurological Surgery: A Comprehensive Reference Guide to the Diagnosis and Management of Neurosurgical Problems.** 3rd ed. Philadelphia, Pa: WB Saunders, 1990, pp 4227-4262
64. Patil AA, Gelber B: Accuracy of thalamotomy target determination using axial images only. **Stereotact Funct Neurosurg 56:**104-108, 1991
65. Pinder RM, Brogden RN, Sawyer PR, et al: Levodopa and decarboxylase inhibitors: a review of their clinical pharmacology and use in the treatment of parkinsonism. **Drugs 11:**329-377, 1976
66. Rea GL, Goodman JH, Davis JR: Interactive computer graphic image analysis for functional neurosurgery. **Appl Neurophysiol 50:**42-44, 1987
67. Richardson RR: Rehabilitative neurosurgery: posttraumatic syndromes. **Stereotact Funct Neurosurg 53:**105-112, 1989
68. Riechert T: Stereotaxic surgery for treatment of Parkinson's syndrome. **Progr Neurol Surg 5:**1-78, 1973
69. Rinne UK: Recent advances in research on parkinsonism. **Acta Neurol Scand Suppl 57:**77-113, 1978
70. Rosenfeld JV, Barnett GH, Palmer J: Computed tomography guided stereotactic thalamotomy using the Brown-Roberts-Wells system for nonparkinsonian movement disorders. Technical note. **Stereotact Funct Neurosurg 56:**184-192, 1991
71. Rossitch E Jr, Zeidman SM, Nashold BS Jr, et al: Evaluation of memory and language function pre- and postthalamotomy with an attempt to define those patients at risk for postoperative dysfunction. **Surg Neurol 29:**11-16, 1988
72. Sano K, Yashioka M, Ogashiwa M, et al: Central mechanisms of neck movements in the human brain stem. **Confin Neurol 29:**107-111, 1967
73. Schad L, Lott L, Schmitt F, et al: Correction of spatial

distortion in MR imaging: a prerequisite for accurate stereotaxy. **J Comput Assist Tomogr 11**:499-505, 1987
74. Schaltenbrand G, Bailey P: **Introduction to Stereotaxis with an Atlas of the Human Brain.** New York, NY: Grune & Stratton, 1959
75. Schaltenbrand G, Wahren W: **Atlas for Stereotaxy of the Human Brain.** 2nd ed. Stuttgart: Thieme, 1977
76. Selby G: Treatment of parkinsonism. **Drugs 11**:61-70, 1976
77. Spiegel EA, Wycis HT, Szekely EG, et al: Campotomy in various extrapyramidal disorders. **J Neurosurg 20**: 871-884, 1963
78. Struppler A, Lipinski HG: Computer processing and anatomic correlation of somatosensory evoked potentials in the ventrolateral (VL) thalamus, in Kelly PJ, Kall BA (eds): **Computers in Stereotactic Neurosurgery.** Boston, Mass: Blackwell, 1992, pp 165-174
79. Taira T, Kawamura H, Tanikawa T, et al: Unexpected movement disorders in neurosurgical practice: report of three cases. **Surg Neurol 38**:135-140, 1992
80. Taren J, Guiot G, Derome P, et al: Hazards of stereotaxic thalamectomy. Added safety factor in corroborating X-ray target localization with neurophysiological methods. **J Neurosurg 29**:173-182, 1968
81. Tasker RR, Doorly T, Yamashiro K: Thalamotomy in generalized dystonia. **Adv Neurol 50**:615-631, 1988
82. Tasker RR, Dostrovsky JO: Computers in functional stereotactic surgery, in Kelly PJ, Kall BA (eds): **Computers in Stereotactic Neurosurgery.** Boston, Mass: Blackwell, 1992, pp 155-164
83. Tasker RR, Dostrovsky JO, Dolan EJ: Computerized tomography (CT) is just as accurate as ventriculography for functional stereotactic thalamotomy. **Stereotact Funct Neurosurg 57**:157-166, 1991
84. Tasker RR, Kiss ZHT: The role of the thalamus in functional neurosurgery. **Neurosurg Clin North Am 6**:73-105, 1995
85. Tasker RR, Organ LW, Hawrylyshyn P: Investigation of the surgical target for alleviation of involuntary movement disorders. **Appl Neurophysiol 45**:261-274, 1982
86. Tomlinson FH, Jack CR Jr, Kelly PJ: Sequential magnetic resonance imaging following stereotactic radiofrequency ventralis lateralis thalamotomy. **J Neurosurg 74**:579-584, 1991
87. Uematsu S, Delong M, Jankel W, et al: Microphysiological recordings at CT gantry site during stereotactic thalamotomy. **Stereotact Funct Neurosurg 52**: 183-190, 1989
88. Uematsu S, Rosenbaum AE, Delong MR, et al: Magnetic resonance planned thalamotomy followed by X-ray/CT-guided thalamotomy. **Acta Neurochir Suppl 39**:21-24, 1987
89. Van Buren J, Li C, Shapiro DY, et al: A qualitative and quantitative evaluation of parkinsonians three to six years following thalamotomy. **Confin Neurol 35**: 202-235, 1973
90. Van Buren JM, Bourke RC: **Variations and Connections of the Human Thalamus.** New York, NY: Springer, 1972
91. van Manen J: Indications for stereotaxic operations in cerebral palsy. **Confin Neurol 26**:254-257, 1965
92. van Manen J: Long-term results of stereotactic operations for Parkinson's disease. **Psychiatry Neurol Neurochir 73**:365-374, 1970
93. van Manen J, Speelman JD: Thalamotomy for tremor after a vascular brain stem lesion. **Acta Neurochir Suppl 39**:70-72, 1987
94. Velasco F, Velasco M, Ogarrio C, et al: Neglect induced by thalamotomy in humans: a quantitative appraisal of the sensory and motor deficits. **Neurosurgery 19**:744-751, 1986
95. Yamashiro K, Tasker RR: Stereotactic thalamotomy for dystonic patients. **Stereotact Funct Neurosurg 60**: 81-85, 1993
96. Yoshida M: Electrophysiological characterization of human subcortical structures by frequency spectrum analysis of neural noise (field potential) obtained during stereotactic surgery. Preliminary presentation of frequency power spectrum of various subcortical structures. **Stereotact Funct Neurosurg 52**:157-163, 1989
97. Yoshida M: Three-dimensional maps by interpolation from the Shaltenbrand and Bailey atlas, in Kelly PJ, Kall BA (eds): **Computers in Stereotactic Neurosurgery.** Boston, Mass: Blackwell, 1992, pp 143-152

CHAPTER 9

PALLIDOTOMY: INDICATIONS AND TECHNIQUES

ANDRES LOZANO, MD, PHD, FRCS(C), AND WILLIAM D. HUTCHISON, PHD

There are at least four reasons why we are now experiencing a rebirth of pallidotomy in the treatment of Parkinson's disease. First, medications have shortcomings and there continues to be a large number of patients who are disabled despite optimal medical therapy. Second, advances in neurosurgery, in imaging the brain, and in neurophysiological monitoring make functional procedures more accurate and safer. Third, advances in the understanding of basal ganglia circuitry, function, and pathophysiology, based largely on experiments conducted on the MPTP (1-methyl-4-phenyl-1,2,3,6-tetrahydropyridine) primate model of parkinsonism, now provide a solid scientific rationale for intervening at the level of the basal ganglia. Finally, the recent preliminary clinical results of pallidotomy suggest that this procedure can provide striking benefits.

The tremor, bradykinesia, rigidity, and postural and gait disturbances that characterize Parkinson's disease are initially quite responsive to pharmacotherapy. However, with progression of the illness and chronic medical treatment, the response to levodopa (L-DOPA) is less predictable and less sustained, leading to wide fluctuations in motor function, from an "on" state in which function may be relatively preserved to a disabling, akinetic/rigid "off" state. With time, several additional complications commonly arise. First, the duration and severity of the off state increase. Second, there is the appearance of drug-induced involuntary movements (dyskinesias), of both the slow, twisting dystonic variety and the faster, choreiform type. Their relationship to drug ingestion can be complex; they can occur near the onset of the dose, at the peak dose, or at the end of the dose, or can be present throughout these periods. The antiparkinsonian drugs also may produce psychiatric and cognitive impairments and gastrointestinal disturbances, which are sometimes difficult to distinguish from non-drug-related complications that accompany the natural course of the illness. When patients have reached these endpoints, other strategies clearly have to be considered.

Together with the pars reticulata of the substantia nigra, the internal segment of the globus pallidus (GPi) constitutes the final output of the basal ganglia. The current understanding is that, as the result of the dopamine deficiency present in parkinsonism, the level of activity in the gamma-aminobutyric acid (GABA)ergic (and inhibitory) GPi is heightened. It is believed that two factors contribute to this: 1) increased drive from the excitatory glutamatergic subthalamic nucleus; and 2) decreased inhibition from the motor striatum.[7] The hyperactive GPi is thought to exert an excessive inhibitory influence on the thalamus and downstream cortical motor system to produce the disordered and impoverished movement that is characteristic of Parkinson's disease. The surgical strategy is to place lesions selectively in the GPi to relieve the disturbance in the motor system function. The lesions should be limited to the sensorimotor portions of the GPi as defined by the area populated by neurons that respond to movement. To avoid unwanted complications, lesions should spare the limbic and associative territories of the GPi and should avoid injury to the adjacent external segment of the globus pallidus (GPe) and nearby important axonal pathways, the optic tract, and the internal capsule.

Indications for Pallidotomy

The indications for stereotactic pallidotomy are rapidly evolving. Functional neurosurgery should be directed toward alleviating the patient's most disabling symptoms on the most affected side of the body. With advanced neuroimaging and neurophysiological techniques, it is possible to accurately reach all components of the basal ganglia circuitry and to choose the most appropriate target for the patient's symptoms. Our current understanding is that certain parkinsonian features may respond to surgery better than others. Features that may respond to surgery are tremor, rigidity, bradykinesia, postural and gait disturbances, and drug-induced involuntary movements. Features that are resistant to surgery include cognitive deficits, psychiatric disorders, and autonomic disturbances.

For patients with Parkinson's disease in whom tremor is the dominant feature, the ventral intermediate (VIM) nucleus of the thalamus or its afferent axonal projections is still the most commonly chosen surgical target.[17] Both thalamotomy and chronic electrical stimulation of the thalamus are being used with a high degree of success.[12,25,27,33] It should be noted, however, that pallidotomy also has beneficial effects on parkinsonian tremor[3,24] and that as the role of the pallidum in the genesis of tremor is better defined, some of the enthusiasm for the thalamic target to treat tremor may shift to the pallidum. Patients with tremor-dominant parkinsonism, however, constitute a small minority. More common are patients with akinetic/rigid parkinsonian syndromes with fluctuating on/off periods and drug-induced dyskinesias. For this larger group of patients, the GPi is a more appropriate surgical target. The VIM thalamic target is largely ineffective for the nontremor components.[4]

The ideal pallidotomy patient is one who: 1) has Parkinson's disease; 2) is young; 3) has symptoms responsive to L-DOPA, but who, despite this, continues to have significant parkinsonian motor impairment; 4) is disabled by (in approximate order of most to least responsive to pallidotomy) drug-induced dyskinesias, rigidity, tremor, bradykinesia, and gait/postural disturbances; 5) is cognitively intact; and 6) has reasonable expectations of the effects of surgery. Because pallidotomy benefits predominantly the contralateral side, patients with asymmetric symptoms are the ideal candidates (see below).

A thorough neurological investigation is required to identify the patients who are referred with a presumptive diagnosis of Parkinson's disease but who actually have other syndromes. At the authors' institution, on the order of approximately 15% of referred patients are ultimately diagnosed as having something other than idiopathic Parkinson's disease. The most common among these diagnoses are multiple system atrophies and diffuse Lewy body disease. This distinction is important because, in the authors' limited experience, four patients with striatonigral degeneration who were unresponsive to antiparkinsonian medications did not significantly benefit from pallidotomy, nor did one patient in whom the diagnosis of progressive supranuclear palsy was made 2 years after his surgery.

Age is not an absolute selection criteria, although preliminary analysis at the authors' institution[19] and that of others[3] suggests younger patients derive more benefit from pallidotomy than do older patients. This also raises the controversial issue of when in the course of the illness surgery is best used. At the authors' institution, surgery is generally reserved for patients in whom medical therapy has failed and who have reached a level of impairment that prevents them from carrying out important activities of daily living (for example, work or self-care). Pallidotomy is not usually offered to end-stage (Hoehn and Yahr Stage 5) wheelchair- or bed-bound patients, based on the early experience of the limited benefits they derive and their often disabling associated features that are unresponsive to surgery.

The cognitive assessment of potential surgical candidates is important. As an office screening test, patients who score 25 or less out of 30 on the Folstein mini-mental status examination[11] are not considered good candidates. These patients may not be fully cooperative for the surgery, may perhaps be more prone to cognitive side effects with pallidal lesions, and, because of their cognitive impairment, may derive less overall benefit associated with an improved motor status. At the authors' institution, all patients undergo pre- and postoperative neuropsychological testing as part of a research protocol.

Because the benefits of pallidotomy are predominantly unilateral, surgery is directed first toward the patient's worst side. When the disease is symmetrical, the dominant hemisphere is surgically treated. The efficacy and safety of bilateral pallidal lesions is under active investigation. There has been a worrisome number of anecdotal reports of complications involving speech (Burchiel KJ, Favre J, Taha JM, et al: Risk of speech deterioration after pallidotomy. Poster presentation at the Congress of Neurological Surgeons Annual Meeting, Montreal, 1996) and cognitive function with bilateral procedures. While some of these may be related to suboptimal placement of lesions, perhaps encroaching on the internal capsule or nonmotor portions of the GPi, it is prudent to proceed carefully and to rigorously assess both the benefits and side effects of bilateral lesions.

By far the most striking effect of pallidotomy is the near complete (>90%)[24] elimination of drug-induced involuntary movements on the contralateral side. The appearance of this complication often sets the limit on the dosage of L-DOPA that patients can tolerate. Patients oscillate between being undermedicated, akinetic, and rigid to being in an on but dyskinetic state. After pallidotomy, patients can better tolerate similar or even higher doses of medication because of the striking diminution in contralateral and, to a lesser extent, ipsilateral dyskinesias. This translates into more dyskinesia-free on time and a striking improvement in their quality of life. The effects of pallidotomy on rigidity, tremor, and bradykinesia are also quite significant, with improvement in off-period scores, using validated rating scales, of 30%-70%.[3,8,24] The gait and postural instability score improvements are more modest.[24] Further, there is now evidence that the gains in postural and gait function provided by unilateral pallidotomy are less sustained than those for the other parkinsonian features.[19] For this reason, patients whose primary disability is gait and postural disturbance are less suitable candidates for unilateral pallidotomy and should be considered for alternative surgical approaches, including staged bilateral pallidotomy and other emerging surgical strategies such as bilateral chronic electrical stimulation of the GPi or subthalamic nucleus.[20,21,30]

It is important that the patient have realistic expectations of the surgery. Much optimism has been generated by the lay media showing spectacular effects of surgery. The surgery can indeed restore a higher level of function and independence. Pallidotomy improves symptoms; however, it is not a cure. Patients continue to have Parkinson's disease, they continue to require medications, and the illness continues to progress.

Surgical Technique for Pallidotomy

The surgical procedure is divided into three phases. First is stereotactic imaging; second, neurophysiological mapping; and third, lesion-making.

Imaging

Imaging is used to obtain the location of the tentative surgical target in three-dimensional (3-D) stereotactic space. Three methods of imaging are currently being used: ventriculography, computed tomography (CT), and magnetic resonance imaging (MRI). Whichever method is chosen, the first step is to apply the stereotactic frame to provide the terms of reference for the target in stereotactic space. The target can in some cases be directly visualized (using MRI, for example). More commonly, because of the difficulties in accurately identifying the desired target directly, the position of the target is derived as a function of its relationship to established brain landmarks, such as the anterior and posterior commissures. Ventriculography provides a high degree of resolution of the position of the commissures and the ventricular system. The position of the pallidal target is inferred from these landmarks. Because of the invasive nature of ventriculography, however, it is gradually being replaced by CT and MRI. CT has the advantages of being less invasive, rapid, and relatively free of image distortion, but the resolution of certain targets and the anterior commissure is suboptimal. With MRI, most structures, including the commissures, are readily identified. However, MRI has associated problems, including gradient field nonlinearity and magnetic field inhomogeneity; these can lead to image distortion that can affect spatial accuracy. A number of strategies are emerging to deal with these difficulties, including image-correction computer algorithms and CT and MRI fusion to increase both image quality and spatial resolution. Further aspects of MRI guidance for surgery of Parkinson's disease are discussed in Chapter 14, "Magnetic Resonance Imaging Guidance for Parkinson's Disease Surgery."

At the authors' institution, patients have the stereotactic frame applied under local anesthesia on the morning of surgery. The protocols for CT scan and MRI acquisition are quite similar, but the authors use MRI almost exclusively. MRI is used to localize the coordinates of the anterior and posterior commissures and to visualize the pallidal complex. The authors routinely use 1-mm slices without skip to increase the spatial accuracy. The 1.5-T MRI computer software is used to determine the coordinates of the anterior and posterior commissures in 3-D stereotactic space. These coordinates are then entered into a computer program containing digitized sagittal stereotactic maps from the Schaltenbrand and Wahren stereotactic atlas.[29] The map is shrunk or stretched in relation to the length of the patient's intercommissural line. From this map, a tentative target is chosen within the globus pallidus. This usually corresponds quite closely to the target described by Laitinen[18] and is often 2-3 mm anterior to the midcommissural point, 3-6 mm below the intercommissural line, and 20-21 mm from the midline.

Mapping

The patient undergoes surgery while in the off state, after medications have been withheld for 12 hours. The reason for this is to accentuate the pathophysiological cellular activity in the basal ganglia and to directly observe the effects of incremental lesions in the pallidum on motor function. If the patient is already in a good on state, one would be unlikely to perceive any additional motor benefits with pallidotomy in the intraoperative setting. The details of the neurosurgical procedure have been described elsewhere.[22] Briefly, a burr hole or a twist drill opening is made at the coronal suture on the side opposite the worse parkinsonian symptoms. The twist drill opening used by the authors measures 4 mm in diameter and allows the introduction of a macroelectrode or cannula to guide a microelectrode.

The optimal target within the pallidum and the optimal size of the pallidal lesion have not been systematically determined. The location of the most effective and safest target within the pallidum cannot be recognized by imaging alone. The globus pallidus and its neighboring structures, like all brain regions, show anatomical variability in size and shape. Using a standard target without taking these variations into account would be fraught with danger. This provides a strong argument for the individualization of target location. There is, in addition, variability in the functional organization of brain areas, which cannot be discriminated on the basis of conventional imaging. For these reasons, and because of intrinsic error with any imaging modality used alone, physiological corroboration of the target is essential.

There are currently two widely used alternate techniques for physiological mapping: 1) either macroelectrode stimulation or microelectrode recording; and 2) stimulation mapping. Macroelectrodes allow mapping based on the interpretation of macrostimulation responses (μA currents).

The technique of macroelectrode mapping is rapid and requires minimal equipment but does not allow neuronal activity recording.

Microelectrodes, on the other hand, allow the acquisition of direct measures of cellular activity from individual neurons. These recordings offer exquisite physiological resolution of nuclei based on the pattern of neuronal activity and the determination of receptive fields. Further, microelectrode recordings allow the unequivocal identification of and distinction between axons and neurons. These advantages come at the price of extra time, extra equipment, and a higher level of expertise required for the procedures. The next section comments on macroelectrode stimulation mapping but emphasizes the microelectrode technique utilized at the authors' institution.

Macroelectrode Mapping

Stimulation mapping can be carried out through the lesioning macroelectrode. The dimensions of this electrode and the stimulation parameters used to select the final lesion target, based on the patient's reaction to the stimulation, vary from surgeon to surgeon (Table 1).

With macroelectrode stimulation, three pieces of information can be obtained: 1) an assessment of the position of the corticospinal tract; 2) the location of the optic tract; and 3) a prediction of the beneficial effects and possible side effects of lesioning at that site. One surgical approach that has been used is to introduce the lesioning/stimulating macroelectrode to the calculated target, and then stimulate to determine the threshold for the production of undesirable side effects, most commonly visual or capsular. If the threshold currents are too low, indicating close proximity to important structures, the surgeon withdraws or repositions the electrode and repeats the stimulation. This process is repeated until a lesioning target that is considered safe is reached.

The corticobulbar and corticospinal tracts lie immediately medial and posterior to the GPi. With the macroelectrode introduced in the vicinity of the desired target, progressively higher electrical stimuli are given to determine the threshold voltage or current required to elicit a contraction in orofacial axial structures or limbs, indicating spread of the current to the motor fibers. Using a frequency of 50-100 Hz, tetanization is produced. At low frequencies, for example, 2-5 Hz, the contractions follow the stimulation frequency. The lower the threshold required to elicit this response, the closer the electrode lies to the corticospinal or corticobulbar tract. The relationship between the stimulation thresholds and the distance to the motor tracts varies with several parameters and in general has not been systematically studied or validated. Factors that influence this motor response include electrode size, stimulation frequency, pulse width, duration of the stimulus train, electrode position (for example, in cerebrospinal fluid or gray or white matter), and individual patient variation. Macroelectrodes are usually 1-1.8 mm in diameter and have an exposed tip 1-3 mm in length (see Table 1). Stimulation frequencies are usually 2-300 Hz. Pulse widths vary from 50 to 200 msec and stimulus trains can be 1 second or longer.

The threshold that indicates that it is "safe" to place a lesion at that particular site has to be determined empirically and individualized according to the stimulation technique. While the threshold current required to elicit the motor response provides some information about the distance from corticospinal and corticobulbar fibers, it cannot distinguish in which direction they lie. An important feature of the macrostimulation-induced motor response, however, is that it does not require the patient's cooperation.

The optic tract lies ventral to the GPi and is also susceptible to injury with pallidotomy. As with the motor axons, the smaller the distance separating the macroelectrode from the optic tract, the lower the threshold of current required to elicit a response, in this case, the report of stimulation-evoked perceptions of light in the contralateral visual field. Obtaining information on the position of the optic tract with this approach can be problematic, however, because it relies on the patient's verbal report. This introduces the possibility of false-positive and false-negative responses. False-positive responses may lead to inappropriate readjustment of the desired target for fear of producing an optic tract injury. False-negative responses are particularly worrisome because they may lead to visual field deficits. Indeed, false-negative reports with macrostimulation are likely the cause of the reports of a high incidence of visual field defects (2%-14%) associated with pallidotomy.[16,18] The authors have direct evidence that such false-nega-

TABLE 1

SURVEY OF LESIONING PARAMETERS

	Macroelectrode Parameters		Macrostimulation Parameters		Lesioning Parameters		Lesion Features	
Authors & Year	Diameter (mm)	Exposed (mm)	Frequency (Hz)	Current	Temp. (°C)	Time (sec)	Multiple Lesions	Size
Laitinen et al,[18] 1992	1.8	2	6-60	2-8 μA	72-82	60-90	yes	7 × 6 mm
Dogali et al,[8] 1995	1.1	3	5-50	up to10 V	80	60	yes	60-90 mm^3
Iacono et al,[16] 1995	1.6	2	2-100	0.2-3 V	65-80	30-60	yes	
Sutton et al,[32] 1995	1.2	2	2-50	low voltage	72-80	60	yes	
Baron et al,[16] 1996	1.1-1.8	3-5	100-300	0.1-2 μA			yes	65-181 mm^3
Lozano et al,[22] 1996	1	3			90	60	no	6 × 4 mm

tive reports occur. Up to 15% of the Parkinson's disease patients at the authors' institution fail to report seeing light flashes with electrical stimulation, even though microelectrode recordings unequivocally identify light flash-induced axonal action potentials in the optic tract at the exact same site.

Macroelectrode stimulation may also be used to predict the beneficial effects of the proposed pallidotomy lesion. Continuous stimulation at current intensities set below the threshold to elicit unwanted side effects is used. Patients are monitored for improvement in their parkinsonian signs with stimulation. This approach may help in choosing the optimal target.

Microelectrode Mapping

Mapping via microelectrode recording is more complex but permits the acquisition of detailed physiological measures of neuronal and axonal position and activity in the basal ganglia. A hydraulic microdrive is used to push a microelectrode in submillimeter steps along the desired trajectory. This electrode has an exposed tip of 15-30 μm and a high electrical impedance, in the range of 0.5-1 MΩ at 1000 kHz. The signal is amplified, filtered, and displayed on an oscilloscope and fed into an audio monitor. This technique not only allows the recording and distinction of individual neuronal units, but also allows the passing of electrical current (1-100 μA) through the tip of the electrode for microstimulation mapping. A window discriminator is used to determine the discharge frequency of the units that are encountered.

Typical trajectories through the pallidal complex are shown in Figure 1. The electrode courses through the GPe and across the medial pallidal lamina to enter the GPi. The GPi is itself subcompartmentalized into an external segment and internal segment by the incomplete pallidal lamina. Ventrally, beyond the internal GPi, the electrode enters the pallidofugal axons to reach the optic tract, which lies approximately 2 mm beyond the base of the pallidal complex. Each of these structures can be distinguished with pallidal microrecordings.

GPe neurons have characteristic discharge rates and patterns that are distinct from those neurons that populate the GPi.[5,14,31] The pattern of neuronal discharge in the pallidal complex in parkinsonian patients is strikingly similar to that seen in the monkey.[6,9,10,26] Particular attention must be paid to identifying the pallidal

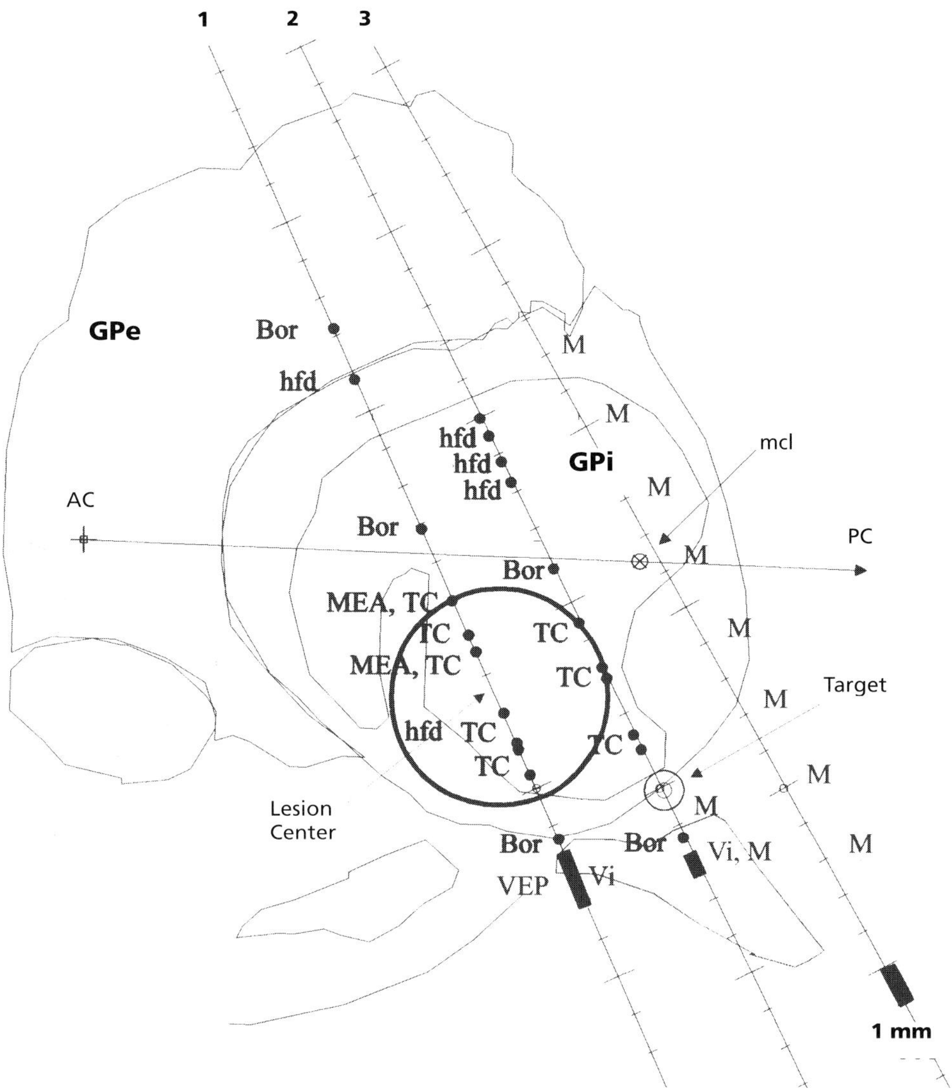

Figure 1: Physiological map for a patient with Parkinson's disease undergoing pallidotomy. Three sequential electrode trajectories were chosen. Illustrated are the major findings, superimposed on a sagittal map of the globus pallidus 20 mm lateral to the midline. The position of isolated single units are denoted by black dots along the trajectories. Tract 1 contained cells that responded to movements in the upper extremity and cells whose discharge was related to arm tremor. Tract 2 had several high-frequency discharging cells characteristic of GPi and tremor-related cells. Tract 3 was devoid of neurons and ran through the motor internal capsule. The optic tract was identified in tracts 1 and 2. There is an important discrepancy between the atlas-derived sagittal map and the intraoperatively acquired physiological data. The findings suggest that the microelectrode trajectories are in reality approximately 3 mm more posterior than anticipated; this emphasizes the need for physiological corroboration of the target. Note that in this case, the recommended target site determined by anatomical localization methods alone (denoted by the word "Target") was too close to both the internal capsule and the optic tract. Based on the physiological findings, to avoid capsular and optic tract injury, the final lesion site was modified to a location 3 mm more anterior and 3 mm superior to the original target. Microrecording results are shown to the left of the tracts; microstimulation results to the right. Bor = border cell; hfd = high-frequency discharge cell; mcl = midcommissural line; MEA = movement-evoked activity; TC = tremor cell. The optic tract located ventral to the GPi, was found by recording visual evoked potentials (VEP) and by the patient's reports of visual responses (Vi) to microstimulation (< 100 μA). The internal capsule (posterior to the GPi) was located by observation of motor (M) responses to microstimulation and the absence of somatodendritic action potentials. The *large circle* shows the estimated final lesion position and size. (Reproduced from Lozano and Hutchison[23] with permission.)

units that respond to kinesthetic inputs. This confirms the location of the sensorimotor territory, which occupies the most posterior and ventral portion of the GPi and which is functionally and anatomically distinct from the associative and limbic portions of the pallidum.

The pattern of neural activity in the parkinsonian pallidal complex is shown in Figure 2. The GPe is characterized by large, spontaneously active units firing in two distinct patterns: 1) low-frequency discharges (10-20 Hz) punctuated by rapid bursts; or 2) slow-frequency discharges (mean rate approximately 40-60 Hz) with occasional pauses. As the electrode advances more ventrally to leave the GPe, the transition from GPe to GPi is marked by a 1- to 2-mm wide band of fibers, the medial pallidal lamina, which is identified in microelectrode recordings by the absence of somatodendritic action potentials. This lamina is lined on both dorsal and ventral aspects by so-called "border cells." The border cells, described in primates over 25 years ago,[6] are cholinergic, have diffuse cortical projections, and are characterized by a more regular and slow discharge rate and a wider action potential. The border cells are believed to be displaced neurons from the nucleus basalis of Meynert. The entry into the GPi from the medial pallidal lamina is characterized by the sudden appearance of high-activity, rapidly firing neurons. The mean discharge rate is 80-90 Hz in the GPi, considerably higher than that in the GPe. At approximately the midpoint of the GPi, the incomplete pallidal lamina, can often be identified. Border cells are also found along this lamina, which compartmentalizes the GPi, as well as at the ventral border of the pallidum adjacent to the pallidofugal outflow axons.

In Parkinson's disease patients at the authors' institution, approximately 25% of neurons in the caudal ventral portion of the GPi respond to kinesthetic movements. The representation of the upper and lower limbs, the face, and extraocular muscles can be found. Certain neurons increase while others decrease their discharge rates with passive movements. Some neurons do so in a reciprocal fashion, increasing their firing rates with movement in one direction and decreasing in the other direction. The responses seen in patients with Parkinson's disease resemble those of parkinsonian MPTP-treated monkeys.[9,10] As in the animal model, GPi neuronal responses to kinesthetic inputs appear to be exaggerated and to lack specificity, with several units responding to movement at multiple joints, including not only the contralateral but also the ipsilateral side. Further, the sensorimotor territory in parkinsonian patients with tremor is populated by cells that fire in synchrony with the occurrence of tremor.[15,22] The possibility that these cells are involved in the generation of tremor is supported by the often marked amelioration in tremor that is seen with pallidotomy. The identification of the tremor and kinesthetic responses is important for identifying the sensorimotor territory of the GPi.

As the electrode is moved ventroposteriorly to leave the GPi, it encounters the pallidofugal outflow fibers. With microelectrode recordings, this encounter is characterized by an abrupt decrease or indeed absence of somatodendritic action potentials. By driving the electrode another 1-2 mm further, the optic tract is often reached. Here flashes of light produce action potentials in optic tract axons, which can be recorded.[22] Microstimulation is used to identify the optic tract with currents as low as 1 μA and 300 Hz. The perception of phosphenes in the contralateral visual field is most often described as white dots or sparkles of light.

A more posterior electrode trajectory is used to identify the internal capsule (see Figure 1). The position of the capsule is determined with microelectrodes, by its characteristic absence of somatodendritic action potentials, and the tetanization produced by stimulating corticospinal tract fibers. The known somatotopic organization of the corticospinal system (the face is medial, followed by the upper limb and leg most laterally) provides useful information on the laterality of the trajectory.

A sufficient number of microelectrode trajectories should be made to identify the position of three important landmarks: 1) the sensorimotor (kinesthetic responsive) portion of the GPi; 2) the optic tract; and 3) the internal capsule (see Figure 1). The average number of trajectories per patient is three to four. These physiological maps provide a good appreciation of the volume of the sensorimotor portion of the pallidal complex and its important borders, as well as the optic tract, which lies ventral to the

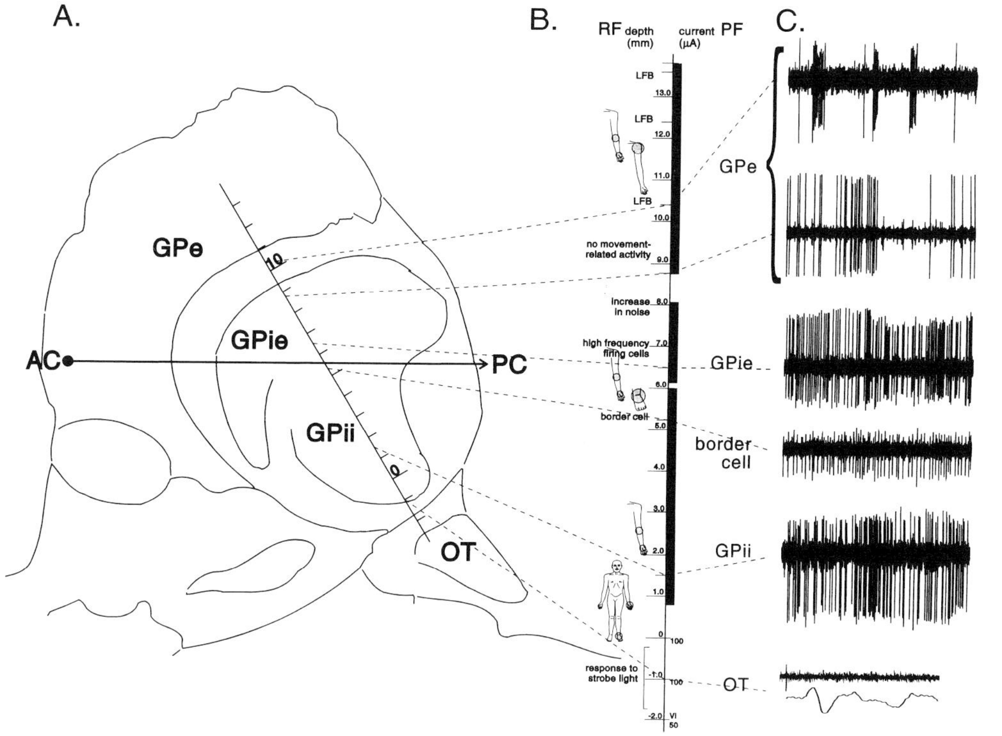

Figure 2: A) Physiological data obtained from one trajectory through the globus pallidus and optic tract (OT), plotted on the 20-mm sagittal map from the Schaltenbrand and Wahren stereotactic atlas.[29] **B)** The locations of neurons and their responses, as well as intraoperative observations of the characteristics of recordings, can be seen. **C)** Oscilloscope traces of representative examples of the neuronal type described in the text. At the bottom is a single sweep of the filtered trace where the optic tract field potential to visual stimuli was heard, but not readily seen. With appropriate filter settings for visual evoked potential measurement from the optic tract, the visual evoked potential can be seen, as illustrated below (the smooth trace). LFB = low-frequency burst neuron; RF = receptive field; PF = projected field; AC = anterior commissure; PC = posterior commissure; GPie = external segment of the GPi; GPii = internal segment of the GPi. (Reproduced from Lozano et al[22] with permission.)

target, and the internal capsule, which lies medial and posterior to the target. Using this mapping approach, the surgical target is modified from the tentative image-derived target in the majority of cases.[22]

Lesioning

Once the mapping is complete, a lesion site is chosen within the sensorimotor territory of the GPi and at least 3 mm away from the optic tract and internal capsule. The lesioning electrode used at the authors' institution has a 1-mm diameter and 3-mm exposed tip, which is thermistor coupled. Macrostimulation with the lesioning electrode can also provide some predictive information regarding the possible benefits and potential side effects of lesioning. Various lesioning protocols are used (see Table 1). At the authors' institution, a single lesion is made in increments of 10°C, starting at 60°C for 60 seconds. During lesion-making, the patient is tested for speech, sensory, motor, and visual function. After the initial lesion, the process is repeated at 70°C, 80°C, and finally 90°C for 60 seconds. This produces a lesion that measures approximately 6 mm in height and 4 mm in diameter on the T1-weighted MRI obtained 24 hours after surgery (Figure 3). Others make multiple smaller lesions based on the somatotopic localization within the GPi,[3] while still others make a series of vertically stacked lesions.[8,18] The optimal lesion size and location have yet to be determined. The lesion has to be sufficiently large to produce a long-

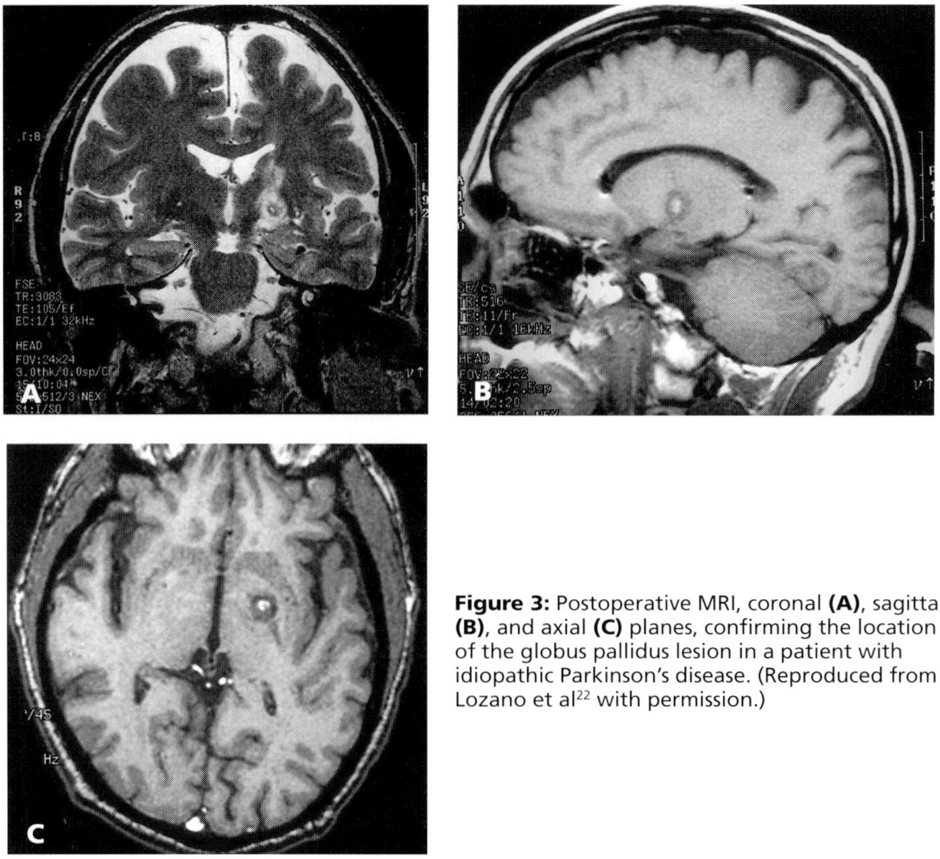

Figure 3: Postoperative MRI, coronal **(A)**, sagittal **(B)**, and axial **(C)** planes, confirming the location of the globus pallidus lesion in a patient with idiopathic Parkinson's disease. (Reproduced from Lozano et al[22] with permission.)

standing clinical benefit but small enough to avoid unwanted side effects.

The benefits of pallidotomy are seen immediately in the operating room, often with the mere introduction of the mapping electrode and invariably as the lesion is being made. A significant number of patients experience transient choreiform or dystonic movements with lesioning, which are most often seen contralaterally but which can be bilateral and resemble their customary drug-induced dyskinesias. The authors consider this to be a good prognostic sign. There is immediate relief of rigidity and improvement in bradykinesia at operation.

Future Directions in Pallidotomy

Among the most fundamental issues that remain to be resolved regarding pallidotomy are the determination of the best location for the lesion and the optimal lesion volume. Given the organization of the basal ganglia and the globus pallidus as segregated circuits,[1,2] it is logical to assume that lesions are best placed in the sensorimotor territory, sparing the limbic and associative regions of the GPi.[28] Indeed, there is now evidence of several subcircuits within the sensorimotor area of the GPi, with segregated pallidal outputs through the thalamus to the premotor cortex, motor cortex, and supplementary motor cortex.[13] The role of each of these subcircuits in normal motor control and in the pathogenesis of parkinsonism has yet to be determined. It may be possible to restrict or tailor surgical interventions to individual GPi motor subcircuits. An important issue in the future will be the relative role of GPi versus other basal ganglia targets and the role of lesion versus nonlesion surgery in the treatment of Parkinson's disease. Whatever target and surgical procedure are ultimately chosen, an important component in assessing the effects of specific lesions is the use of standardized measures of motor function in Parkinson's disease. In this way, we will learn to correlate lesion size and location with surgical outcome.

REFERENCES

1. Alexander GE, Crutcher MD: Functional architecture of basal ganglia circuits: neural substrates of parallel processing. **Trends Neurosci 13:**266-271, 1990
2. Alexander GE, DeLong MR, Strick PL: Parallel organization of functionally segregated circuits linking basal ganglia and cortex. **Annu Rev Neurosci 9:** 357-381, 1986
3. Baron MS, Vitek JL, Bakay RAE, et al: Treatment of advanced Parkinson's disease by posterior GPi pallidotomy: 1-year results of a pilot study. **Ann Neurol 40:**355-366, 1996
4. Benabid AL, Pollak P, Gao D, et al: Chronic electrical stimulation of the ventralis intermedius nucleus of the thalamus as a treatment of movement disorders. **J Neurosurg 84:**203-214, 1996
5. Beric A, Sterio D, Dogali M, et al: Characteristics of pallidal neuronal discharges in Parkinson's disease patients. **Adv Neurol 69:**123-128, 1996
6. DeLong MR: Activity of pallidal neurons during movement. **J Neurophysiol 34:**414-427, 1971
7. DeLong MR: Primate models of movement disorders of basal ganglia origin. **Trends Neurosci 13:**281-285, 1990
8. Dogali M, Fazzini E, Kolodny E, et al: Stereotactic ventral pallidotomy for Parkinson's disease. **Neurology 45:**753-761, 1995
9. Filion M, Tremblay L: Abnormal spontaneous activity of globus pallidus neurons in monkeys with MPTP-induced parkinsonism. **Brain Res 547:** 142-151, 1991
10. Filion M, Tremblay L, Bédard PJ: Abnormal influences of passive limb movement on the activity of globus pallidus neurons in parkinsonian monkeys. **Brain Res 444:**165-176, 1988
11. Folstein MF, Folstein SE, McHugh PR: "Mini -mental state." A practical method for grading the cognitive state of patients for the clinician. **J Psychiatr Res 12:** 189-198, 1975
12. Goldman MS, Ahlskog JE, Kelly PJ: The symptomatic and functional outcome of stereotactic thalamotomy for medically intractable essential tremor. **J Neurosurg 76:**924-928, 1992
13. Hoover JE, Strick PL: Multiple output channels in the basal ganglia. **Science 259:**819-821, 1993
14. Hutchison WD, Lozano AM, Davis KD, et al: Differential neuronal activity in segments of globus pallidus in Parkinson's disease patients. **Neuroreport 5:** 1533-1537, 1994
15. Hutchison WD, Lozano AM, Kiss ZHT, et al: Identification and characterization of neurons with tremor-related activity in human globus pallidus. **Exp Brain Res 113:** 557-563, 1997
16. Iacono RP, Shima F, Lonser RR, et al: The results, indications, and physiology of posteroventral pallidotomy for patients with Parkinson's disease. **Neurosurgery 26:**1118-1125, 1995
17. Laitinen LV: Brain targets in surgery for Parkinson's disease. Results of a survey of neurosurgeons. **J Neurosurg 62:**349-351, 1985
18. Laitinen LV, Bergenheim AT, Hariz MI: Leksell's posteroventral pallidotomy in the treatment of Parkinson's disease. **J Neurosurg 76:**53-61, 1992
19. Lang AE, Lozano AM, Montgomery EB, et al: Posteroventral pallidotomy in Parkinson's disease. **N Engl J Med 337:**1036-1042, 1997
20. Limousin P, Pollak P, Benazzouz A, et al: Bilateral subthalamic nucleus stimulation for severe Parkinson's disease. **Mov Disord 10:**672-674, 1995
21. Limousin P, Pollak P, Benazzouz A, et al: Effect of parkinsonian signs and symptoms of bilateral subthalamic nucleus stimulation. **Lancet 345:**91-95, 1995
22. Lozano A, Hutchison W, Kiss Z, et al: Methods for microelectrode-guided posteroventral pallidotomy. **J Neurosurg 84:**194-202, 1996
23. Lozano AM, Hutchison WD: Microelectrode-guided pallidotomy, in Rengachary SS, Wilkins RH (eds): **Neurosurgical Operative Atlas.** Park Ridge Ill: American Association of Neurological Disorders, 1997, Vol 6, pp 27-32
24. Lozano AM, Lang AE, Galvez-Jimenez N, et al: Effect of GPi pallidotomy on motor function in Parkinson's disease. **Lancet 346:** 1383-1387, 1995
25. Matsumoto K, Shichijo F, Fukami T: Long-term follow-up review of cases of Parkinson's disease after unilateral or bilateral thalamotomy. **J Neurosurg 60:** 1033-1044, 1984
26. Mitchell SJ, Richardson RT, Baker FH, et al: The primate globus pallidus: neuronal activity related to direction of movement. **Exp Brain Res 68:**491-505, 1987
27. Ohye C, Hirai T, Miyazaki M, et al: Vim thalamotomy for the treatment of various kinds of tremor. **Appl Neurophysiol 45:**275-280, 1982
28. Parent A, Hazrati LN: Functional anatomy of the basal ganglia. I. The cortico-basal ganglia-thalamo-cortical loop. **Brain Res Rev 20:**91-127, 1995
29. Schaltenbrand G, Wahren W: **Atlas for Stereotaxy of the Human Brain.** Stuttgart: Georg Thieme, 1977
30. Siegfried J, Lippitz B: Bilateral chronic electrostimulation of ventroposterolateral pallidum: a new therapeutic approach for alleviating all parkinsonian symptoms. **Neurosurgery 35:**1126-1133, 1994
31. Sterio D, Berić A, Dogali M, et al: Neurophysiological properties of pallidal neurons in Parkinson's disease. **Ann Neurol 35:**586-591, 1994
32. Sutton JP, Couldwell W, Lew MF, et al: Ventroposterior medial pallidotomy in patients with advanced Parkinson's disease. **Neurosurgery 36:**1112-1117, 1995
33. Tasker RR, Siqueira J, Hawrylyshyn P, et al: What happened to VIM thalamotomy for Parkinson's disease? **Appl Neurophysiol 46:**68-83, 1983

CHAPTER 10

PALLIDOTOMY: CLINICAL RESULTS

PHILIP A. STARR, MD, PHD, JERROLD L. VITEK, MD, PHD, AND ROY A.E. BAKAY, MD

Pallidotomy is the surgical destruction of portions of the globus pallidus. Although often considered a standardized procedure, throughout its 50-year history the practice of pallidotomy has varied greatly with respect to the selection of patients, the intended lesion location, the surgical techniques used to place the lesion, and the methods used to assess outcome. These differences must be considered in order to interpret the wide variation in reported clinical results.

While pallidotomy has been performed mainly for Parkinson's disease, it has also been used to treat hemiballismus, dystonia, and Huntington's disease. The clinical results of pallidotomy for each of these conditions are described in this chapter.

STANDARD RATING SCALES

To objectively quantify the clinical results of pallidotomy, patients must be assessed before and after the procedure using standard rating scales of motor function and disability. The most commonly used set of rating scales for evaluating treatments of Parkinson's disease is the Core Assessment Program for Intracerebral Transplantation (CAPIT).[45] The major rating scale in the CAPIT protocol is the Unified Parkinson's Disease Rating Scale (UPDRS). This scale has four subscales: I, mentation, behavior, and mood; II, activities of daily living (ADL); III, motor examination; and IV, complications of therapy (see Table 4 in Chapter 3, "Clinical Characteristics of Parkinson's Disease: Diagnosis and Assessment"). The ADL and motor examination subscores are often reported separately from the total score. The total UPDRS score may vary from 0 (no signs or symptoms) to 199 (most disabled). Because motor signs in parkinsonian patients typically fluctuate widely between the "on" and "off" states, ratings must be performed in both states at multiple time points.

Other standard rating scales for Parkinson's disease included in the CAPIT battery are: the Hoehn and Yahr staging scale, which measures overall disability from the disease on a scale of 1 to 5, with 5 being the worst (see Table 5 in Chapter 3); the dyskinesia rating scale, which measures both the intensity and the duration of dyskinesias on a scale of 0 to 5, with 5 corresponding to violent dyskinesias 100% of the day; and the CAPIT timed motor tests (pronation-supination, hand/ arm movement between two points, finger dexterity, and the stand-walk-sit test).[45] An additional scale commonly used to measure overall disability in Parkinson's disease is the Schwab and England score, which measures functional independence on a scale from 0% (totally dependent) to 100% (totally independent).[64]

For surgical intervention in dystonia and Huntington's disease, the results may be quantified using the Fahn-Marsden Dystonia Rating Scales[82] or the Unified Huntington's Disease Rating Scale, respectively.[34] Other measures that may be included are the Sickness Impact Profile and the Medical Outcome Score, both of which assess quality-of-life measures.

Pallidotomy for Parkinson's Disease

Parkinson's disease is a progressive, degenerative disease involving the basal ganglia. The fundamental biochemical defect is loss of dopamine in the striatum and in other basal ganglia nuclei, due to loss of the dopaminergic cells of the pars compacta of the substantia nigra.[32] The cardinal clinical signs of Parkinson's disease are resting tremor, rigidity, bradykinesia, and postural instability.

Early Work Versus Contemporary Pallidotomy

The literature on pallidotomy for Parkinson's disease can be divided into two groups: 1) the older literature, dating from the 1940s to the introduction of levodopa (L-DOPA) in the 1960s; and 2) the contemporary literature, which begins with the 1992 report of Laitinen et al[41] on the clinical results of posterolateral pallidotomy.

H. Russell Meyers,[55] in the 1940s, was the first to describe surgery in the region of the globus pallidus for Parkinson's disease, showing that lesions of the globus pallidus or its outflow tracts could reduce rigidity and tremor without causing paresis. In the 1950s, several others confirmed this using a variety of techniques, including open surgical intervention,[29] anterior choroidal artery ligation,[13,60] closed stereotactically guided procedures,[56,69-71,75] and closed procedures without stereotactic guidance, i.e., freehand.[14] Closed procedures generally used ventriculography to define the anterior commissure-posterior commissure line as a landmark for target localization, and lesions were made by chemical infusion or thermal injury.

The patient population in the 1950s probably included many patients with "Parkinson's plus" syndromes, such as postencephalitic parkinsonism, in addition to patients with idiopathic Parkinson's disease. Because computed tomography (CT) and magnetic resonance imaging (MRI) were not available, lesion location could not be routinely confirmed. Those using stereotactic techniques often reported target coordinates to be 0-5 mm behind the anterior commissure and 15-17 mm lateral to the midline, which would have placed lesions in the anterodorsal internal segment of the globus pallidus (GPi).[69] A small number of autopsy reports from the pre-L-DOPA era showed that the location of the pallidal lesion was highly variable, but confirmed that most lesions involved the anterodorsal portion of the GPi.[26,68,84] The only major exception to this is the series by Leksell's group in the 1950s, who systematically varied the target in the GPi from the anterodorsal region to the posterolateral region. Symptoms were more consistently improved with more posteriorly placed lesions.[75] In addition, Spiegel et al[71] noted five cases in which tremor recurred following pallidal lesions placed 0-3 mm behind the anterior commissure, but could be abolished for long time periods (1-5 years follow-up) by enlarging the lesion to 6-9 mm behind the anterior commissure.

Overall, the clinical results of pallidotomy in the 1950s were unpredictable and were not reported in terms of objective, standardized rating scales. Improvements in tremor and rigidity were frequently noted, but effects on bradykinesia were less consistent.[71] The advent of L-DOPA for treatment of Parkinson's disease in the late 1960s resulted in a decrease in enthusiasm for any surgical treatment.

In the decades following the introduction of

L-DOPA, however, it was recognized that long-term medical therapy for Parkinson's disease is often unsatisfactory, with patients eventually suffering from drug-induced dyskinesias, motor fluctuations, and variable responses to medications. At the same time, surgical techniques improved and the theoretical and experimental bases for several surgical interventions, including pallidotomy, were developed. In this setting, in 1992, Laitinen et al[41] published a seminal paper describing the results of posterolateral GPi pallidotomy in 38 patients, confirming the earlier result of Leksell's group[75] that all four cardinal signs of the disease can be relieved by this procedure. Dramatic benefit for drug-induced dyskinesias was also reported. As a result, pallidotomy re-emerged as one of several surgical procedures for the treatment of Parkinson's disease, and is now being investigated for the treatment of other movement disorders as well.

It is important to note the differences between pallidotomy in the 1990s and pallidotomy in the 1950s. In contemporary series, patients largely suffer from idiopathic Parkinson's disease that has become refractory to medications, while surgery in "Parkinson's plus" syndromes is ineffective[22] and thus contraindicated. Target localization is based on CT- or MRI-guided stereotaxis. Nearly all groups utilize physiological confirmation of lesioning probe placement, by macrostimulation, prior to lesioning. Many groups, in addition to stimulation with the lesioning electrode, also localize the GPi and surrounding structures using microelectrode recording techniques. Lesions are usually generated by radiofrequency thermocoagulation. Postoperative confirmation of lesion location by CT or MRI and the use of rating scales to objectively quantify outcome are used by most groups. Finally, the portion of the GPi targeted for lesion placement has changed substantially. Unlike the anterodorsal GPi lesions of most older series, the target for pallidotomy is now considered by most to be the posterolateral portion of the GPi. This target choice is supported both experimentally and clinically. Anatomically segregated subregions of the GPi, which mediate different functions (including motor, limbic, and associative), have now been defined.[1] Electrophysiological studies in humans[51,73,80] and in nonhuman primates[16] have shown that the posterolateral GPi is the part containing neurons whose discharge is modulated by joint movements, demonstrating that the posterolateral GPi is the portion of the nucleus participating in motor function. Thus, lesions in this area are likely to be more efficacious in treating motor signs than lesions in other, nonmotor areas of the GPi. This concept is supported by Leksell's series, in which the clinical results of posterolateral lesions were superior to those of anterodorsal lesions.[75]

Because of the many changes in the indications and techniques for pallidotomy, the clinical results of contemporary pallidotomy can be assessed only from relatively recent studies.

Contemporary Clinical Results of Unilateral Pallidotomy for Parkinson's Disease

Overview of Clinical Results Assessed by Standard Rating Scales

Only a small number of groups have published the results of unilateral pallidotomy using standard rating scales in both the on and off periods.[4,19,44,52,74,81] These studies are summarized in Table 1. In all of these studies, lesions were made by radiofrequency thermocoagulation, and all but one[74] used microelectrode recording to guide lesion placement.

UPDRS total and motor scores improved in all but one study. In the Toronto study by Lozano et al,[52] UPDRS rating was performed by blinded investigators based on videotaped examinations. At 6 months follow-up, UPDRS total scores in the off state had improved by 25% (from 74 to 55.2) and UPDRS motor scores in the off state by 30% (from 33 to 23). Motor scores in the on state did not change significantly. Results of the Emory study by Baron et al[4] (at 1 year) were similar to those of the Toronto study. The UPDRS total score improved by 19% (from 98.6 to 79.5) while UPDRS motor scores improved by 17% (from 55.4 to 46). Changes in the on state were again not significant. At 2-year evaluations, improvements in UPDRS motor scores over baseline remained significant, but were quantitatively less than at 1-year evaluations.[81] The New York University (NYU) study by Dogali et al[19] (at 1 year follow-up) showed an

TABLE 1

Effect of Unilateral Pallidotomy as Measured By Standard Parkinsonian Rating Scales*

Authors & Year	Mean Follow-up Time (mos)	No. of Patients	Age Range (mean)	Change in Disability Scales, Off Period, pre⇒post	Change in UPDRS Total, Off Period, pre⇒post	Change in UPDRS Motor, Off Period, pre⇒post	Change in UPDRS Motor, On Period
Dogali et al,[19] 1995	12	18	42-79 (59.8)	ADL 18⇒8 (55%)		35⇒13 (63%)	Improved; numbers not reported
Lozano et al,[52] 1995	6	14	44-71 (58.9)	ADL 26.8⇒19.3 (28%) S&E 30⇒55	74⇒55.2 (25%)	33⇒23 (30%)	None
Sutton et al,[74] 1995	2	5[+]	60-75 (67.0)	ADL none S&E none	None	None	None
Baron et al,[4] 1996	12	15	38-71 (57.0)	ADL 30.2⇒25.7 (15%) S&E 49⇒69	98.6⇒79.5 (19%)	55.4⇒46 (17%)	None
Vitek et al,[81] 1996	24	8		S&E 51⇒67	92⇒77 (16%)	51⇒42 (18%)	

*Includes only studies that employed standard rating scales in both the on and off states; ADL = activities of daily living in UPDRS; pre = preoperative; post = postoperative (at the end of the evaluation period); S&E = Schwab and England scale.

improvement in UPDRS motor scores in the off state of over 60% (from 35 to 13). UPDRS motor score improvement in the on state was stated to be "significant."

Scales that measure overall functional disability, such as the Schwab and England scale and the ADL subscale of the UPDRS, also showed significant improvement in most reports, varying from 15% to 55% (see Table 1).[4,19,52]

Only the University of Southern California (USC) group (Sutton et al)[74] reported no improvement following pallidotomy. In five patients with advanced Parkinson's disease followed for 2 months, none showed a significant reduction in the total score or the subscores of the UPDRS. Factors contributing to the lack of significant improvement may have been the relatively high mean age of the patients and the choice of surgical technique (microelectrode recording was not used for localization, so lesioning may not have included the sensorimotor GPi).

Effects on Cardinal Motor Signs in the Off State

Pallidotomy consistently improves contralateral tremor, rigidity, and bradykinesia in the off state. In the Emory series,[4] tremor was nearly eliminated in seven of eight patients (87.5%) who had significant tremor preoperatively. Similar effects on tremor have been observed by others.[19,52] Blinded evaluations of bradykinesia have shown contralateral improvements of 37% (CAPIT timed motor tasks) in the NYU study[19] and 26% (UPDRS akinesia score) in the Toronto study.[52] In the Toronto series, UPDRS rigidity scores improved 30%. Improvements in axial symptoms (gait, posture, falling, and freezing) have been observed by many,[19,36,41,62] but in some studies failed to reach statistical significance at the longest evaluation times.[4,52] Thus, patients should be counseled that significant improvement in axial symptomatology is less predictable than that for tremor, rigidity, bradykinesia, and drug-induced dyskinesias.

Effects During the On State and On-Off Fluctuations

Pallidotomy is reported to increase the amount of time spent in the on state[4,36] and to decrease motor fluctuations.[4] Virtually all of the groups reported dramatic and sustained amelioration of peak dose L-DOPA-induced dyskinesias on the contralateral side, with ipsilateral improvements in some.[4,19,36,38,41,52,74] This is the only consistently reported benefit in the on state. While some have reported dramatic[36] or significant[19] improvements in UPDRS motor subtest scores in the on state, most report only modest improvements that may not reach statistical significance.[4,38,52]

Effects on Medication Dosage

At 2-year evaluations, the Toronto group[44] reported a significant (22%) decrease in dopaminergic drug use. In most studies in which this was examined, however, intake of L-DOPA did not change significantly.[19,52] Because patients may increase L-DOPA usage, due to amelioration of rate limiting side effects of dyskinesias, while others may reduce their intake due to improved off-periods.[19]

Ipsilateral Effects

Multiple reports agree that there is a modest ipsilateral benefit of pallidotomy on bradykinesia.[4,19,41,52] The NYU group[19] reported a 24.2% improvement in ipsilateral bradykinesia by standard CAPIT timed movement tasks (pronation-supination, finger dexterity, and hand/arm movement between two points), as compared with 38.2% contralateral improvement for the same set of tasks. Ipsilateral improvements in motor signs other than bradykinesia have not been consistently observed.

Complications

Reported complications of GPi pallidotomy from contemporary series are listed in Table 2. Because of its proximity to the inferior border of the GPi, optic tract injury is one of the major potential complications of pallidotomy. In the first 38 patients in the series of Laitinen et al,[41] there was a 14% incidence of visual field deficits, presumably due to injury to the optic tract. However, this group later reported only 3 additional field cuts in over 200 additional patients.[40] In studies utilizing microelectrode recording, few field cuts have been reported.[4,19,52] In the authors' own series,[80] 4 of 160 patients (2.5%), all from early in the series, developed partial visual field cuts.

Most series report isolated cases of hypophonia or worsened speech articulation. The incidence of mild hypophonia following pallidotomy may be higher. In one study based on patient questionnaires, 8 of 22 patients (36%) reported worsening of speech volume (K Burchiel, personal communication, 1996). Two studies, however, note that on rare occasions the volume and articulation of speech improves.[4,41]

In the Emory series of 160 cases,[80] in addition to the visual field cuts reported above, postoperative weakness developed in the face in 8 patients (5%) and in the limb in 3 patients (2%), most of which resolved completely. Other major complications included symptomatic intraparenchymal hemorrhages along the lesioning tract in two patients, a subdural hematoma at a site distant from the surgical intervention, a subdural empyema requiring drainage, and a postoperative encephalopathy in an elderly patient. Although there were no immediate deaths, two of these patients died several months after surgery.[80]

The Emory study[4] has reported detailed neuropsychological testing. In 12 patients tested, there were no significant changes in 21 of 25 neuropsychological variables. Four variables relating to frontal lobe function did change between the preoperative and the 1-year assessments, but there was no significant change on the initial postoperative assessment, indicating that the declines may have been unrelated to surgery.

Long-Term Outcome

At the present time, no published study in the contemporary literature has examined the outcome for longer than 2 years, using standard rating scales.

Predictors of Outcome

Age and Mental Status

In the Emory pilot study,[4] patients with dementia (2 of 15) showed markedly less overall

TABLE 2

COMPLICATIONS OF UNILATERAL PALLIDOTOMY IN CONTEMPORARY SERIES*

Authors & Year	No. of Patients	Visual Field Cut	Worsened Speech	Symptomatic Hemorrhage	Miscellaneous
Laitinen et al,[40,41] 1992 and 1995	259 (12 bilat)	9 (3.5%)	1	0	2 foot apraxia 2 transient facial weakness 1 seizure 1 delayed stroke (1 week postop)
Dogali et al,[19] 1995	18	0	0	0	1 transient disinhibition
Iacono et al,[36] 1995	126 (68 bilat)	3 (2.4%)	0	3	1 abscess 1 transient hemiparesis unrelated to bleed
Lozano et al,[52] 1995	14	0	0	0	3 transient facial weakness 4 transient euphoria
Sutton et al,[74] 1995	5 (2 bilat)	2 (40%)	1	0	2 transient worsening depression 2 transient facial weakness 1 worse swallowing
Baron et al,[4] 1996, and Vitek et al,[80] 1998	160 (6 bilat)	4 (2.5%)	1	3	1 subdural empyema requiring drainage 3 capsular lacunae (0-14 days postop) 3 asymptomatic hemorrhages 8 facial weakness (6 transient, 2 persistent) 3 limb weakness (1 transient, 2 persistent) 3 postop seizures
Shima et al,[66] 1996	86 (28 bilat)	0	3[+]	1	Not detailed
Johansson et al,[38] 1997	22	1 (4.5%)	1	0	2 pyschoses (1 transient, 1 persistent)

* Bilat = bilateral surgery.
[+] All cases of worsened speech in the Japanese series were bilateral pallidotomies.

benefit. Age correlated inversely with outcome, including or excluding the two demented patients. UPDRS total scores decreased by an average of 52.2% in six patients aged 38-52 years, and 13.8% in seven patients aged 58-69 years.[4] However, older patients also had significant benefit and thus should not be excluded based on age alone. Other studies have shown a trend toward less benefit in older patients, although the trend was not statistically significant.[19] Duration of parkinsonian symptoms does not appear to correlate with outcome.[4]

Lesion Location and Size

Based upon current understanding of basal ganglia physiology,[1,15] the location and size of the lesion within the pallidal complex would be predicted to affect clinical outcome. Most modern series attempt to target the posterolateral, sensorimotor portion of the GPi. Lesions in other, nonmotor regions of the GPi might be expected to give some benefit by extension of edema into, or partial lesioning of, the motor territory; however, such benefit would not be expected to be as robust as lesions of the motor territory. Evaluating 11 patients from early in the series, the authors subdivided patients into two groups based upon lesion location as determined on thin-cut, volumetrically acquired postoperative MRI.[79] Patients with lesions clearly centered in the sensorimotor (posterolateral) portion of the GPi had sustained improvement in UPDRS scores at 18 months. Patients with lesions that involved only a portion of this area or that encroached substantially upon the external segment of the globus pallidus (GPe) sustained significantly less benefit. One of the authors' early patients presented following a pallidotomy performed elsewhere, with a lesion anterior to the sensorimotor part of the GPi. The patient reported immediate resolution of all parkinsonian motor signs; however, she experienced a gradual return of symptoms after 2 weeks. Repeat pallidotomy in this patient, with lesion placement posterior and lateral to the first lesion, has provided sustained benefit at 3 years.[79]

However, there is not yet general agreement on the optimal lesion location for long-term benefit. It is not known whether lesions that include the ansa lenticularis would provide greater improvement than pure GPi lesions. Laitinen et al[40,42] have advocated inclusion of the GPe within the lesion. Postoperative MRI in the series by Laitinen et al, however, clearly shows the lesion involving the posterolateral GPi as well as the GPe. It is not clear whether inclusion of the GPe enhances or detracts from the effect of the GPi lesion. In the 1-methyl-4 phenyl-1,2,3,6-tetrahydropyridine (MPTP)-treated primate model of Parkinson's disease, pure GPe lesions do not relieve L-DOPA-induced dyskinesias,[7] whereas dyskinesias in the patients reported by Laitinen et al are clearly relieved, supporting the idea that this therapeutic benefit derives from the GPi component of the lesion.

Ideal lesion size is also unclear. Where reported, mean lesion size has varied. Using early postoperative MRI, mean lesion sizes have been reported to range from 75 mm^3 (in the NYU study[19]) to 127 mm^3 (in the Emory study[4]) or 6-8 mm in diameter (in the Toronto study[52]). The mean lesion volume in the study by Laitinen et al[41] was 95 mm^3, as measured by CT scans obtained 3-12 months postoperatively. These variations probably correspond to variable technique: some groups make multiple lesions along multiple tracks, while others generally use one track. Radiographic measurements of lesion size are inherently approximate because the precise boundaries of the lesion are subject to interpretation. In only one case from the contemporary literature has lesion size by postoperative MRI been confirmed by autopsy.[80] In this report, physiological, radiological, and histological approximation of lesion size showed good correspondence. Anecdotal cases indicate that enlarging a lesion, when the patient has had initial benefit followed by relapse, may improve long-term results.[74] However, the reason for improvement with a second surgery could be either suboptimal size or suboptimal location of the original lesion. More reports of clinical results after repeat operation for pallidotomy, in which lesions are enlarged or generated in new locations, are needed and will provide useful information about the best lesion size and location for the best long-term outcome.

Techniques Used

The technique used for target localization may affect clinical outcome. Virtually all groups use image-guided stereotaxis for target localization, and most confirm the position of the lesioning electrode by macrostimulation, that is, passing current through the lesioning probe to check for activation of neighboring white matter pathways.[21,51,80] However, there is not yet a clear consensus as to whether microelectrode recording, as an additional aid to target localization, is necessary.[21] Nearly all published studies that utilized standard parkinsonian rating scales (see Table 1) employed this technique. The one study that did not use microrecording techniques was the only study that observed no changes in UPDRS scores following pallidotomy.[74] The theoretical accuracy of standard stereotactic systems, with 1-mm thick slice imaging, is approximately 1.5 mm at the 95% confidence limit,[53] while the resolution of microelectrode mapping is significantly more precise.[51,80] The authors believe that the use of microelectrode mapping significantly increases the precision of lesion placement. Because the precise position of the lesion affects outcome,[79] it is likely that the use of microelectrode techniques will lead to improved outcome.

The technique used for lesion generation may also affect outcome. In the majority of published cases in the modern era, the lesion is created by radiofrequency thermocoagulation. Other techniques, however, are being explored. Radiosurgical pallidotomy for Parkinson's disease, using the Leksell Gamma Knife, has been reported.[24,61,85] In two small series, symptomatic improvement was seen in only four of eight[61] and one of four[24] patients. Young et al,[85] in a series of 15 parkinsonian patients, reported that Gamma Knife pallidotomy was effective for drug-induced dyskinesias in all patients and for bradykinesia and rigidity in 77% of patients. No complications were reported. However, patient assessment by standardized Parkinson's disease rating scales was not performed, so it is impossible to compare these results with those of radiofrequency pallidotomy. At this time, without documentation of results by standardized rating scales, radiosurgical pallidotomy cannot be recommended. Chemical pallidotomy by infusion of excitotoxins has been successful in a primate model of parkinsonism.[48] This technique has the theoretical advantage of being axon-sparing, thus potentially avoiding damage to the corticospinal tract, the optic tract, and to fibers passing through the GPi. The size of the lesion made using chemical infusion techniques, however, may be difficult to control.[25,84] Also, it is unknown whether sparing fibers within the GPi would be beneficial or detrimental to outcome.

Summary

Based upon these studies, the authors can conclude that unilateral, microelectrode-guided pallidotomy is relatively safe and effective for at least 2 years, for moderate to advanced idiopathic Parkinson's disease, when lesions include the posterolateral portion of the GPi. There are consistent, sustained improvements in off-period contralateral rigidity, bradykinesia, and tremor, and in some patients, moderate improvement in ipsilateral bradykinesia. Dystonia, when present, appears to improve. Improvements in off-period gait, posture, freezing, and painful cramping have been reported but are more variable. On periods appear to be prolonged and motor fluctuations decreased. In the on state, contralateral L-DOPA-induced dyskinesias are greatly improved, although UPDRS motor scores in the on state, in most studies in which they are reported, are not generally changed significantly.

Bilateral Pallidotomy for Parkinson's Disease

Because the major benefit of pallidotomy is contralateral and because most parkinsonian patients have bilateral disease, some groups are investigating bilateral pallidotomy for Parkinson's disease.[36,40,66] The results, even in the short term, of bilateral pallidotomy are not yet well documented. Iacono et al[36] have published 68 cases of bilateral pallidotomy, with many "good" or "excellent" results. However, the effects in the off state are not quantified by standard rating scales, and their series lumps together the results of unilateral and bilateral pallidotomy. Shima et al[66] have reported 28 cases of bilateral pallidotomy, but without quantification of the results. In 11 staged bilateral pallidotomies performed by the NYU group, the incremental benefit of the additional lesion in UPDRS and CAPIT movement times was only 10% (R Kim, personal communication, 1996).

From a small number of published reports, bilateral pallidotomy probably carries a higher complication rate than unilateral surgery. Following simultaneous or staged bilateral pallidotomy, the likelihood of significant speech deterioration (based on questionnaire data) has been reported as 53% to 60% (K Burchiel, personal communication, 1996). The Toronto group[43] has reported that bilateral pallidotomy produced major cognitive deficits in two of two patients treated. Of 11 staged bilateral pallidotomies by the NYU group, discussed above, four patients had worsened speech (R Kim, personal communication, 1996). The authors have performed six staged bilateral pallidotomies, and although the majority of patients are hypophonic to varying degrees, patients experienced significant motor benefits (unpublished data). The safety of bilateral pallidotomy needs closer scrutiny before it can be recommended.

Pallidotomy Versus Other Surgical Procedures for Parkinson's Disease

Thalamotomy

Ablation of the motor thalamus, or thalamotomy, has been performed for parkinsonism since it was introduced by Hassler et al[30,31] in the 1950s. Ventral intermediate nucleus thalamotomy has well documented effectiveness for parkinsonian tremor.[18,23,37] If the lesion involves the ventral oral posterior nucleus, thalamotomy may be effective for rigidity[30] and for drug-induced dyskinesias.[57] However, there is little evidence that thalamotomy improves bradykinesia. Because pallidotomy is more effective for bradykinesia and is also effective for rigidity and tremor, it is currently the ablative technique of choice for most Parkinson's disease patients.

GPi Stimulation

A small number of reported cases suggest that GPi stimulation has effects similar to pallidotomy for rigid/bradykinetic Parkinson's disease, and may be safe for bilateral use.[58,67] It is possible that pallidal stimulation contralateral to a previous pallidotomy would benefit patients with bilateral disease, while avoiding the potential complications associated with bilateral pallidotomy, but this remains to be confirmed in clinical trials.

Subthalamic Nucleus Stimulation

Based on work in parkinsonian monkeys showing substantial benefit of subthalamic nucleus (STN) lesions,[6] Limousin and colleagues[49] have implanted bilateral stimulators in the STN in patients with predominantly rigid/bradykinetic Parkinson's disease. In the first three patients, UPDRS motor scores were improved by 42%-82% 3 months after surgery. Akinesia and rigidity were the motor signs that improved the most. These results are comparable to the best reported results of pallidotomy. In two of five patients, dyskinesias could be induced by STN stimulation, but were alleviated by reducing the stimulation voltage.[50] In those two patients, antiparkinsonian benefit remained at stimulation voltages that did not produce dyskinesias.

Pallidotomy for Other Movement Disorders

While medically intractable Parkinson's disease is the predominant indication for GPi pallidotomy, the operation has been applied to other movement disorders, including hemiballismus, dystonia, and Huntington's disease. The literature on pallidotomy in these conditions is summarized in Table 3.

Hemiballismus

Hemiballismus is characterized by violent, uncontrollable movements of the proximal extremities. It is usually due to ischemic lesions involving the subthalamic nucleus and/or its efferent pathways.[17]

Early literature suggested that pallidotomy may be effective for alleviation of hemiballismus. In 1966, Gioino et al[26] described four of their own cases and reviewed seven previous case reports. Only one had anatomical verification of lesion location. This patient had developed hemiballismus subsequent to a thalamotomy for Parkinson's disease, in which the thalamic lesion had extended into the zona incerta. The patient had "complete" resolution of hemiballismus following chemical pallidotomy by alcohol injections, but died of pneumonia 9 weeks after pallidotomy. Autopsy showed the lesion was within the anterodorsal portion of the GPi. One report has described lesions in the GPe in two cases of hemiballismus, with a good clinical result at 2 years.[78] Anatomical verification of lesion location was not available and the etiology of the hemiballismus was not reported. The authors recently performed a posterolateral GPi pallidotomy in a patient with hemiballismus due to a brain stem hemorrhage involving the STN. Following pallidotomy, there was complete and immediate resolution of hemiballismus, which has persisted over the follow-up period of 2 years.[83]

Caution is advised before embarking on surgical treatment of hemiballismus. The appropriate lesion target is still unclear, because thalamotomy has also been reported to relieve hemiballismus.[10,47] Patients who have hemiballismus on the basis of cerebral infarction may have chronic hypertensive changes in the brain,

TABLE 3

PALLIDOTOMY FOR DISORDERS OTHER THAN PARKINSONISM*

Author(s) & Year	Disease Treated	No. of Cases	Region Targeted	Lesion Location Verifed?	Reported Clinical Results
Tailarach et al,[76] 1950	HB, postencephalitic	1	GPi and ansa	No	Partial recurrence after a few wks
Spiegel et al,[70-72] 1952 and 1958	HD	4	GPi, possibly including GPe (bilat)	No	Relief of chorea in 3 of 4 at 9-10 yrs f/u
Andy,[3] 1962	HB, postinfarction	1	Anterodorsal GPi	No	Good relief at 5.5 yrs
Gioino et al,[26] 1966	HB (1 posttraumatic, 2 postencephalitic, 1 postsurgical)	4	Various pallidal regions	Autopsy (1 case) (anterodorsal pallidum)	Good relief in 4 of 4, 9 wks-7 yrs postop
Tsubokawa and Moriyasu,[78] 1975	HB, origin not stated	2	Ventral GPe	No	Excellent relief at 2 yrs
Cooper,[12] 1976	Gen dystonia	13	GPi, some bilat, exact location unclear	No	1 detailed case report shows resolution of all symptoms except torticollis; 19 yrs f/u
Burzaco,[9] 1985	Gen dystonia Focal dystonia	10 8	Posterolat GPi	No	Satisfactory in 8 of 10 Satisfactory in 6 of 8
Vitek et al,[83] 1995	HB (STN hemorrhage)	1	Posterolat GPi	MRI	Complete relief; short f/u
Iacono et al,[35] 1996	Gen dystonia	1	Posterolat GPi (bilat)	MRI	Sustained relief at 1 yr
Laitinen and Hariz,[42] 1996	HD	1	Posterolat GPi and GPe	Yes	Relief of chorea, short f/u
Vitek et al,[82] 1998	Gen dystonia	3	Posterolat GPi	MRI	72%-80% improvement in FMDRS at 1 wk-2 mos

* Bilat = bilateral; FMDRS = Fahn-Marsden Dystonia Rating Scales; f/u = follow-up; gen = generalized; HB = hemiballismus; HD = Huntington's disease; posterolat = posterolateral.

increasing the risk of surgery. In addition, many cases of hemiballismus resolve spontaneously without surgical intervention.[17]

Dystonia

Dystonia refers to a symptom rather than to a particular disease, and a heterogeneous group of disorders may have dystonia as the primary manifestation. Dystonia is characterized by sustained muscle contractions leading to twisting, repetitive movements and abnormal postures. Primary (idiopathic) forms of dystonia are often inherited. Dystonia may also be secondary to traumatic, neoplastic, or infectious lesions involving the basal ganglia (usually the putamen) or less commonly the motor thalamus.[46,54,59]

Clinical results of pallidotomy for idiopathic generalized dystonia were originally reported by Spiegel et al,[71] who treated two cases using thermocoagulative lesions, and by Cooper,[12] who treated 13 cases using chemical infusion (see Table 3). Documentation of lesion location in these cases is not available, but based on intended stereotactic coordinates[69] or autopsy data[26] from other pallidotomies by the same authors, lesions may have been in the anterodorsal GPi. One of the cases in the series of Spiegel and Wycis had "elimination of the abnormal posture" at 2 years postoperatively. One of Cooper's cases had well-documented long-term outcome. This patient underwent bilateral pallidotomy at age 12 years, 3 years after the onset of severe generalized dystonia. Nineteen years after surgery, dystonic signs remained relatively mild, except for persistent torticollis. Burzaco[9] reported 18 cases of pallidotomy for dystonia, with the intended target in the posterolateral GPi at Leksell's coordinates.[75] Results were "satisfactory" in 8 of 10 cases of generalized dystonia and 6 of 8 cases of focal dystonia, although the length of follow-up was not reported.

Several recent reports have favorably reexplored pallidotomy for generalized dystonia, with short follow-up times (see Table 3). In four cases, one bilateral[35] and three unilateral,[82] the lesion was documented radiographically to be in the posterolateral GPi. One case of radiosurgical (Gamma Knife) pallidotomy for dystonia resulted in symptomatic improvement but produced a homonymous hemianopsia.[39] Careful clinical follow-up is needed to document long-term effectiveness before the use of pallidotomy in the treatment of dystonia can be recommended.

The neurosurgical treatment of dystonia is evolving rapidly. Thalamotomy for dystonia has been performed more frequently than pallidotomy, although the results are highly variable.[2,10,12,28,77] Generalized dystonia is bilateral; however, bilateral lesions may have unacceptable risks. Deep brain stimulation techniques may prove to be the most appropriate surgical treatment of this condition.[5,8,65]

Huntington's Disease

Huntington's disease is an autosomal dominant degenerative brain disease. In the early stages, its cardinal motor sign is chorea, whereas later stages are often characterized by an akinetic rigid state. Its pathophysiological hallmark is degeneration of striatal output neurons. Huntington's disease is due to expansion of a trinucleotide repeat region on chromosome 4 that encodes for the protein Huntingtin, but it is not known how this gene defect produces the observed pathology and clinical signs.[33]

The first use of stereotactic pallidotomy for a movement disorder was for Huntington's disease.[70] In three of four reported patients, bilateral pallidotomy decreased choreiform movements at follow-up times of 9-10 years.[71] The location of the lesions in these cases is unclear. While lesions for parkinsonism performed by the same group targeted the anterodorsal pallidum,[69] lesions for Huntington's disease were reportedly placed more laterally, and may have involved the GPe.[72] More recently, Laitinen and Hariz[42] reported complete relief of contralateral chorea in a patient with Huntington's disease, following lesioning of the "ventroposterolateral" pallidum, which probably included portions of both the GPe and the GPi. It is unclear whether this procedure could provide meaningful functional benefit to patients, because chorea is more prominent earlier in the disease and because nonmotor signs such as depression, psychotic behavior, and dementia often result in greater disability than do the motor signs.

Results of Pallidotomy: Theoretical Aspects

Effect of Pallidotomy on Cortical Function in Parkinson's Disease

According to the model of DeLong,[15] the GPi in the parkinsonian state is overactive and cortical regions involved in motor control are inhibited. Lesions in the sensorimotor region of the GPi decrease the inhibitory influence of the GPi on the motor thalamus, and restore thalamocortical activity. Based on this model of Parkinson's disease, normalization of thalamocortical activity should in turn lead to amelioration of the motor signs associated with parkinsonism. In support of this theory, pallidotomy in parkinsonian patients is associated with increased activation of cortical motor areas, as determined by positron emission tomography. Following pallidotomy, metabolic activity in the supplementary motor area is increased during performance of timed motor tasks, as compared with the preoperative state.[11,27] The metabolic activity of motor and premotor cortex in the resting state is increased as well.[20]

Unexplained Effects of Pallidotomy

Not all clinical effects of pallidotomy can be explained by this model. Because hyperkinetic disorders are presumably due to increased thalamocortical activity,[15] it is unclear why pallidotomy simultaneously improves bradykinesia and dyskinesias. One possibility is that hypokinetic and hyperkinetic signs are mediated by different pallidal output pathways. The pedunculopontine nucleus receives major output from the GPi and probably plays an important, although poorly understood, role in motor control.[63,86] It has been speculated that hyperkinetic signs of movement disorders are mediated by the ascending thalamocortical projections, while bradykinetic signs are mediated by the descending projections from the GPi and pars reticulata of the substantia nigra to the pedunculopontine nucleus.[36,66]

An alternative explanation is that the current model[15] considers abnormal motor function to result from alterations in mean discharge rates within the basal ganglia-thalamocortical circuit. In the pathophysiology of movement disorders, however, alterations in the pattern of action potential firing may be much more important than alterations in mean rates. Recent observations of the altered patterns of neuronal activity in patients with dystonia[82] and hemiballismus[83] support this hypothesis. As understanding of these altered patterns is gained, the role of thalamocortical pathways in mediating different types of movement disorders may be clarified.

Conclusions

Surgery for movement disorders is a rapidly advancing area. While pallidotomy has been performed for over 40 years, changes in the patient population, surgical techniques, and standards for quantitative motor assessment have changed, mandating a thorough reassessment of this technique. At 24-month evaluations, unilateral posterolateral GPi pallidotomy for Parkinson's disease offers significant benefit for most motor signs, as assessed by standard parkinsonian rating scales, and is relatively safe. The safety of bilateral pallidotomy requires further scrutiny. The best reported results of some other surgical procedures for Parkinson's disease, such as bilateral STN stimulation, are comparable to the best reported results of pallidotomy. In a small number of short-term studies, pallidotomy offers benefit in other movement disorders, including hemiballismus and dystonia. Even as the reassessment of ablative techniques progresses, nonablative and restorative techniques offer promise for the future treatment of movement disorders.

References

1. Alexander GE, Crutcher MD, DeLong MR: Basal ganglia-thalamocortical circuits: parallel substrates for motor, oculomotor, "prefrontal" and "limbic" functions. **Prog Brain Res 85:**119-146, 1990
2. Andrew J, Fowler CJ, Harrison MJG: Stereotaxic thalamotomy in 55 cases of dystonia. **Brain 106:** 981-1000, 1983
3. Andy OJ: Diencephalic coagulation in the treatment of hemiballismus. **Confin Neurol 22:**346-350, 1962
4. Baron MS, Vitek JL, Bakay RAE, et al: Treatment of advanced Parkinson's disease by posterior GPi pallidotomy: 1-year results of a pilot study. **Ann Neurol 40:**355-366, 1996
5. Benabid AL, Pollak P, Gao D, et al: Chronic electrical stimulation of the ventralis intermedius nucleus of the thalamus as a treatment of movement disorders. **J Neurosurg 84:**203-214, 1996
6. Bergman H, Wichmann T, DeLong MR: Reversal of experimental parkinsonism by lesions of the subthalamic nucleus. **Science 249:**1436-1438, 1990
7. Blanchet PJ, Boucher R, Bédard PJ: Excitotoxic lateral pallidotomy does not relieve L-DOPA-induced dyskinesia in MPTP parkinsonian monkeys. **Brain Res 650:**32-39, 1994
8. Blond S, Siegfried J: Thalamic stimulation for the treatment of tremor and other movement disorders. **Acta Neurochir Suppl 52:**109-111, 1991
9. Burzaco J: Stereotactic pallidotomy in extrapyramidal disorders. **Appl Neurophysiol 48:**283-287, 1985
10. Cardoso F, Jankovic J, Grossman RG, et al: Outcome after stereotactic thalamotomy for dystonia and hemiballismus. **Neurosurgery 36:**501-508, 1995
11. Ceballos-Baumann AO, Obeso JA, Vitek JL, et al: Restoration of thalamocortical activity after posteroventral pallidotomy in Parkinson's disease. **Lancet 344:**814, 1994 (Letter)
12. Cooper IS: 20-year followup study of the neurosurgical treatment of dystonia musculorum deformans. **Adv Neurol 14:**423-452, 1976
13. Cooper IS: Ligation of the anterior choroidal artery

for involuntary movements of parkinsonism. **Psychiatr Q 27**:317-319, 1953
14. Cooper IS, Bravo G: Chemopallidectomy and chemothalamectomy. **J Neurosurg 15**:244-250, 1958
15. DeLong MR: Primate models of movement disorders of basal ganglia origin. **Trends Neurosci 13**: 281-285, 1990
16. DeLong MR, Crutcher MD, Georgopoulis AP: Primate globus pallidus and subthalamic nucleus: functional organization. **J Neurophysiol 53**:530-543, 1985
17. Dewey RB Jr, Jankovic J: Hemiballism-hemichorea. Clinical and pharmacologic findings in 21 patients. **Arch Neurol 46**:862-867, 1989
18. Diederich N, Goetz CG, Stebbins GT, et al: Blinded evaluation confirms long-term asymmetric effect of unilateral thalamotomy or subthalamotomy on tremor in Parkinson's disease. **Neurology 42**: 1311-1314, 1992
19. Dogali M, Fazzini E, Kolodny E, et al: Stereotactic ventral pallidotomy for Parkinson's disease. **Neurology 45**:753-761, 1995
20. Eidelberg D, Moeller JR, Ishikawa T, et al: Regional metabolic correlates of surgical outcome following unilateral pallidotomy for Parkinson's disease. **Ann Neurol 39**:450-459, 1996
21. Favre J, Taha JM, Nguyen TT, et al: Pallidotomy: a survey of current practice in North America. **Neurosurgery 39**:883-892, 1996
22. Fazzini E, Dogali M, Berich A, et al: Ventral pallidotomy operations in patients with Parkinson's plus syndromes: lack of significant symptomatic benefit. **Ann Neurol 34**:266, 1993 (Abstract)
23. Fox MW, Ahlskog JE, Kelly PJ: Stereotactic ventrolateralis thalamotomy for medically refractory tremor in post-levodopa era Parkinson's disease patients. **J Neurosurg 75**:723-730, 1991
24. Freidman JH, Epstein M, Sanes JN, et al: Gamma knife pallidotomy in advanced Parkinson's disease. **Ann Neurol 39**:535-538, 1996
25. Gildenberg PL: Studies in stereoencephalotomy VIII. Comparison of the variability of subcortical lesions produced by various procedures. **Confin Neurol 17**: 299-309, 1957
26. Gioino CG, Dierssen G, Cooper IS: The effect of subcortical lesions on production and alleviation of hemiballic or hemichoreic movements. **J Neurol Sci 3**: 10-36, 1966
27. Grafton ST, Waters C, Sutton J, et al: Pallidotomy increases activity of motor association cortex in Parkinson's disease: a positron emission tomographic study. **Ann Neurol 37**:776-783, 1995
28. Gros C, Frerebeau P, Perez-Dominquez E, et al: Long term results of stereotaxic surgery for infantile dystonia and dyskinesia. **Neurochirurgia 19**:171-178, 1976
29. Guiot G, Brion S: Traitement des mouvements anormaux par la coagulation pallidale. Technique et résultats. **Rev Neurol 89**:578-580, 1953
30. Hassler R, Mundinger F, Riechert T: **Stereotaxis in Parkinsonian Syndrome.** New York, NY: Springer-Verlag, 1979, pp 183-196
31. Hassler R, Riechert T: Indikationen und Lokalisations-methode der gezielten Hirnoperationen. **Nervenarzt 25**:441-447, 1954
32. Hornykiewicz O, Kish SJ: Biochemical pathophysiology of Parkinson's disease. **Adv Neurol 45**:19-34, 1986
33. The Huntington's Disease Collaborative Research Group: A novel gene containing a trinucleotide repeat that is expanded and unstable on Huntington's disease chromosomes. **Cell 72**:971-983, 1993
34. The Huntington's Study Group: Unified Huntington's Disease Rating Scale: reliability and consistency. **Mov Disord 11**:136-142, 1996
35. Iacono RP, Kuniyoshi SM, Lonser RR, et al: Simultaneous bilateral pallidoansotomy for idiopathic dystonia musculorum deformans. **Pediatr Neurol 14**: 145-148, 1996
36. Iacono RP, Shima F, Lonser RR, et al: The results, indications, and physiology of posteroventral pallidotomy for patients with Parkinson's disease. **Neurosurgery 36**:1118-1127, 1995
37. Jankovic J, Cardoso F, Grossman RG, et al: Outcome after stereotactic thalamotomy for Parkinsonian, essential, and other types of tremor. **Neurosurgery 37**: 680-687, 1995
38. Johansson F, Malm J, Nordh E, et al: Usefulness of pallidotomy in advanced Parkinson's disease. **J Neurol Neurosurg Psychiatry 62**:125-132, 1997
39. Kwon Y, Whang CJ: Stereotactic Gamma Knife radiosurgery for the treatment of dystonia. **Stereotact Funct Neurosurg 64 (Suppl 1)**:222-227, 1995
40. Laitinen LV: Pallidotomy for Parkinson's disease. **Neurosurg Clin N Am 6**:105-112, 1995
41. Laitinen LV, Bergenheim AT, Hariz MI: Leksell's posteroventral pallidotomy in the treatment of Parkinson's disease. **J Neurosurg 76**:53-61, 1992
42. Laitinen LV, Hariz MI: Movement disorders, in Youmans JR (ed): **Neurological Surgery.** Philadelphia, Pa: WB Saunders, 1996, pp 3575-3609
43. Lang AE: Medial pallidotomy. **Mov Disord 11 (Suppl 1)**:12, 1996 (Abstract)
44. Lang AE, Lozano A, Galvez-Jiménez N, et al: Posteroventral-medial pallidotomy for late-stage Parkinson's disease: a 2-year follow-up. **Ann Neurol 40**: 538, 1996 (Abstract)
45. Langston JW, Widner H, Goetz CG, et al: Core assessment program for intracerebral transplantations (CAPIT). **Mov Disord 7**:2-13, 1992
46. Lee MS, Marsden CD: Movement disorders following lesions of the thalamus or subthalamic region. **Mov Disord 9**:493-507, 1994
47. Levesque MF, Markham C, Nakasato N: MR-guided ventral intermediate thalamotomy for post-traumatic hemiballismus. **Stereotact Funct Neurosurg 58**:88, 1992 (Abstract)
48. Lieberman DM, Oldfield EH, Corthesy ME: Selective lesioning of large brain structures using high-flow microfusion of neurotoxins: chemopallidotomy reverses experimental parkinsonism. **J Neurosurg 84**: 333A, 1996 (Abstract)
49. Limousin P, Pollak P, Benazzouz A, et al: Effect on parkinsonian signs and symptoms of bilateral subthalamic nucleus stimulation. **Lancet 345**:91-95, 1995
50. Limousin P, Pollak P, Hoffman D, et al: Abnormal involuntary movements induced by subthalamic nucleus stimulation in parkinsonian patients. **Mov Disord 11**:231-235, 1996
51. Lozano A, Hutchison W, Kiss Z, et al: Methods for microelectrode-guided posteroventral pallidotomy. **J Neurosurg 84**:194-202, 1996
52. Lozano AM, Lang AE, Galvez-Jimenez N, et al: Effects of GPi pallidotomy on motor function in Parkinson's disease. **Lancet 346**:1383-1387, 1995

53. Maciunas RJ, Galloway RL Jr, Latimer JW: The application accuracy of stereotactic frames. **Neurosurgery 35:**682-695, 1994
54. Marsden CD, Obeso JA, Zarranz JJ, et al: The anatomical basis of symptomatic dystonia. **Brain 108:** 463-483, 1985
55. Meyers HR: Surgical procedures for postencephalitic tremor, with notes on the physiology of premotor fibers. **Arch Neurol Psychiatry 44:**455-459, 1940
56. Narabayashi H, Okuma T: Procaine oil blocking of the globus pallidus for the treatment of rigidity and tremor of parkinsonism. **Psychiatr Neurol Japonica 56:**471-495, 1954
57. Narabayashi H, Yokochi F, Nakajima Y: Levodopa-induced dyskinesias and thalamotomy. **J Neurol Neurosurg Psychiatr 47:**831-839, 1984
58. Pahwa R, Wilkinson S, Smith D, et al: High-frequency pallidal stimulation in Parkinson's disease. **Ann Neurol 40:**533, 1996 (Abstract)
59. Pettigrew LC, Jankovic J: Hemidystonia: a report of 22 patients and a review of the literature. **J Neurol Neurosurg Psychiatry 48:**650-657, 1985
60. Rand RW, Brown WJ, Stern WE: Surgical occlusion of anterior choroidal arteries in parkinsonism. Clinical and neuropathologic findings. **Neurology 6:** 390-401, 1956
61. Rand RW, Jacques DB, Melbye RW, et al: Gamma Knife thalamotomy and pallidotomy in patients with movement disorders: preliminary results. **Stereotact Funct Neurosurg 61 (Suppl 1):**65-92, 1993
62. Roberts-Warrior D, Overby AS, Orr D, et al: Postural control in patients with Parkinson's disease after pallidotomy. **Ann Neurol 40:**534, 1996 (Abstract)
63. Rye DB, Turner RS, Vitek JL, et al: Anatomical investigations of the pallidotegmental pathway in monkey and man, in Ohye C (ed): **The Basal Ganglia V.** New York, NY: Plenum, 1996, pp 59-75
64. Schwab RS, England AC: Projection technique for evaluating surgery in Parkinson's disease, in Gillingham FJ, Donaldson IML (eds): **Third Symposium on Parkinson's Disease.** Edinburgh: E & S Livingstone, 1969, pp 152-157
65. Sellal F, Hirsch E, Barth P, et al: A case of symptomatic hemidystonia improved by ventroposterolateral thalamic electrostimulation. **Mov Disord 8:**515-518, 1993
66. Shima F, Ishido K, Sun S, et al: Surgical control of akinesia in Parkinson's disease. **Eur Neurol 36 (Suppl 1):**55-61, 1996
67. Siegfried J, Lippitz B: Bilateral chronic electrostimulation of ventroposterolateral pallidum: a new therapeutic approach for alleviating all Parkinsonian symptoms. **Neurosurgery 35:**1126-1130, 1994
68. Smith MC: Pathological findings subsequent to stereotactic lesions. **J Neurosurg 24:**443-445, 1966
69. Spiegel EA, Wycis HT: Ansotomy in paralysis agitans. **Arch Neurol Psychiatry 71:**598-614, 1954
70. Spiegel EA, Wycis HT: Thalamotomy and pallidotomy for treatment of choreic movements. **Acta Neurochir 2:**417-422, 1952
71. Spiegel EA, Wycis HT, Baird HW III: Long-range effects of electropallidoansotomy in extrapyramidal and convulsive disorders. **Neurology 8:**734-740, 1958
72. Spiegel EA, Wycis HT, Freed H: Stereoencephalotomy. Thalamotomy and related procedures. **JAMA 148:**446-451, 1952
73. Sterio D, Berić A, Dogali M, et al: Neurophysiological properties of pallidal neurons in Parkinson's disease. **Ann Neurol 35:**586-591, 1994
74. Sutton JP, Couldwell W, Lew MF, et al: Ventroposterior medial pallidotomy in patients with advanced Parkinson's disease. **Neurosurgery 36:**1112-1117, 1995
75. Svennilson E, Torvik A, Lowe R, et al: Treatment of parkinsonism by stereotactic thermolesions in the pallidal region. A clinical evaluation of 81 cases. **Acta Psychiatry Neurol Scand 35:**358-377, 1960
76. Talairach J, Paillas JE, David M: Dyskinésie de type hémiballique traitée par cortectomie frontale limitée, puis par coagulation de l'anse lenticulaire et de la portion interne du globus pallidus. Amélioration importance depuis un an. **Rev Neurol 83:**440-451, 1950
77. Tasker RR, Doorly T, Yamashiro K: Thalamotomy in generalized dystonia. **Adv Neurol 50:**615-631, 1988
78. Tsubokawa T, Moriyasu N: Lateral pallidotomy for relief of ballistic movement—its basic evidences and clinical application. **Confin Neurol 37:**10-15, 1975
79. Vitek JL, Bakay RAE, DeLong MR: Microelectrode guided GPi pallidotomy for medically intractable Parkinson's disease. **Adv Neurol 74:**183-198, 1997
80. Vitek JL, Bakay RAE, Hashimoto T, et al: Microelectrode-guided pallidotomy: Technical approach and application for medically intractable Parkinson's disease. **J Neurosurg** (In press)
81. Vitek JL, Baron M, Bakay RAE, et al: Pallidotomy for medically intractable Parkinson's disease: 2 year followup. **Ann Neurol 40:**488, 1996 (Abstract)
82. Vitek JL, Evatt M, Zhang J, et al: Treatment of dystonia with GPi pallidotomy: neuronal activity and clinical outcome. **Dystonia** (In press)
83. Vitek JL, Kaneoke Y, Hashimoto T, et al: Neuronal activity in the pallidum of a patient with hemiballismus. **Ann Neurol 38:**296-297, 1995 (Abstract)
84. White RJ, MacCarty CS, Bahn RC: Neuropathologic review of brain lesions and inherent dangers in chemopallidectomy. **Arch Neurol 2:**12-18, 1960
85. Young RF, Vermeulen SS, Grimm P, et al: Electrophysiological target localization is not required for the treatment of functional disorders. **Stereotact Funct Neurosurg 66 (Suppl 1):**309-319, 1997
86. Zweig RM, Jankel WR, Hedreen JC, et al: The pedunculopontine nucleus in Parkinson's disease. **Ann Neurol 26:**41-46, 1989

PART C

Treatment of Parkinson's Disease: Restorative Surgical Procedures

CHAPTER 11

CHRONIC DEEP BRAIN STIMULATION: INDICATIONS AND TECHNIQUES

ISABELLE M. GERMANO, MD

The concept of high-frequency electrical stimulation to ameliorate parkinsonian tremor was recognized by Hassler[10] and numerous other groups,[2,11,26] who used electrical stimulation instead of or together with microrecording to map the areas surrounding the ventral intermediate (VIM) nucleus of the thalamus while performing thalamotomy. These authors observed that high-frequency (>100 Hz) stimulation of the VIM suppressed parkinsonian rest tremor and that this was reversible, as the effects would stop as soon as the stimulation was discontinued. The first report of an implanted deep brain stimulator in the VIM providing significant amelioration of parkinsonian tremor led to subsequent clinical trials.[1-4,14]

The aim of this chapter is to review indications, contraindications, anatomical targets, and surgical techniques of deep brain stimulation (DBS) for surgical teatment of Parkinson's disease.

PATIENT SELECTION

Indications

The key to successful neurosurgical treatment of movement disorders rests on careful patient selection. Prior to consideration for surgery, all patients should have adequate trial of medical therapy, as reviewed in Chapter 7, "Pharmacological Treatment of Movement Disorders." When medical treatment is unsuccessful, as measured by lack of amelioration of symptoms and/or occurrence of side effects (mostly dyskinesias), surgery is indicated. Naturally, the diagnosis of Parkinson's disease must be confirmed and the patient must have shown responsiveness to levodopa (L-DOPA).

There have been no studies directly comparing indications and benefits of chronic brain stimulation to those of conventional ablative procedures for treatment of Parkinson's disease. Currently, there is no clear evidence that DBS results in superior amelioration of Parkinson's disease symptoms or decreased morbidity compared to ablative procedures. Although ablative procedures can be very successful in suppressing parkinsonian tremor, a high rate of symptom recurrence over time is reported. Furthermore, tissue ablation may be associated with transitory or permanent deficits, such as motor deficit, dystonia, speech disturbance, sensory loss, and visual field cuts (see Chapter 10, "Pallidotomy: Clinical Results").

The theoretical advantage of restorative over ablative procedures is the lack of tissue destruction, especially with DBS. This is particularly appealing for patients needing bilateral procedures. Furthermore, DBS may be reversible. In two thirds of patients with a VIM deep brain stimulator, the stimulator could be turned off at night, with return to pre-implant conditions. On the other hand, in one third of patients, discontinuation of the VIM stimulation resulted in a rebound effect with increased intensity of the tremor.[2] When reversibility is possible, the opportunity to employ future therapies, if proven to be efficacious, exists. Furthermore, DBS provides adaptability, as stimulation parameters can be adjusted to optimize resolution of symptoms while minimizing side effects.

The disadvantages of DBS include side effects associated with any implantable device, such as mechanical failure and infections. Furthermore, the system is costly. Additionally, at the present time, further surgery is necessary to replace the batteries of the pulse generator every 2-4 years. Finally, a high percentage of patients may experience transient side effects after chronic stimulation.[2]

Currently, the only DBS procedure for movement disorders approved by the Food and Drug Administration (FDA) in the United States is chronic stimulation of the VIM for essential or parkinsonian tremor. The choice of DBS over a standard ablative procedure should be discussed by the surgeon with the patient in each case. Until more clinical data on the use of DBS are acquired, the ultimate decision whether to perform an ablative or restorative procedure will continue to rely on the physician-patient discussion.

Contraindications

Contraindications for DBS include those of any stereotactic procedure. Coagulopathy, the use of antiplatelet agents, and uncontrolled hypertension are contraindications to surgical stereotactic procedures, as they increase the risk of intraoperative hemorrhage. If a patient is on a course of aspirin, typically it is discontinued at least 10 days prior to surgery. Ipsilateral hemianopsia is a contraindication for pallidotomy or pallidal stimulation, as contralateral hemianopsia may be a complication of this procedure. There is no unanimous consent on age limits. At the author's institution, procedures are generally limited to patients in the seventh decade.

Patients with Parkinson's plus syndromes respond poorly to DBS, presumably because the underlying pathophysiology is not the same as for idiopathic Parkinson's disease. This spectrum of diseases includes Shy-Drager syndrome, striatonigral degeneration, progressive supranuclear palsy, and olivopontocerebeller atrophy. In these syndromes, observation of autonomic dysfunction, cerebellar signs, lack of response to L-DOPA are used to differentiate them from Parkinson's disease.

The role of surgical procedures in patients with Hoehn and Yahr Stage 5 is not clear, as it appears that symptomatic improvement may not translate into functional improvement. Similarly, dementia is a contraindication to surgery.

Selecting the Target

Clinical and laboratory data support the concept that Parkinson's disease is associated with increased basal ganglia output, as described in detail in Chapter 4, "Pathophysiology of Movement Disorders and Basal Ganglia." The goal of ablative procedures is to destroy the center responsible for this increased output by targeting different nuclei, depending on the predominant symptom. The best target is the VIM when the predominant symptom is tremor, and the globus pallidus when the predominant symptoms are dyskinesia and rigidity.[24] The straightforward mechanism of action for ablative procedures is neuronal demise as a result of thermocoagulation. Similarly, chronic high-frequency brain stimulation results in a decreased output of the targeted nucleus. However, its mechanisms of action remain speculative.

In general terms, the effects of chronic stimulation can be described as a change in the proportion of the excitatory and inhibitory drives to a neural network and the corresponding neurotransmitter levels, thereby changing the response of this network to physiological input signals. A well-known example is the modulation of pain signals in the "gate control" theory of Melzack and Wall.[20] According to this theory, activity in large-caliber, primary afferent nerves evokes inhibitory synaptic potentials in spinal neurons that are part of the pain transmission pathway. Therefore, the transmission of pain signals to the brain can be blocked by the electrical stimulation of these large fibers. The basis for the mechanism of DBS for Parkinson's disease seems, however, more complex. In fact, only high frequencies (>100 Hz) reduce tremor, while frequencies of <100 Hz generally increase tremor. This suggests that the therapeutic effect is due to an inhibition of neuronal activity.[6,8] Other mechanisms are also advocated and include depolarization blockade, stimulation of inhibitory interneurons, and jamming of neuronal activity.[2,5,9] Furthermore, it is not clear whether the cells are stimulated directly by the electrical impulse or synaptically through other elements.[22]

Irrespective of its mechanisms of action, chronic high-frequency stimulation results in amelioration of Parkinson's symptoms. Different basal ganglia nuclei can be targeted depending on the predominant parkinsonian feature. Similarly to ablative procedures, the VIM nucleus of the thalamus is chosen when the predominant symptom is contralateral tremor.[2,14] This could be essential or parkinsonian tremor.[12] In patients selected to undergo a VIM procedure, the tremor should constitute a significant functional disability and be refractory to pharmacological therapies.

Recent advances in the understanding of the pathophysiological mechanisms underlying Parkinson's disease suggest that different targets—in particular, the globus pallidus and the subthalamic nucleus (STN)—may be used to treat other features of Parkinson's disease. The author and colleagues have recently completed a multicenter clinical study to assess the effects of DBS for treatment of Parkinson's disease with implants in the internal segment of the globus pallidus (GPi) and STN. Although the results of this study will be reported elsewhere in detail, the globus pallidus seems to be a promising target for amelioration of contralateral dyskinesias and rigidity. Furthermore, levodopa-induced dyskinesias seem to be improved by chronic GPi stimulation. The STN seems to be an excellent target for contralateral rigidity and dyskinesias, and to ameliorate problems in other areas caused by Parkinson's disease, including rapid alternating movements, gait, postural stability, and daily activities.[21] Further studies are warranted to corroborate these and other preliminary observations.[16,17]

Target Localization

At the author's institution, all stereotactic procedures for implantation of DBS electrodes are performed with local anesthesia and minimal sedation as needed. The Cosman-Roberts-Wells (CRW) stereotactic system (Radionics, Burlington, Massachusetts) is applied with a local anesthetic, supplemented with short-acting anxiolytic agents the morning of the procedures. The base of the frame should be below the orbitomeatal line (under the tip of the nose) to assure accurate targeting of deep targets. Anti-parkinsonian medications are usually withheld the day before surgery in order to accentuate the symptoms.

The standard, FDA-approved target site for DBS implants for control of tremor is the VIM nucleus of the thalamus. This nucleus is bounded laterally by the internal capsule and posteriorly by the ventral posterolateral (VPL) nuclei of the thalamus. The VIM can be localized using magnetic resonance imaging (MRI), computed tomography, and ventriculography. Different measurement techniques can be used to locate the VIM on images. One method for its localization is based on Guiot's diagram, which divides the anterior commissure (AC)-posterior commissure (PC) line in twelfths.[2] The VIM is located 2/12 to 3/12 of the distance from the PC and 11 mm from the lateral wall of the third ventricle in the plane of the AC-PC line. The author uses MRI localization. Axial T1-weighted images are meticulously acquired in the plane of the AC-PC line (GE 1.5-T scanner, General Electric, Milwaukee, Wisconsin; spin echo; TR 600; TE 14; thickness 2 mm; interspace 0, matrix 256 × 256; 2 NEX).The VIM is located 3 mm posterior to the midcommissural point, 2.5 mm superior to the intercommissural line, and 14 mm lateral to the lateral wall of the third ventricle.[13]

Similarly, MRI targeting may be used for the GPi (Figure 1). Laitinen et al[15] have provided widely used coordinates for the GPi. The ideal target is 2-3 mm anterior, 18-22 mm lateral, and 6 mm inferior to the AC-PC. These coordinates

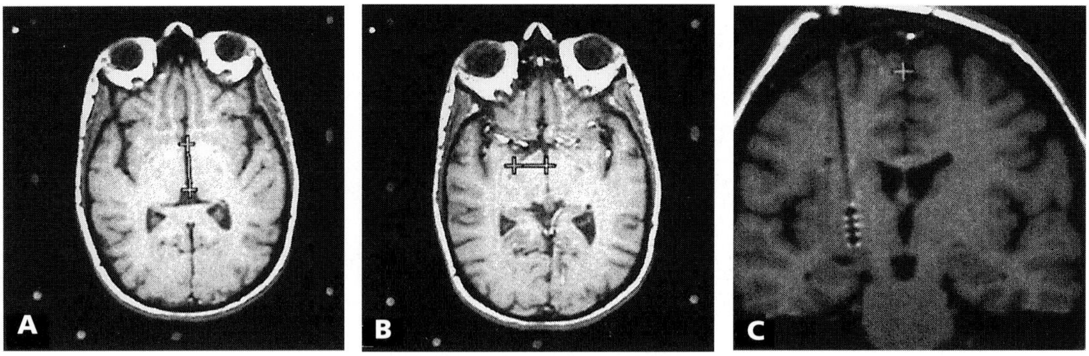

Figure 1: Axial T1-weighted brain MRIs used to target the GPi for chronic DBS. **A)** Image at the level of the AC-PC plane. The length of the midcommisural line is first measured; here it is 29 mm. **B)** Image at 6 mm inferior to the AC-PC line. The medial cross is 2 mm anterior to the midcommissure and the lateral cross is 19 mm lateral to it. These arbitrary measurements, based on work by Laitinen et al,[15] were adjusted after projecting them onto the image. It is indeed obvious that the arbitrarily chosen target is 1 mm too lateral and 1 mm too inferior. **C)** Postoperative MRI showing a deep brain electrode in the globus pallidus. The four contacts are seen as signal voids due to metallic artifact. The MRI- based target was intraoperatively confirmed by microrecording and stimulation (see text).

are projected onto the MRIs and the final location of the chosen target is adjusted based on recognition of the internal capsule, which is medial to the GPi and the optic tract, inferior to the GPi, and readily seen on the sequences used. When targeting the ventrolateral GPi, the ideal target is 2 mm superior and just lateral to the optic tract, to include the junction of the ansa lenticularis with the GPi.

The STN, or corpus luysi, can be easily localized on T1-weighted coronal images (GE 1.5-T scanner; spin echo; TR 800; TE 50; thickness 2 mm; interspace 0, matrix 256 × 256; 2 NEX). Other sequences can be used to localize the STN, including fast spin echo inversion recovery, T2-weighted images, and gradient echo acquisitions. In the author's experience with phantoms, however, these sequences result in a greater distortion of the stereotactic coordinates than the sequence reported above. The STN is a small (approximately 1 cm), almond-shaped nucleus that lies ventral to the thalamus, medial to the posterior limb of the internal capsule, and lateral to the red nucleus. It is caudal and slightly lateral to the pars reticulata of the substantia nigra (SNr), and rostral to the STN is the zona incerta (Figures 2 and 3).

After the desired target is localized, computer-assisted technology, as described in Chapter 16, "Interactive Computer-Assisted Image-Guided Technology as an Adjuvant to Neurosurgery for Movement Disorders," is used to choose a trajectory avoiding sulci and ventricular cavities.

Intraoperative Procedure

Burr Hole and Placement of Recording Electrode

The patient is positioned supine on the operating table with the head fixed in a Mayfield adapter for the CRW frame. Attention to neck position and the use of an indwelling urinary catheter is important to optimize comfort, which is necessary for a meaningful intraoperative neurological examination. The hair is shaved over the frontotemporal area, a linear paramedial skin incision approximately 3 cm long is marked and infiltrated with local anesthetic, and a clear drape is used. Intravenous sedation is used to supplement the local anesthetic. This includes intravenous midazolam supplemented by fentanyl and/or propofol. A burr hole is then made with a power drill using a disposable 14-mm perforator (Acra-Cut, Codman, Philadelphia, Pennsylvania). After generous irrigation is used to wash out all the bony debris, a burr hole ring is placed on the burr hole. This will allow the surgeon to

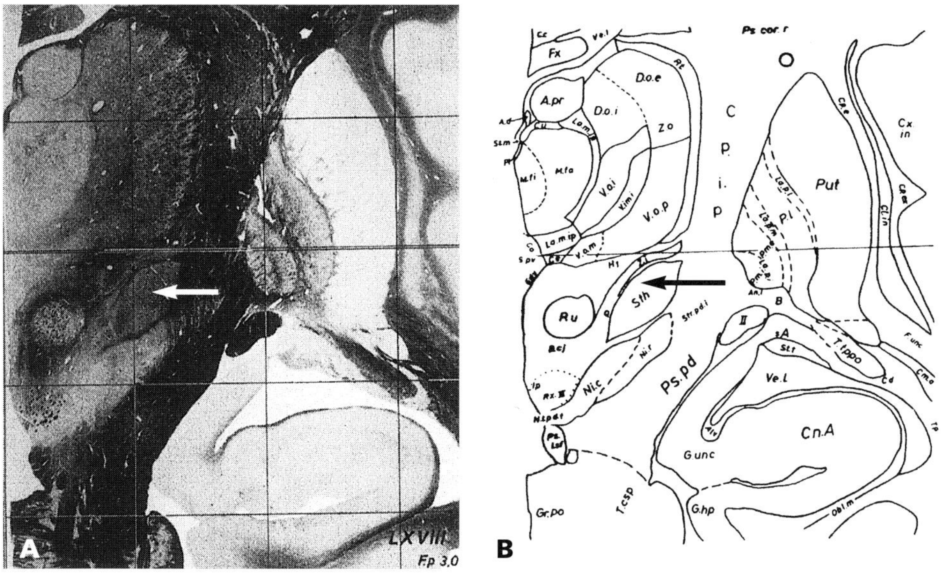

Figure 2: Coronal views of the brain through the STN: **A)** Myelin-stained brain section; **B)** Diagram of the brain. The STN *(arrow)* is ventral to the thalamic nuclei and the zona incerta (Zi), dorsal to the substantia nigra reticulata (Nir), medial to the internal capsule (Cpip), and lateral to the red nucleus (Ru). (Reproduced from Schaltenbrand and Wahren,[23] Plate 27, Figure LXVIII, with permission.)

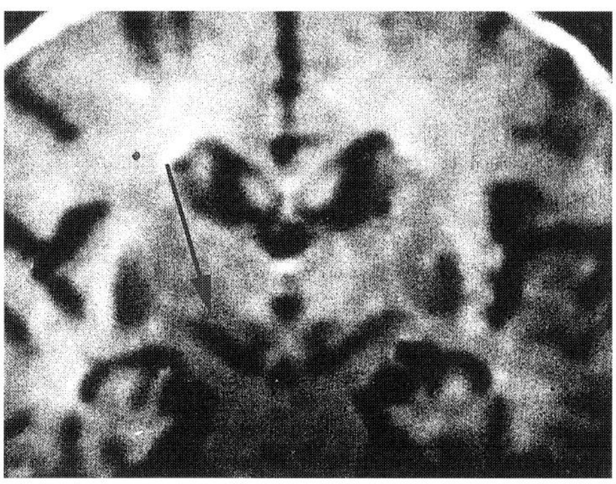

Figure 3: Coronal T1-weighted brain MRI with appropriate windowing used to target the STN for chronic DBS. The STN *(arrow)* is located caudal and slightly lateral to the SNr, easily seen as a band of decreased signal intensity.

secure the electrode in place at the end of the procedure; however, the author prefers to place it before the permanent electrode is passed to avoid its manipulation. At the author's institution, intraoperative electrophysiological microrecording is used to optimize the MRI-selected target. The guiding cannula is then inserted to 10 mm above the target under stereotactic guidance and microrecording, as described in Chapter 15, "Intraoperative Electrophysiological Recording Techniques." Advancement of the microrecording electrode is done using a digital microdriver at 0.25-mm increments. When electrophysiological localization of the target is satisfactory, as confirmed by microrecording, a stimulating test electrode is inserted to perform macrostimulation.

Clinical Assessment of Electrode Placement

The Ventral Intermediate Nucleus

Stimulation is performed while neurological assessment of the tremor is obtained. Typically, the author's stimulation parameters consist of an amplitude of <3 V, a pulse width of 60-120 μsec, and a frequency of 130 Hz. The amplitude is gradually increased until there is suppression of tremor. Tremor suppression occurs at low voltage, <3 V. All types of tremors are assessed: resting, postural, and action tremor. Resting tremor is present when the limb is fully supported against gravity and the relevant muscles are not voluntarily activated. Resting tremor is tested by observing the hand resting on the thigh. Postural tremor is apparent during the voluntary maintenance of a particular posture against gravity. This is tested by asking the patient to hold the hands prone in front of the nose. Action tremor is evident during any type of movement; typically it is assessed with the finger-to-nose test. If tremor suppression does not occur or occurs only at amplitudes of >3 V, placement of the electrode in the VIM is suboptimal. The author then proceeds to stimulate at changing frequencies and voltage to rule out the presence of side effects. Contralateral paresthesia, contralateral contractions, and ocular phenomena are the three most common side effects observed when the location of the electrode is suboptimal.

At low voltage, paresthesia in the contralateral hand or the corner of the mouth suggests that the electrode is placed close to the border of the VPL sensory thalamus. Contralateral tonic contraction with high-frequency stimulation or contralateral twitching synchronous with stimulation at low frequency indicates that the electrode is placed too laterally near the internal capsule. Ocular phenomena, fear, and dizziness may occur when the electrode is placed in the mesencephalon.

The Internal Segment of the Globus Pallidus

While the effects on tremor are clearly seen with stimulation of the VIM, clinical evaluation of symptom resolution is more complex for the GPi. This includes assessment of "cogwheel rigidity" and dyskinesia.

The strategy for implantation of a permanent electrode in the GPi includes finding its lateral boundary, the internal capsule, and its inferior boundary, the optic tract. Tonic movements at low voltage (<3 V) is evidence that the electrode tip is too close to the internal capsule and should be moved 1-2 mm laterally. When aiming for placement of the permanent electrode to involve the ansa lenticularis, visual stimulation is performed.[18] The operating room is darkened, as most patients detect stimulation-evoked visual sensation best in the dark. Microstimulation of the optic tract evokes visual sensations at low

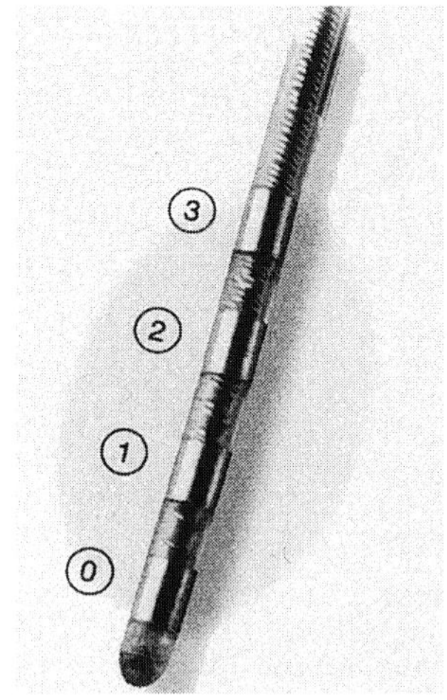

Figure 4: Tetrapolar deep brain electrode. Each number indicates a contact; contact 0 is the most distal. The shaded area indicates the amount of tissue that can be electrically stimulated using different bipolar and monopolar combinations. In reality, the amount of tissue stimulated at any given time is smaller, as bipolar stimulation usually occurs at two adjacent contacts.

amplitude. Patients report seeing flashing lights, white stars, or colored bands (phosphenes) in the contralateral visual field. The visual sensations usually increase with increased current amplitude; the author does not exceed 6 V. The depth of the stimulating electrode when visual sensations are reported is noted. Calculations are then made to position the most distal contact (contact "0") of the permanent electrode 1.5 mm rostral to where the visual sensations were elicited.

The Subthalamic Nucleus

Similarly to the GPi, clinical evaluation of the resolution of Parkinson's disease symptoms following stimulation in the STN includes assessment of cogwheel rigidity, dyskinesia, and tremor. Side effects after stimulation to map the boundaries of the STN include tonic movements when the electrode is too lateral and involves the internal capsule. On the other hand, mydriasis may be seen if the electrode is placed too far medially.

Permanent Electrode Implantation

After adequate placement of the electrode is

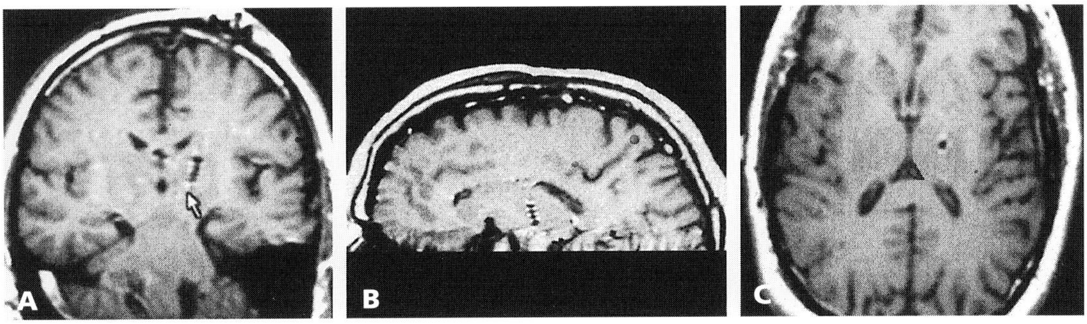

Figure 5: Postoperative coronal **(A)**, sagittal **(B)**, and axial **(C)** brain MRIs showing a tetrapolar deep brain electrode *(arrow)* for chronic stimulation of the VIM. The four contacts are seen as signal voids due to metallic artifact in A and B. On the axial image (C), only contact 0 is seen as a signal void in the VIM.

confirmed by microrecording and stimulation testing and the presence of side effects is ruled out, the permanent electrode is implanted. The electrode is a 1.2-mm diameter, tetrapolar electrode with four contacts, each 1.5 mm long, at a 1.5-mm distance from each other (Figure 4). Using the four contacts in combination, the electrical stimulus can be directed within a range of 10.6 mm with different bipolar or monopolar stimulation modes. Stimulation is briefly repeated to confirm correct positioning of the permanent electrode. The aim is for placement of contact 0 (the most distal) at the target, selected by electrophysiological recording and clinical assessment.

The stylet is then removed from the electrode while stabilizing it with a lead holder and rubber-shod forceps. The electrode is then secured to the burr hole ring by placing a burr hole cap. The distal part of the electrode is buried under the skin and the incision closed in anatomical layers. The patient then undergoes MRI to confirm accurate electrode placement and to rule out the presence of intracranial hemorrhage (Figures 5 and 6).

Technical Pitfalls

The currently FDA-approved permanent deep brain electrode (Model 3387 Lead, Medtronic, Minneapolis, Minnesota) is very soft and the author would not recommend inserting it without a guiding cannula, as this could result in a curved placement. However, because the guiding cannula is larger, this should not be inserted into the target, to avoid a "microthalamotomy" effect. Typically, the guiding cannula is inserted to 10 mm above the target.

Removal of the stylet from the electrode is a very delicate maneuver and can easily result in movement of the electrode. This is a problem common to other types of electrode placement, such as those used for epilepsy, and experience in refining the movements and techniques of removing the stylet without disturbing the electrode is necessary. If the surgeon is not familiar with these techniques, the use of intraoperative skull x-rays, to be obtained before and after the stylet is removed, is recommended.

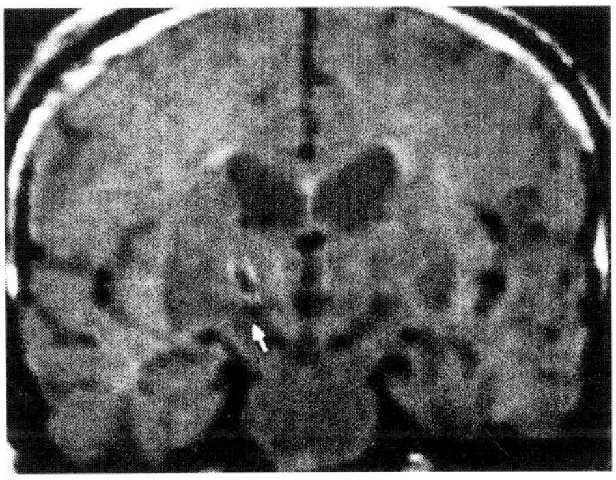

Figure 6: Postoperative coronal brain MRI showing placement of a tetrapolar deep brain electrode for chronic stimulation of the STN. The most distal contact (contact 0, *arrow*) is seen as signal void in the STN.

Placement of a Pulse Generator

The patient is returned to the operating room the same day and general anesthesia is induced for placement of the pulse generator (ITREL II, Model 7424, Medtronic). The pulse generator is placed below the clavicle in a subcutaneous pocket, and is connected with the intracranial electrode by an extension wire tunneled under the skin. Care is taken to place the connector between the electrode and the wire on the convexity of the skull. The connector is indeed relatively bulky and, if placed on the side of the head, it would be uncomfortable and prone to skin erosion. Alternatively, the electrode could be externalized and external stimulation performed until optimal parameters are achieved. At that point (2-7 days after implantation), the electrode is internalized and the pulse generator placed. It is the author's preference to implant the pulse generator on the same day as the implant because it is believed that this decreases the risk of infection.

Chronic Stimulation

Stimulation is usually begun 24-48 hours after the procedure, when the "microthalamotomy" or "micropallidotomy" effects have resolved. This is done by telemetry. Optimal parameters are determined by varying the electrode contact (monopolar/bipolar) and pulse (msec), frequency (Hz), and amplitude (V). In general, good results are obtained with stimulation frequencies of 100-180 Hz, a pulse width of 60-210 μsec, and an amplitude of 3-4 V. Reduction of tremor is usually observed 1-3 seconds following activation of the stimulator. Similarly, the effect is lost within seconds of turning it off. Stimulation is usually optimized at 1 month postimplantation.[14]

Although long-term follow-up studies of DBS are currently not available, "tolerance" to the stimulation may develop over time and the stimulation parameters may need to be adjusted, usually by increasing the amplitude. A requirement for increased amplitude postoperatively may also represent migration of the electrode.

Bilateral Procedures

In most cases, patients with Parkinson's disease have bilateral symptoms. There are a few reports on the effects of bilateral pallidotomy.[15,24] Although improvement of Parkinson's disease symptoms is reported, speech deterioration and cognitive impairment are associated with this procedure.[24] Thus, DBS could be a valid alternative.

Siegfried and Lippitz[25] reported on three patients with simultaneous bilateral placement of DBS electrodes in the GPi, with good resolution of Parkinson's disease symptoms and no mention of transient cognitive impairment. On the other hand, the authors and colleagues reported on two patients with simultaneous bilateral placement of DBS electrodes in the STN who had amelioration of Parkinson's disease symptoms but experienced transient postoperative cognitive impairment.[21] Thus, bilateral chronic high-frequency stimulation of the basal ganglia seems to be a promising technique for Parkinson's disease patients. However, the timing of surgery, i.e., simultaneous versus staged, needs to de defined.

Future Directions in Deep Brain Stimulation

The success of DBS in treating essential tremor and Parkinson's disease symptoms (see Chapter 12, "Chronic Deep Brain Stimulation: Clinical Results") opened new horizons to expand this technology for treatment of other movement disorders that are only modestly improved by medical treatments, such as dystonia. Although the pathophysiology of dystonia is poorly understood, there are a few reports suggesting that GPi pallidotomy may result in amelioration of symptoms. Lozano et al[19] reported on a 9-year-old boy who underwent GPi palli166 dotomy, with improvement of both axial and limb dystonia. Vitek et al[27] also reported on good improvement of dystonia after GPi pallidotomy in three cases. In most instances, however, dystonia is bilateral, and bilateral lesions may have unacceptable risks. The author and colleagues are currently investigating the effects of chronic

DBS for treatment of dystonia, with encouraging preliminary results that will be reported in detail elsewhere. DBS is also being investigated for other types of tremor.[7]

Conclusions

Similar to ablative procedures, high-frequency, chronic DBS is a technically challenging procedure that requires stereotactic skills and excellent knowledge of the anatomy and physiology of the basal ganglia. With the presently available implantable equipment, special care should be taken in handling the various components.

Although DBS may have theoretical advantages over ablative procedures, further clinical experience with long-term follow-up is necessary to establish whether these advantages are real. Thus, at the present time the decision to treat a Parkinson's disease patient with an ablative procedure or DBS rests solely on the patient-physician's discussion. The author believes that investigation in this field is very exciting and necessary to allow precise determination of the role of chronic DBS for treatment of Parkinson's disease and other movement disorders.

References

1. Alesch F, Pinter MM, Helscher RJ, et al: Stimulation of the ventral intermediate thalamic nucleus in tremor dominated Parkinson's disease and essential tremor. **Acta Neurochir 136:**75-81, 1995
2. Benabid AL, Pollak P, Gao D, et al: Chronic electrical stimulation of the ventralis intermedius nucleus of the thalamus as a treatment of movement disorders. **J Neurosurg 84:**203-214, 1996
3. Benabid AL, Pollak P, Gervason C, et al: Long-term suppression of tremor by chronic stimulation of the ventral intermediate thalamic nucleus. **Lancet 337:** 403-406, 1991
4. Benabid AL, Pollak P, Louveau A, et al: Combined (thalamotomy and stimulation) stereotactic surgery of the VIM thalamic nucleus for bilateral Parkinson's disease. **Appl Neurophysiol 50:**343-346, 1987
5. Blond S, Caparros-Lefebvre D, Parker F, et al: Control of tremor and involuntary movement disorders by chronic stereotactic stimulation of the ventral intermediate thalamic nucleus. **J Neurosurg 77:**62-68, 1992
6. Blond S, Siegfried J: Thalamic stimulation for the treatment of tremor and other movement disorders. **Acta Neurochir Suppl 52:**109-111, 1991
7. Broggi G, Brock S, Franzini A, et al: A case of post-traumatic tremor treated by chronic stimulation of the thalamus. **Mov Disord 8:**206-208, 1993
8. Burleigh AL, Horak FB, Burchiel KJ, et al: Effects of thalamic stimulation on tremor, balance, and step initiation: a single subject study. **Mov Disord 8:** 519-524, 1993
9. Deiber MP, Pollak P, Passinghan R, et al: Thalamic stimulation and suppression of parkinsonian tremor: evidence of a cerebellar deactivation using positron emission tomography. **Brain 116:**267-279, 1993
10. Hassler R: The influence of stimulations and coagulations in the human thalamus on the tremor at rest and its physiopathologic mechanism. **Excerpta Media Foundation 2:**637-642, 1955
11. Hirai T, Miyazaki M, Nakajima H, et al: The correlation between tremor characteristics and the predicted volume of effective lesions in stereotaxic nucleus ventralis intermediate thalamotomy. **Brain 106:** 1001-1018, 1983
12. Hubble JP, Busenbar KL, Wildinson S, et al: Effects of thalamic deep brain stimulation based on tremor type of diagnosis. **Mov Disord 12:**337-341, 1997
13. Kelly PJ: Stereotactic thalamotomies, in: Koller WC, Paulson G (eds): **Therapy of Parkinson's Disease.** New York, NY: Marcel Dekker, 1990, pp 415-441
14. Koller W, Pahwa R, Busenbark K, et al: High-frequency unilateral thalamic stimulation in the treatment of essential and parkinsonian tremor. **Ann Neurol 42:**292-299, 1997
15. Laitinen LV, Bergenheim AT, Hariz MI: Leskell's posteroventral pallidotomy in the treatment of Parkinson's disease. **J Neurosurg 76:**53-61, 1992
16. Limousin P, Greene J, Pollak P, et al: Changes in cerebral activity pattern due to subthalamic nucleus or internal pallidum stimulation in Parkinson's disease. **Ann Neurol 42:**283-291, 1997
17. Limousin P, Pollak P, Benazzouz A, et al: Effect on parkinsonian signs and syptoms of bilateral subthalamic nucleus stimulation. **Lancet 345:**91-95, 1995
18. Lozano A, Hutchinson W, Kiss Z, et al: Methods for microelectrode-guided posteroventral pallidotomy. **J Neurosurg 84:**194-202, 1996
19. Lozano AL, Kumar R, Gross RE, et al: Globus pallidus internus pallidotomy for generalized dystonia. **Mov Disord 12:**865-870, 1997
20. Melzack R, Wall PD: Pain mechanisms: a new theory. **Science 150:**971-978, 1965
21. Olanow CW, Germano IM, Brin MF, et al: Deep brain stimulation of the subthalamic nucleus for Parkinson's disease. **Mov Disord 11:**598-599, 1996
22. Ranck JB Jr: Which elements are excited in electrical stimulation of mammalian central nervous system: a review. **Brain Res 98:**417-440, 1975
23. Schaltenbrand G, Wahren W: **Atlas for Stereotaxy of the Human Brain.** New York, NY: Thieme, 1977
24. Shima F, Ishido K, Sun S, et al: Surgical control of akinesia in Parkinson's disease. **Eur Neurol 36 (Suppl 1):**55-61, 1996
25. Siegfried J, Lippitz B: Bilateral chronic electrostimulation of ventroposterolateral pallidum: a new therapeutic approach for alleviating all parkinsonian symptoms. **Neurosurgery 35:**1126-1130, 1994
26. Tasker RR, Organ LW, Hawrylyshyn P: Investigation of the surgical target for alleviation of involuntary movement disorders. **Appl Neurophysiol 45:**261-274, 1982
27. Vitek JL, Kaneoke Y, Hashimoto T, et al: Neuronal activity in the pallidum of a patient with hemiballismus. **Ann Neurol 38:**296-297, 1995 (Abstract)

CHAPTER 12

Chronic Deep Brain Stimulation: Clinical Results

Giovanni Broggi, MD

The efficacy of chronic deep brain stimulation (DBS) in the treatment of movement disorders led to renewed interest in surgical therapy for Parkinson's disease. Chronic stimulation of deep brain targets started in the early 1960s,[8] inspired by the experiments of Olds and Milner[15] showing beneficial effects after stimulation of the septal area in animals. In the 1970s, the development and refinement of implantable electrodes and pulse generators allowed broader use of this procedure, including stimulation of the thalamus.[11]

The resurgence of interest in ablative procedures for surgical treatment of Parkinson's disease, together with a better understanding of the pathophysiology underlying this disease, has prompted the search for targets for DBS. The purpose of DBS is to interrupt the circuits involved in the pathogenesis of the cardinal symptoms of Parkinson's disease; preferred targets include the ventral intermediate (VIM) nucleus of the thalamus, the internal segment of the globus pallidus (GPi), and the subthalamic nucleus (STN). Combining chronic DBS with new targets for surgical treatment of Parkinson's disease allows for continued advances in this field.[3,4,17]

In contrast to ablative procedures, the literature on the clinical outcome of DBS is limited and has a short-term follow-up. The aim of this chapter is to review the currently available literature and combine it with the author's clinical experience with outcome and complications of DBS.

Clinical Experience and Techniques

The techniques used for target localization and intraoperative procedures may affect clinical outcome. Therefore, a few technical aspects that the author believes are essential to optimize placement of DBS in the desired target are reviewed.

For the period January 1991-June 1997, 40 patients at the author's institution were treated using DBS for medically refractory Parkinson's disease. Targets are selected using computed tomography for localization of the CRW (Cosman-Roberts-Wells) stereotactic system (Radionics, Burlington, Massachusetts) fiducials, fused with magnetic resonance images (MRIs) for anatomical detail and on-line anatomical atlases. After anatomical neuroradiographic identification, neurophysiological/clinical confirmation is man-

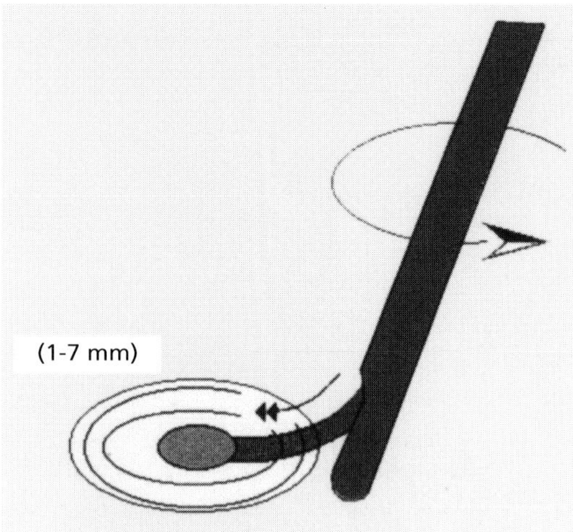

Figure 1: Rigid electrode with flexible side port (Medtronic, Minneapolis, Minnesota) used to perform macrostimulation prior to permanent implantation of a deep brain electrode. The side port can be extruded up to 7 mm. By rotating the needle shaft, brain tissue can be stimulated for a diameter of 14 mm.

datory due to great interindividual variability of the basal ganglia functional anatomy. Intraoperative validation of the anatomically selected target is achieved by first using a rigid electrode with a flexible side port (Figure 1). This electrode allows macrostimulation over a radius of 1-7 mm, depending on the extrusion of the flexible side tip. Thus, with a single pass through the cortex, a very large volume of deep brain can be tested. Macrostimulation is performed by connecting the electrode to a radiofrequency stimulator (RF-G5, Radionics). Low-frequency (2- to 10-Hz) and high-frequency (130- to 160-Hz) stimulation are performed to detect amelioration of symptoms, i.e., tremor arrest, decreased rigidity, and improved motor performance, and to check for adverse effects such as capsular and psychic responses (Table 1). When mapping the VIM boundaries, the somatosensory ventral posterolateral nuclei of the thalamus can be mapped by noting the presence of paresthesias or with somatosensory evoked potentials. Electrophysiological microrecording is not performed.

When satisfactory neurological improvement is achieved, a tetrapolar permanent electrode is implanted (Quad electrode, Medtronic, Minneapolis, Minnesota). Contact "0" (the most distal) is placed at the desired target. The electrode is then connected with a temporary stimulation cable, tunneled under the skin, and externalized. Intravenous prophylactic antibiotics are administered until the electrode is internalized. Postoperatively, patients undergo MRI to confirm adequate placement of the electrode. Neurostimulation through the externalized cables is started as soon as the "microthalamotomy" effects have worn off. In the author's experience, this is usually within 48 hours of the surgery, but it can last as long as 7 days. Monopolar stimulation is performed with the following parameters: amplitude 0.6-2.0 V, frequency 130-160 Hz, and pulse width 90-270 µsec. Data pertinent to the author's clinical experience are summarized in Table 2.

TABLE 1

Intraoperative Macrostimulation of the VIM

Low frequency (2-10 Hz)	Motor effects (internal capsule)
High frequency (70-120 Hz)	Tetanic contraction (internal capsule)
	Psychic disturbance (medial nuclei)
	Speech disturbances Anomia (anterior nuclei) Speech arrest (medial nuclei)
	Sensory disturbances (posterolateral nuclei)
	Oculomotor effects (STN)

TABLE 2

CLINICAL EXPERIENCE WITH DBS IN 40 PATIENTS

No. of Patients	Nucleus	Symptom	Duration (yrs)	No. of Bilateral Implants
28	VIM	tremor	3-4	2
9	GPi	dyskinesia	9-10	3
3	STN	tremor/rigidity	3-6	3

CLINICAL OUTCOME

Chronic Stimulation of the VIM Nucleus

There is a body of evidence indicating that high-frequency chronic stimulation of the VIM nucleus provides excellent control of essential and parkinsonian tremor. Benabid et al[2] reported on 80 patients with Parkinson's disease, 20 patients with essential tremor, and 17 patients with other dyskinesias. In Parkinson's disease patients, tremor was suppressed for as long as 8 years after surgery. Furthermore, in 50% of the Parkinson's disease patients, levodopa (L-DOPA) dosage was decreased by one third compared to presurgical intake. Bradykinesia and rigidity, on the other hand, were not affected by chronic stimulation of the VIM. In the 20 patients with essential tremor, the tremor was satisfactorily controlled; however, there was deterioration over time in 19% of patients.

Koller et al[12] reported on 24 patients who underwent electrode implantation in the VIM for chronic DBS and had a 1-year follow-up. In 31% of patients with essential tremor and 58% of patients with Parkinson's disease, there was total resolution of tremor. Only 3.4% and 4.2% of patients, respectively, did not experience changes in their tremor. Blond and Siegfried[5] reported tremor reduction in 11 of 14 patients. In the author's series of 28 patients who underwent DBS of the VIM for parkinsonian tremor, complete resolution of the tremor was observed in 100% of patients, with a clinical follow-up of 20 months. The author believes that this high success rate depends on correct anatomical/functional placement of the electrode (Figure 2). Longer follow-up times may change this percentage of excellent results.

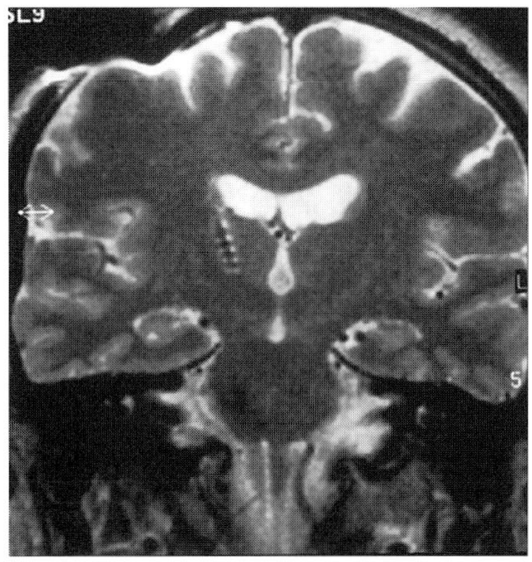

Figure 2: Coronal T2-weighted brain MRI showing a deep brain electrode in the right VIM nucleus of the thalamus. The four contacts of the electrode are seen as focal signal void (black dots) due to metallic artifact. The most distal contact (contact 0) is in the VIM. This patient experienced total resolution of left-handed parkinsonian tremor after DBS at the following settings: 1.9 V, 90 μsec, 160 Hz.

Thus, chronic high-frequency stimulation of the VIM is a promising technique for surgical treatment of essential tremor and parkinsonian tremor, provided that patient selection and surgical techniques are rigorous.

Chronic Stimulation of the GPi

Whereas tremor is best controlled by targeting the thalamus, according to the ablative literature, bradykinesia and rigidity are best controlled by targeting the GPi. There are only a few reports on the use of this target for DBS. In

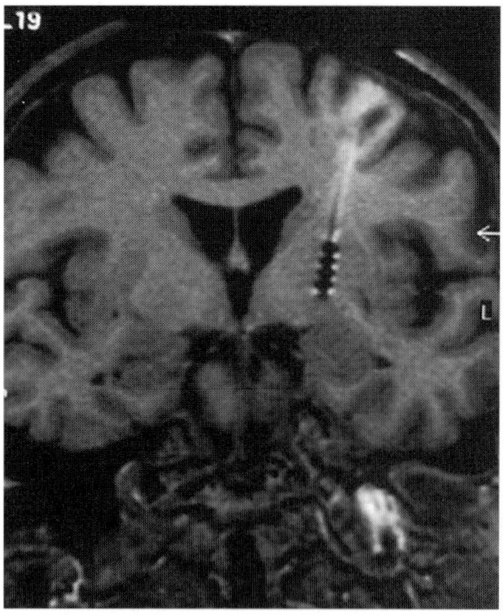

Figure 3: Coronal brain MRI showing a deep brain electrode in the left GPi. The four contacts of the electrode are seen as focal signal void (black dots) due to metallic artifact. The most distal contact (contact 0) is in the GPi. This Parkinson's disease patient experienced total resolution of right-sided dyskinesia and rigidity after DBS at the following settings: 2.2 V, 120 μsec, 150 Hz.

1994, Siegfried and Lippitz[16] reported on three patients who underwent implantation of DBS electrodes in the GPi, with good resolution of bradykinesia and rigidity. Gross et al[9] reported on seven patients who underwent unilateral implantation of DBS electrodes in the GPi. In all cases, DBS alleviated dyskinesia and rigidity. Furthermore, improvements in gait and speech disturbances were noted. On the other hand, Tronnier et al[18] reported on seven Parkinson's disease patients who underwent bilateral implantation of DBS electrodes in the GPi, with no improvement in six of the seven patients. In the author's series, nine patients underwent high-frequency stimulation of the GPi, with good resolution of dyskinesia and rigidity in five patients (Figure 3). The other four patients had fair or minimal benefit from the procedure.

The discrepancy in the results of GPi stimulation may be secondary to different effects of stimulating different parts of the globus pallidus. Bejjani et al[1] reported on five patients who underwent implantation of deep brain electrodes in the globus pallidus. Stimulation of the distal contact, located in the dorsal pallidum, resulted in improvements in gait, dyskinesia, and rigidity, whereas stimulation of the posteroventral contact resulted in worsened gait and dyskinesia. Recently, Siegfried reported on 55 cases of DBS of the GPi, with good results in amelioration of Parkinson's disease symptoms (personal communication, 1998). After electrode implantation, a few patients were able to decrease their daily L-DOPA intake.

Thus, chronic high-frequency stimulation of the GPi is a promising technique for providing resolution of levodopa-induced dyskinesia and rigidity in Parkinson's disease patients. However, in view of the discrepancy in results currently reported in the literature, further clinical investigation is warranted.

Chronic Stimulation of the STN

The literature on DBS of the STN shows the technique to be still in its embryonic phase. In 1995, Limousin et al[13] reported on three patients who underwent chronic stimulation of the STN. These patients showed improvement in activities of daily living scores of 58%-88% and motor score improvement of 42%-84%. In 1996, Olanow et al[14] reported on two patients with improvement of their Unified Parkinson's Disease Rating Scale motor score after high-frequency stimulation of the STN.

Benabid reported on 40 cases of STN stimulation (personal communication, 1998). Excellent results in amelioration of Parkinson's disease symptoms were observed in 80% of cases. Furthermore, approximately 30% of patients who underwent high-frequency stimulation of the STN were able to decrease their daily dose of L-DOPA. In the author's clinical series, three patients underwent bilateral simultaneous implantation of deep brain stimulators in the STN (Figure 4). Good resolution of symptoms was seen in all three patients, with a 40% decrease in L-DOPA treatment.

Thus, chronic high-frequency stimulation of the STN seems to provide the best control of akinesia, levodopa–induced dyskinesia, and rigidity in Parkinson's disease patients. Further clinical experience to corroborate these exciting preliminary results is needed.

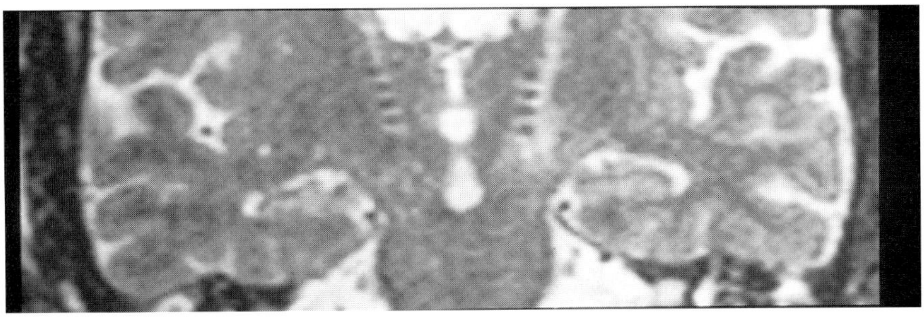

Figure 4: Coronal T2-weighted brain MRI showing bilateral deep brain electrodes in the STN. The four contacts of the electrode are seen as focal signal void (black dots) due to metallic artifact.The most distal contact (contact 0) is in the STN. This patient experienced total resolution of bilateral parkinsonian dyskinesia and rigidity after DBS at the following settings: 0.7 V, 90 μsec, 150 Hz.

COMPLICATIONS

Theoretically, the complication rate associated with DBS should be higher than that associated with ablative procedures because, in addition to acute surgical complications, difficulties secondary to malfunction of the equipment and side effects of the stimulation can occur. Furthermore, just as with any other implantable device, infection can occur at any time. On the other hand, because there is minimal tissue destruction, the morbidity of surgical complications should be less. Before reviewing the scarce literature reporting on complications of DBS for treatment of movement disorders, a few words on the experience with DBS for pain are warranted. Hosobuchi[10] reported a series of 122 patients in which there were 5 hemorrhages (2 deaths), 1 case of ventriculitis, 1 subdural empyema, and 4 subgaleal infections complicating electrode implantation. Young[19] reported on 300 patients with electrode implantation for pain; 2 patients had subdural hematomas requiring surgical intervention, 4 patients developed hemiparesis unrelated to hemorrhage, and an unspecified number of infections occurred.

As with implantation of any other mechanical device, complications of DBS may be surgical, equipment-related, and secondary to application of the device (stimulation). The recent literature on complications following DBS is reported below and summarized in Table 3.

TABLE 3

COMPLICATIONS OF CHRONIC HIGH-FREQUENCY DEEP BRAIN STIMULATION*

		No. of	Complications		
Author(s)	Year	Cases	Surgical	Mechanical	Stimulation
Benabid et al[2]	1996	117	5%	4%	46.5%‡
Gross et al[9]	1997	7	0	0	NR
Koller et al[12]	1997	59	5%	5%	24%
Tronnier et al[18]	1997	6	0	0	NR
Broggi	1998+	40	0	12%	5%
Germano	1998+	10	0	0	TBR

* NR = not reported; TBR = to be reported elsewhere.
+ Personal communication.
‡ See text.

Surgical Complications

Benabid et al[2] reported six intracerebral hematomas complicating VIM stimulation (5%). The hematomas were asymptomatic in three patients and resulted in a transient deficit in the other three patients. Koller et al[12] reported surgical complications in 3 of 59 patients: intracranial hemorrhage, subdural hematoma, and seizure.

In the author's series of 40 patients, there was no surgical morbidity. This is in agreement with other series. Germano (personal communication, 1988), Tronnier et al,[18] and Gross et al[9] reported no surgical morbidity in 10, 6, and 7 patients, respectively.

Mechanical Complications

Benabid et al[2] reported a 5% incidence of "skin-related" problems: in three cases skin erosion over the cable connector occurred, in two other patients a granuloma formed over the wires, and one patient had seroma formation over the pulse generator. In the series of Koller et al,[12] there were three equipment-related complications: a malfunctioning pulse generator, a malfunctioning wire, and dislodgment of the electrode. In the author's series, in 4 of 40 patients the electrode placement was not ideal and required repositioning. This could have been secondary to movement during positioning and securing of the permanent electrode, or due to migration after surgery. In one patient the pulse generator had to be replaced after 6 months due to battery failure.

Stimulation-Related Side Effects

In the series of Koller et al,[12] complications related to the stimulation were seen in 20% of cases and consisted of paresthesias that resolved with adjustment of the stimulating parameters. In 4% of patients, dysequilibrium, gait disorders, dystonia, dysarthria, or paresis was seen. Blond and Siegfried[5] reported stimulation-related complications, namely, paresthesia and dystonia, in 2 of 14 patients who underwent DBS. Benabid et al[2] reported that 37 of 117 patients (31.6%) had side effects as a result of DBS. However, the combined rate of side effects after stimulation was 46.5%. Paresthesias occurred in 9% of 117 patients. These were induced at intensities of stimulation higher than those that suppressed the tremor. In 9% of patients, dystonic movements of the foot were observed. Dysarthria was seen in 23 patients (20%), 14 of whom had a bilateral implant or a contralateral ablative procedure. In patients who underwent bilateral DBS electrode implantation, 14 of 51 bilaterally implanted patients had dysarthria. Dysequilibrium was observed in 8.5% of patients. Furthermore, neuropsychological testing showed a decrease in performance, as did spatial testing.

In the author's series, stimulation-related complications were observed in two patients. These included speech disturbances and visual hallucination. A decrease in amplitude and an increase in pulse width resulted in resolution of the symptoms.

Thus, the current clinical experience with DBS suggests that the surgical morbidity with electrode implantation is similar to that of ablative procedures in the occurrence of symptomatic hemorrhage (see Chapter 10, "Pallidotomy: Clinical Results"). Unlike ablative procedures, there is no morbidity related to the lesioning itself, i.e., visual field cuts or dysarthria. On the other hand, chronic high-frequency DBS has further complications related to the equipment and stimulation itself. Whereas most of the equipment-related complications require further surgery, the stimulation-induced side effects are generally reversible by changing the stimulation parameters.

Long-Term Effects

A present concern in counseling a patient regarding ablative procedures versus DBS is that of long-term effects. The recurrence of symptoms after ablative procedures is well documented in the literature. With chronic high-frequency DBS, there is a suggestion that tolerance may develop. Koller et al[12] showed that a significant increase in amplitude is necessary to maintain clinical resolution of the symptoms over time. The author's clinical experience concurs with these findings. In most patients, increased amplitude and/or a change from monopolar to bipolar stimulation is necessary to maintain clinical success. The author postulates that this "tolerance" may be due to changes in the thresh-

TABLE 4

REVERSIBILITY OF DBS

Stimulation may be stopped (similar to drug treatment)
Volume of electrical stimulation may be changed (as with daily drug dosage)
Target may be modified (four contacts)
Electrode may be removed at any time
Electrode may be replaced (new target, new surgery)

old of neurons around the electrode tip. Further clinical, histological, and electrophysiological data are necessary to corroborate this hypothesis.

CONCLUSIONS

Based on clinical experience with 145 functional ablative procedures for movement disorders,[6,7] the author currently favors the use of chronic DBS for treatment of Parkinson's disease. The author's clinical experience in 40 cases and review of the literature support the evidence that VIM stimulation provides excellent tremor control. The STN is a very promising target for treatment of dyskinesia and rigidity. Irreversible complications related to DBS are similar to, if not less than, those associated with ablative procedures. Improvements in technology will most likely result in amelioration of currently reported equipment-related complications.

The author's current philosophy on DBS is that it is a reversible treatment, as summarized in Table 4. Nevertheless, when treating patients with Parkinson's disease, it should always be remembered that Parkinson's disease may be associated with two irreversible processes: aging and neurodegeneration. Thus, although there may be improvement of a certain Parkinson's disease symptom, there may be an overall decline in a given patient's condition due to the irreversibility of this complex disease.

REFERENCES

1. Bejjani B, Damier P, Arnulf I, et al: Pallidal stimulation for Parkinson's disease. Two targets? **Neurology 49:**1564-1569, 1997
2. Benabid AL, Pollak P, Gao D, et al: Chronic electrical stimulation of the ventralis intermedius nucleus of the thalamus as a treatment of movement disorders. **J Neurosurg 84:**203-214, 1996
3. Benabid AL, Pollak P, Gervason C, et al: Long-term suppression of tremor by chronic stimulation of the ventral intermediate thalamic nucleus. **Lancet 337:**403-406, 1991
4. Benabid AL, Pollack P, Gross C, et al: Acute and long-term effects of subthalamic nucleus stimulation in Parkinson's disease. **Stereotact Funct Neurosurg 62:**76-84, 1994
5. Blond S, Siegfried J: Thalamic stimulation for the treatment of tremor and other movement disorders. **Acta Neurochir Suppl 52:**109-111, 1991
6. Broggi G, Angelini L, Bono R, et al: Long term results of stereotactic thalamotomy for cerebral palsy. **Neurosurg 12:**195-202, 1983
7. Broggi G, Angelini L, Giorgi C: Neurological and psychological side effects after stereotactic thalamotomy in patients with cerebral palsy. **Neurosurg 7:**127-134, 1980
8. Gol A: Relief of pain by electrical stimulation of the septal area. **J Neurol Sci 5:**115-120, 1967
9. Gross C, Rougier A, Guehl D, et al: High-frequency stimulation of the globus pallidus internalis in Parkinson's disease: a study of seven cases. **J Neurosurg 87:**491-498, 1997
10. Hosobuchi Y: Subcortical electrical stimulation for control of intractable pain in humans. Report of 122 cases (1970-1984). **J Neurosurg 64:**543-553, 1986
11. Hosobuchi Y, Adams JE, Rutkin B: Chronic thalamic stimulation for the control of facial anesthesia dolorosa. **Arch Neurol 29:**158-161, 1973
12. Koller W, Pahwa R, Busenbark K, et al: High-frequency unilateral thalamic stimulation in the treatment of essential and parkinsonian tremor. **Ann Neurol 42:**292-299, 1997
13. Limousin, Pollak P, Benazzouz A, et al: Effect on parkinsonian signs and symptoms of bilateral subthalamic nucleus stimulation. **Lancet 345:**91-95, 1995
14. Olanow CW, Germano IM, Brin MF, et al: Deep brain stimulation of the subthalamic nucleus for Parkinson's disease. **Mov Dis 11:**598-599, 1996
15. Olds J, Milner P: Positive reinforcement produced by electrical stimulation of the septal area and other regions of the rat brain. **J Comp Physiol Psychol 47:**419-427, 1954
16. Siegfried J, Lippitz B: Bilateral chronic electrostimulation of ventroposterolateral pallidum: a new therapeutic approach for alleviating all parkinsonian symptoms. **Neurosurgery 35:**1126-1130, 1994
17. Siegfried J, Lippitz B: Chronic electrical stimulation of the VL-VPL complex and of the pallidum in the treatment of movement disorders: personal experience since 1982. **Stereotact Funct Neurosurg 62:**71-75, 1994
18. Tronnier VM, Fogel W, Kronenbuerger M, et al: Pallidal stimulation: an alternative to pallidotomy? **J Neurosurg 87:**700-705, 1997
19. Young RE: Intracranial procedures for pain management, in Apuzzo MLJ (ed): **Brain Surgery: Complication Avoidance and Management.** New York, NY: Churchill Livingstone, 1993, Vol 2, pp 1497-1508

CHAPTER 13

HUMAN FETAL TISSUE TRANSPLANTATION

THOMAS B. FREEMAN, MD, C. WARREN OLANOW, MD, FRCP(C), ROBERT A. HAUSER, MD, JEFFREY H. KORDOWER, PHD, DOUGLAS A. HOLT, MD, CESAR V. BORLONGAN, PHD, AND PAUL R. SANBERG, PHD

Surgical therapies for the treatment of Parkinson's disease can be divided into two broad categories: ablative and restorative. Ablative surgical therapies include thalamotomy and pallidotomy. Although these procedures can ameliorate some of the symptoms of Parkinson's disease, they do little to change the underlying course of neural degeneration. In the case of Huntington's disease, there are no ablative surgical procedures that provide significant clinical benefit or palliation of the disease. Restorative surgical therapies include deep brain stimulation, transplantation of fetal tissue, cell lines that express trophic factors, or somatically delivered gene therapies.

The first restorative neurosurgical trials utilized human fetal tissue transplantation for the treatment of Parkinson's disease, and more recently for Huntington's disease. Fetal tissue transplantation was first utilized clinically for the treatment of Parkinson's disease for several reasons.[76] Parkinson's disease is primarily caused by the loss of a limited number of nigrostriatal dopaminergic neurons, and symptoms are improved significantly with dopamine replacement therapies. The dopamine neurons work in a modulatory capacity physiologically, and do not carry the highly specific, somatotopically organized information seen in other neural systems. Furthermore, the target area (the striatum) is comparatively small, making it a suitable target for transplantation. Finally, fetal grafts can survive, reinnervate the brain, and improve behavioral deficits in rodent and nonhuman primate models of parkinsonism. Because this field is developing so rapidly, it is necessary to carefully analyze specific transplant variables and their relation to outcomes in order to develop a successful clinical transplant program.

Neural Transplantation

Several clinical studies of fetal tissue transplantation for Parkinson's disease have been performed worldwide. It is difficult to compare many studies directly due to differences in transplant variables, methods, and expertise of clinical analysis, as well as differences in positron emission tomography (PET) technology. However, several generalities can be stated at this time. Transplant protocols appear to be reliable in some centers from patient to patient, as well as reproducible between centers. Proof now exists that grafts can survive and reinnervate the brain and that this survival is associated with graft-induced clinical recovery and increased striatal fluorodopa (F-DOPA) uptake on PET. Finally, no center has "cured" Parkinson's disease. At best, improvement to date is moderate.

Lindvall and colleagues[66] reported the results of their first two patients who received fetal transplants in 1989. Only a small improvement was noted and no changes on F-DOPA-PET were reported. These investigators subsequently stored tissue for a shorter time period (yielding higher viability) and implanted tissue using a smaller gauge transplant needle (which has been shown subsequently to improve graft viability).[18,65] This group has used grafts from multiple donors per side and has transplanted tissue from as many as seven donors into the putamen and caudate.[99] Immunosuppression was gradually tapered over a 5-year period postoperatively.[99] Overall, improvement following unilateral transplants was noted in the percentage of time in the "off" state, Unified Parkinson's Disease Rating Scale (UPDRS) off-period scores (see Chapter 10, "Pallidotomy: Clinical Results," Table 1, for UPDRS), and rigidity and hypokinesia contralateral to the side of the implant. Dyskinesias improved in some patients, but worsened in others. The next two patients in this series experienced more pronounced clinical benefit, which lasted for 4 years, before beginning a gradual deterioration during postoperative years 4 to 6.[65,67,68,91,99] However, these patients received unilateral transplants. Long-term F-DOPA-PET scans demonstrated long-term stability (up to 72 months) in the improvement of F-DOPA uptake in the region of the transplant, with progressive contralateral deterioration consistent with progression of the disease on the nontransplanted side.[67,91,99] This suggests that long-term graft survival is possible, as assessed indirectly with F-DOPA-PET. Five of these unilaterally transplanted patients have subsequently received contralateral transplants,[99] although no clinical data have been reported regarding these patients to date. The early clinical data from the Swedish group has been replicated using a similar protocol by Peschanski and colleagues.[25,81,85]

Freed et al[29,30] also provided early data reporting clinical benefit following fetal tissue transplantation. They transplanted tissue from a single embryonic donor into two patients unilaterally and into five patients bilaterally. They reported statistically significant improvement in activities of daily living in both the on and off states. They also noted some improvement in postural control, gait, and bradykinesia. Spencer and colleagues[95] utilized cryopreserved fetal tissue in a transplantation protocol involving four patients with unilateral transplants into the caudate nucleus. Although mild improvement was noted, the transplant group did not differ significantly from the control group, demonstrating the importance of controlled clinical trials in this field. In addition, one of these four patients died 4 months after surgery, and autopsy demonstrated minimal survival of dopaminergic neurons within the graft.[84]

More pronounced benefit was observed in two patients with parkinsonism induced by exposure to 1-methyl-4-phenyl-1,2,3,6-tetrahydropyridine (MPTP).[101] These patients received bilateral transplants from multiple donors into the caudate and putamen. They demonstrated progressive improvement in motor function and bilateral improvement in F-DOPA uptake on PET beginning 1 year after transplantation. The more robust improvement in these two patients may be due to the use of bilateral transplants, but could also be influenced by the younger age of the patients and differences in the nature of the underlying disease process.

Freeman and colleagues at the University of South Florida[38,44,58] reported on fetal nigral transplantation in six patients with Parkinson's disease. All patients received bilateral transplants utilizing multiple donors (three to four per side). Solid fetal nigral grafts were transplanted stereotactically into the posterior (postcommissural) putamen, with all graft deposits separated by 5 mm in a three-dimensional array.[35] Donor age was restricted to 6.5-9 weeks postconception.[41,42] Immunosuppression was discontinued 6 months postoperatively. All patients experienced meaningful clinical benefit. Significant improvement was observed in the UPDRS score and Schwab-England disability scores in the off state and percentage of time in the on state, as well as in the percentage of on time disabled by dyskinesia. Significant increases in striatal F-DOPA-PET were also noted in all patients at 6-12 months postoperatively. Clinical and PET improvement from bilateral transplants continued for 2 years in the absence of immunosuppression[44] (RA Hauser, TB Freeman, BJ Snow, et al, unpublished data, 1998). At autopsy, two patients from this series had robust graft survival that correlated with these clinical benefits and PET changes (see below).

The largest series reported to date is by Kopyov et al.[55] They claimed substantial variability in outcomes following surgery, ranging from "nominal improvements" to "significant changes that can be classified as altering the overall lifestyle of the patient," although this is difficult to evaluate from the report. They also claimed that improvement was seen primarily in the symptoms of dyskinesia, rigidity, and gait disorders.

Transplant Variables

Donor Age

Perhaps the single most important variable affecting graft survival and clinical outcome is related to the age of the embryonic donor.[8] Embryonic grafts must be obtained after dopamine neurons have first developed within the subventricular zone and before they have extended neuritic processes. After this time, graft viability is decreased, most likely due to axotomy-induced cell death. Before reliable transplantation could be performed clinically, it was therefore necessary to delineate the temporal course of development of the human dopaminergic nigrostriatal system and demonstrate that grafts derived from this optimal period would survive in a xenotransplant model. It has been demonstrated that human dopamine producing neurons first appear in the subventricular zone at 5.5-6.5 weeks postconception.[42,98] Neuritic processes are elaborated and reach the striatum by 8-9 weeks.[42] This led to the hypothesis that the optimal donor age is from 5.5 to 8 weeks postconception.[42]

The authors tested this hypothesis using human dopaminergic neural transplants from different ages transplanted into immunosuppressed rats.[41] Both solid and suspension intraparenchymal grafts survived xenotransplantation equally well, with a donor age "window" that was approximately 1 week older in the case of solid grafts. Optimal donor age for suspension grafts was 5.5-8 weeks postconception, and optimal age for solid grafts was 6.5-9 weeks. In humans, the authors have subsequently observed similar robust graft survival at autopsy in two patients who received fetal nigral allografts using identical donor-aged tissue and transplant techniques.[38,57-60] Of note, transplant protocols using donors older than this have in general resulted in poor survival of dopaminergic neurons within grafts.[3,28,45]

Tissue Storage

Tissue storage before transplantation allows for tissue transportation, screening for possible infectious agents, obtaining multiple donors, elective surgical planning, and possible pretreatment with trophic factors, lazaroids, or pretransplant cell sorting.[36] Spencer et al[95] utilized cryopreservation to store tissue before clinical transplantation. This technique has been subsequently shown to significantly decrease cell viability and neuritic outgrowth following transplantation,[21,84,86] even though in vitro dopamine levels before transplantation are similar to what is seen with fresh tissue.[54] The authors have, therefore, utilized storage of human fetal tissue in "hibernation medium," where excellent postgraft viability has been demonstrated following transplantation into both parkinsonian rats and patients, with storage times of up to 2-4 days.[36,38,41,57-61]

Methods of Graft Preparation

Human fetal nigral grafts can be transplanted intraparenchymally as either a suspension[15] or solid graft.[36,41] Equally robust human fetal grafts have been demonstrated using both techniques.[41] Likewise, clinical benefit has been reported in parkinsonian patients using both techniques.[25,38,65,67,81,85,99,101] Solid grafts have an advantage from the neurosurgical perspective in that no ancillary support staff is necessary for graft preparation. Other advantages of either suspension or solid grafts remain theoretical at this time.[15,36,41,76]

Number of Donors

The number of transplanted neurons necessary to induce clinical benefit in patients with Parkinson's disease remains unknown. It is technically difficult to obtain tissue from multiple donors simultaneously for transplantation.[37,73] Therefore, it is important to define the minimum number of donors necessary to induce clinical benefit before fetal tissue transplantation can be used in a widespread manner. Because Parkinson's disease does not become clinically manifest until there has been a reduction of 50%-80% in nigral neurons and striatal dopamine,[6,53] it may not be necessary to transplant a full complement of dopamine neurons in order to get above the threshold number of dopamine neurons needed to induce clinical improvement. In the two patients in the authors' series who came to autopsy, between 82,000 and 137,000 dopamine neurons per side were found to have survived transplantation.[57-60] This corresponds to approximately a 5% survival rate of transplanted dopamine neurons, which is similar to what has been observed in animal models.[17] The authors are currently evaluating the effect of the "dose" of fetal tissue on clinical response in their ongoing trial. Hopefully this study will help to determine the number of donors required for fetal nigral grafts to be efficacious.

Distribution of Grafted Tissue

Even if enough cells are transplanted, they must be distributed in such a way that the grafts can influence the entire target area. This issue is particularly critical in human trials of fetal tissue transplantation because the human striatum is more than 200 times larger than that of the rodent. Autopsy results from the two patients in the authors' series demonstrated that neuritic outgrowth from grafted neurons extends from 2.5 to approximately 7 mm within the striatum.[58,59] Using deposits that were 5 mm apart in a three-dimensional array,[35,38] the authors were able to achieve confluent reinnervation of up to 78% of the designated target area in the postcommissural putamen.[57,60] With this strategy, the caudate and putamen on one side can theoretically be reinnervated using 16 needle passes separated by 5 mm between the tracts. Based on the extent of neuritic outgrowth observed in these autopsy studies, it may be possible to achieve confluent reinnervation of the striatum using needle tracts that are 7 mm apart, thus using fewer needle penetrations.

The authors currently use a grid array in the shape of the caudate and putamen that allows transplantation into multiple sites in the caudate or putamen using a single stereotactic measurement[35,38] (Figure 1). This is a modification of a design by Breeze et al.[13] The outer cannula of the stereotactic needle is 1.5 mm in diameter, and is passed to the dorsal surface of the putamen. The inner cannula has an outer diameter of 0.91 mm and an inner diameter of 0.60 mm (for solid grafts). It is passed to the ventral edge of the striatum and withdrawn in 3- to 5-mm increments as deposits of tissue are made.[13,38] For suspension transplants, the inner cannula has an outer diameter of 0.71 mm and an inner diameter of 0.41 mm. Although the authors have not used this latter needle clinically, these diameters have been shown to produce robust survival of human suspension xenografts in rats.[18,41] The main advantage of a grid array is that of surgical speed. As targets can shift in the brain during surgery with progressive cerebrospinal fluid loss, it is hoped that a grid array will aid in surgical targeting when multiple needle tracts are utilized. A grid array can also contribute to reproducibility of needle tract localization between centers in a multicenter trial.

Site of Implantation

The behavioral benefits that occur in animals following fetal grafting correlate with the site of the graft within the brain.[2,26] It is necessary to

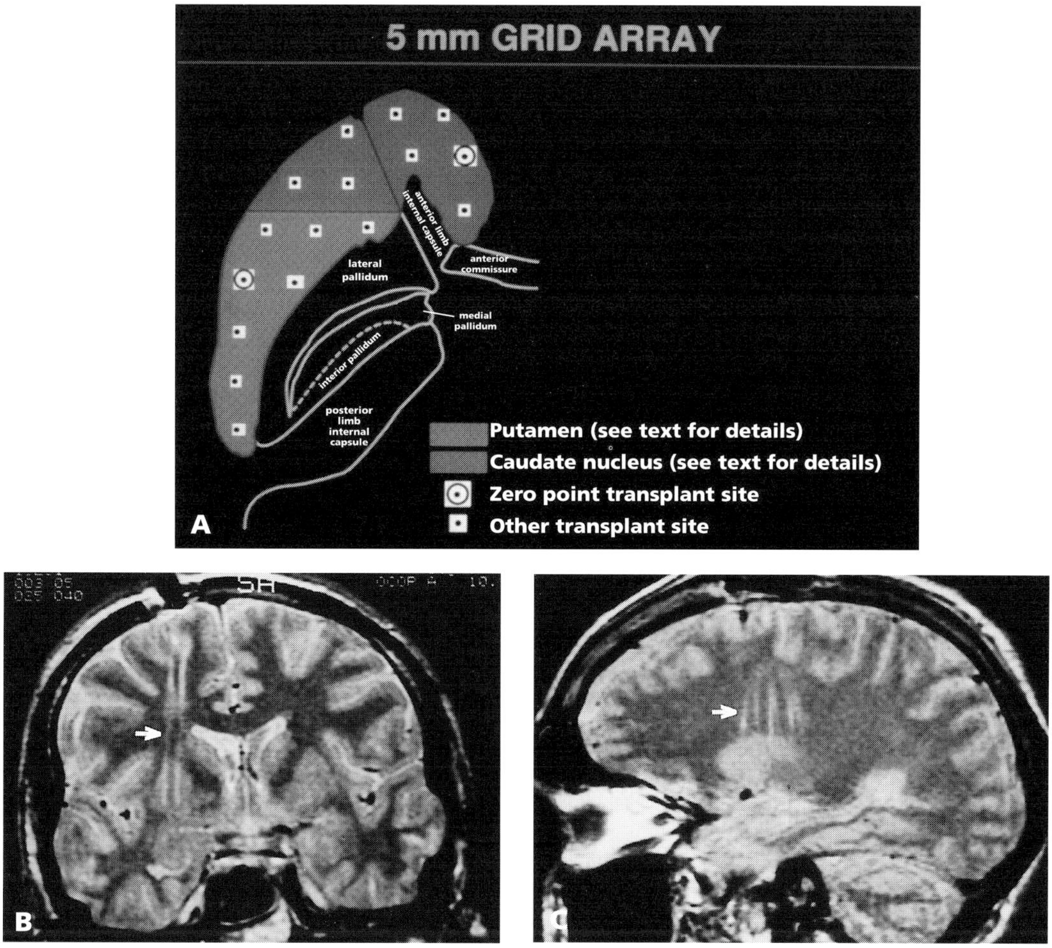

Figure 1: A) Schematic representation of the grid array used for fetal nigral grafting. Although the caudate nucleus and putamen are separate anatomically, the target regions are divided into the postcommissural putamen (shown in lighter gray) and the anterior putamen and caudate nucleus (shown in darker gray), because they are more related structurally, functionally, and embryologically. Parkinson's disease primarily affects the postcommissural putamen, which is the authors' primary surgical target. This grid array allows for graft deposits at 5-mm intervals in three dimensions to facilitate confluent reinnervation of the target area. (Reproduced from Olanow et al[75] with permission.) **B and C)** Coronal **(B)** and sagittal **(C)** magnetic resonance images demonstrating multiple stereotactic needle tracts *(arrows)* entering the postcommissural putamen at 5-mm intervals. The grid array was utilized, with a single cortical entry point.

limit the transplant site within the striatum for patients with Parkinson's disease due to risks associated with multiple needle tracts, as well as technical difficulties in obtaining tissue from multiple donors. The authors have chosen to transplant into the posterior (postcommissural) putamen for several reasons.[38] This is the region that is predominantly depleted of dopaminergic innervation in Parkinson's disease. Furthermore, it is the region that receives primary input from the precentral motor fields.[1,62] However, there is also appealing evidence to suggest that the caudate may be an important target for transplantation in Parkinson's disease.[76] Ongoing studies in Sweden and England will hopefully determine whether transplants into the caudate plus putamen provide additional clinical benefit in comparison to transplants into the putamen alone.[99]

Unilateral Versus Bilateral Transplantation

Unilateral transplantation was utilized in the early transplant protocols of Lindvall et al.[65,67,68] However, long-term follow-up has demonstrated loss of clinical efficacy beginning at 4-6 years, predominantly on the side ipsilateral to the graft.[99] F-DOPA-PET in these patients has demonstrated progressive graft-derived improvement on the side of the transplant, with continued decrease in striatal F-DOPA uptake on the unoperated side of the brain. Also, dyskinesias can become more pronounced following unilateral grafts,[25,99] but improve following bilateral grafts.[38,44] These observations suggest that better results will be obtained with bilateral grafts.

Longevity of Graft Survival

Although the longest autopsy proven graft survival in patients with Parkinson's disease is 18-19 months following transplantation,[57-61] there are several reasons why long-term graft survival can be anticipated. Graft rejection was not seen in either of the two patients in the authors' series who came to autopsy.[61] The disease process has not been seen to affect grafts, as no Lewy bodies or abnormal neuromelanin accumulation were seen within any of these grafts at 18 months.[58,59] Striatal F-DOPA uptake has steadily improved for up to 72 months following transplantation in one patient.[99] At least 15 patients worldwide have been documented to have progressive improvement in striatal F-DOPA uptake on PET at least 6 months after discontinuation of cyclosporine therapy. Therefore, it seems likely that fetal tissue grafts will survive long-term.

Immunological Issues

The need for immunosuppression in neural grafting remains to be delineated.[61,76] However, what is known at this time is that multiple unrelated neural allografts survived in two patients for 18 months. This occurred in the absence of immunosuppression for the last 12 months of their lives.[57-61] However, in these same autopsy cases, immune markers of microglia, macrophages, T-cells, and B-cells were observed within the graft sites in the absence of graft rejection.[61] It is not clear whether this represents an attenuated and ineffective immune response, a reaction to surgical trauma, or an early sign of a chronic rejection process. However, one patient in the Swedish series had progressive improvement in F-DOPA uptake on PET for 72 months, and received cyclosporine for 31 months and prednisolone and azathioprine for 61 and 64 months after surgery, respectively. The authors have also noted progressive bilateral improvement in striatal F-DOPA uptake on PET in one patient for up to 3 years following transplantation, and in the absence of immunosuppression for 30 months.[44] This provides further evidence of long-term survival of neural allografts in the absence of immunosuppression. However, only definitive autopsy data obtained 5-10 years after transplantation will resolve this issue. It also remains to be determined if immunosuppression is required at all. The data regarding this point remain sketchy at best. However, the authors have had a single patient who developed reversible renal complications and could not tolerate cyclosporine after his initial operation. As a result, the contralateral procedure was performed in the absence of cyclosporine. Nonetheless, the patient has improved clinically, and striatal F-DOPA uptake in the region of the second transplant has increased significantly[44] (RA Hauser, TB Freeman, BJ Snow, et al, unpublished data, 1998).

Infection Issues

The risks of infection in the transplant recipient can be grouped into three categories: donor, nosocomial and opportunistic. The infection-related risks to the recipient of fetal neural transplants preliminarily appear to be low following the use of appropriate safeguards.[46] However, the actual risk of infection is still unknown. Elements that combine to improve safety include donor and recipient screening, donor selection, sterile technique to obtain donor tissue, donor storage in antibiotic medium, the use of good laboratory practices, perioperative antibiotics, and short-term low-dose immunosuppression.[46]

Methods of Assessing Grafts in Patients With Parkinson's Disease

One of the major difficulties with comparing results between programs relates to differences in evaluation methods that have been used by the different groups.[76] The Core Assessment Program for Intracerebral Transplantation (CAPIT) was developed to encourage uniformity (and therefore comparability) in clinical assessment methods among transplant programs.[63] Additionally, most transplant programs perform formal neuropsychological testing, and some additionally evaluate neurophysiological measurements of motor function.

Most centers also utilize striatal F-DOPA uptake as measured on PET as a surrogate marker for graft survival. Definitive improvement in F-DOPA uptake following grafting was first reported by Lindvall and colleagues.[65,91] However, increased F-DOPA uptake cannot differentiate between surviving grafted dopamine neurons and graft-induced terminal sprouting of residual dopamine neurons.[58,65] Furthermore, striatal F-DOPA uptake has been found to correlate with the number of dopamine nigral neurons in humans[93] and MPTP-lesioned monkeys.[78] F-DOPA-PET also correlates with clinical benefit following fetal tissue transplantation in some centers.[67,85,94] Significant improvement in F-DOPA uptake has been seen in both of the patients in the authors' series who had robust graft survival at autopsy.[38,44,57-60]

Pathological Analysis of Fetal Grafts

Over 200 patients with Parkinson's disease, MPTP-induced parkinsonism, or spinocerebellar degeneration have received transplants of fetal nigral grafts derived from either human or porcine embryonic sources. Of these patients, 13 have come to autopsy and have been reported at least preliminarily. Two patients died as a direct result of the surgery: one as a consequence of surgical complications[31] and one as a result of probable obstructive hydrocephalus from inadvertent graft migration into the fourth ventricle of tissue derived from multiple germ layers.[28,48,56] The latter patient also may have died from direct brain stem compression by the graft that migrated to the fourth ventricle. This underscores the need for extensive laboratory training in techniques of fetal tissue dissection and grafting for clinicians who perform this procedure. All other patients died of causes unrelated to the operation. Of those patients for whom the etiology of death is known, reasons include pulmonary embolism in two patients[22,58] and aspiration in two patients[57,64] (J Dymecki, personal communication, 1989). Two patients died secondary to cancer,[3,45] three from end-stage parkinsonism,[3,84] one from a motor vehicle accident,[32] and one from an unknown cause.[3] Two of these patients had striatonigral degeneration at autopsy.[31,84]

Survival of dopaminergic neurons in the grafts was poor or nonexistent in 10 of the patients. There are several possible reasons for this, including incorrect donor age,[3,28,41,42] the detrimental use of cryopreservation for storage of tissue,[21,84] poor dissection technique,[28,48,56] possible cross-species immune differences,[22] delayed autolysis time (J Dymecki, personal communication, 1989), anoxic brain injury at time of death[31] (C Freed, personal communication, 1994), and possibly host-related variables in patients without Parkinson's disease.[31,84]

The robust graft survival observed following fetal grafting in the authors' two patients has been described in detail (Figures 2 and 3),[57-61] and a preliminary description of graft survival has been reported recently by Freed and colleagues.[32] Several conclusions can be drawn from these studies:

1. These cases provide definitive proof that fetal nigral grafts survive within the human parkinsonian brain following transplantation.
2. Grafts extend neuritic processes into the recipient's brain and form synaptic connections with the host.
3. Clinical improvement and increased striatal F-DOPA uptake on PET correlates with graft survival and host reinnervation.
4. No host sprouting was observed.
5. There is no evidence that Parkinson's disease adversely affects the grafts in a manner similar to the patient's own nigral neurons.
6. Neuritic outgrowth from grafts is variable,

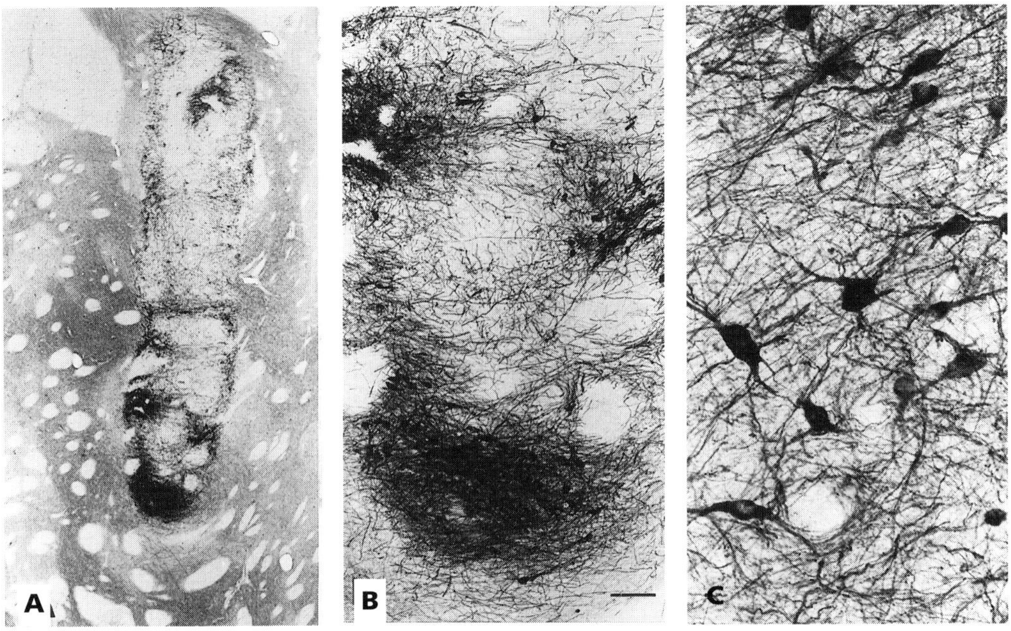

Figure 2: Low- **(A)**, medium- **(B)**, and high- **(C)** powered photomicrographs of tyrosine hydroxylase-immunostained sections illustrating the viability and morphology of a human fetal nigral allograft 18 months after transplantation into a patient with Parkinson's disease. *Scale bar* represents the following magnifications: A, 1000 μm; B, 250 μm; C, 50 μm.

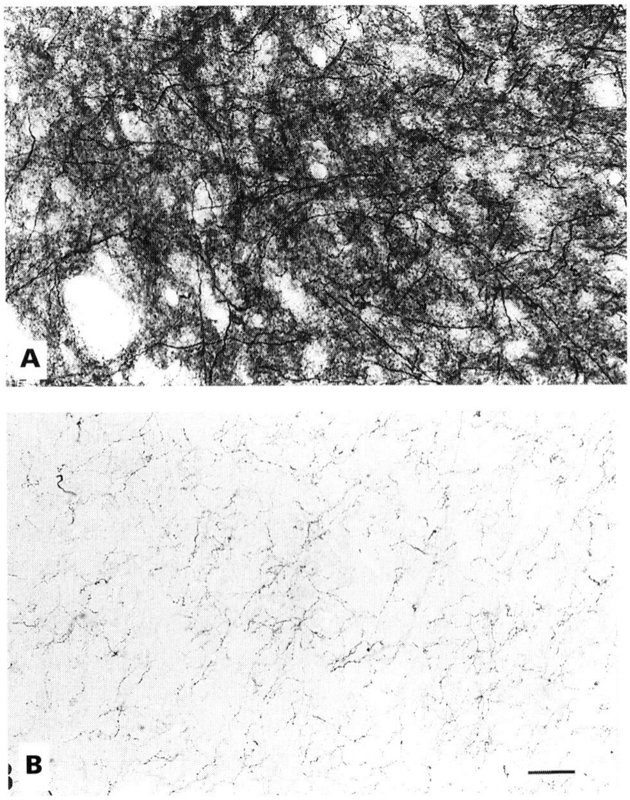

Figure 3: A) Dense tyrosine hydroxylase-immunoreactivity was observed within the putamen proximal to a human fetal nigral allograft. **B)** In contrast, little tyrosine hydroxylase-immunostaining was seen distal to transplants. The few immunoreactive fibers that were seen in these regions likely represent the level of residual host innervation seen in the putamen in Parkinson's disease. *Scale bar* represents 50 μm for both A and B.

ranging from 2.5 to 7 mm within the striatum, and up to 11-12 mm within white matter tracts.

7. Grafting at 5-mm intervals in a three-dimensional array can produce confluent reinnervation of up to 78% of a chosen target area.
8. Host reinnervation occurs in a patch-matrix fashion reminiscent of that seen in the developing nigrostriatal system.
9. Grafts derived from donors aged 6.5-9 weeks postconception, transplanted as solid grafts, can survive transplantation.
10. Graft maturation rate is delayed with respect to the normal developmental rate for dopamine neurons.
11. Multiple unrelated allografts survive in the absence of chronic immunosuppression.
12. Central and peripheral immune markers are activated following grafting.
13. Grafts are metabolically active.
14. Grafts can take up, synthesize, and store dopamine.
15. Grafts have intact blood-brain barriers.
16. Graft survival can be reproduced reliably within and between experienced centers.
17. Virtually all of these findings have correlated to similar findings in animal models of Parkinson's disease.

Future Issues

At this time, preliminary studies of fetal grafts for the treatment of Parkinson's disease have demonstrated that transplants can provide clinical efficacy, induce significant improvement on striatal F-DOPA-PET, and survive and reinnervate the brain in an appropriate manner. However, these patients are not cured of their parkinsonism. There are several possible reasons for this.[34,64,76] As mentioned above, the grafts reinnervate only part of the available target areas due to limitations in the number of needle tracts and tissue availability. Grafting does not complete both the afferent and efferent limbs of the nigrostriatal circuit. The slow maturation of transplanted dopamine neurons, as seen at autopsy in the authors' series of patients, may account for the protracted slow improvement seen in some patients. Only about 5% of transplanted dopamine neurons survive the transplantation process; thus, it may be necessary to increase the number of dopaminergic neurons in grafts. Levodopa (L-DOPA) therapy may adversely affect graft survival. Parkinson's disease involves degeneration in multiple other brain regions besides the striatum, and these regions are not expected to be influenced by grafts placed exclusively into the striatum. Clinical response may be improved if transplants are placed in additional target sites. "Nondopaminergic" symptoms of parkinsonism are not expected to improve following grafts of dopaminergic cells. Finally, the progressive loss of benefit of L-DOPA treatment in both the on and off states of medically treated, unoperated patients with Parkinson's disease may reflect an underlying limitation of all dopamine-replacement strategies in the setting of multisystem degeneration.

In spite of these potential limitations, there remain multiple approaches that might improve the results of fetal tissue grafting based on future advances in the basic sciences. Experimental studies employing xenografts, fetal allografts supplemented by growth factors, genetically modified cells that secrete trophic factors, anti-apoptotic strategies, transplanted cell lines that are transfected to produce dopamine, and antioxidant strategies are all currently being examined either in the laboratory or in the clinic. Prospective randomized placebo-controlled trials are underway to definitively evaluate the safety and efficacy of fetal tissue transplants.[34,43] At this time, however, neural grafting for the treatment of Parkinson's disease continues to be an experimental procedure. Human fetal neural grafts serve as the "gold standard" with which future cellular therapies should be compared.

Neural Transplantation for Huntington's Disease

Recent advances in molecular biology and genetics have elucidated the gene underlying Huntington's disease.[47] The discovery of this gene may lead to treatments based on molecular genetic approaches that replace or delete specific genetic information. However, no such techniques exist at the moment. For patients already carrying the Huntington's disease gene or for those who are clinically symptomatic, no long-term proven treatment exists outside of suboptimal pharmacological intervention for some of the symptoms associated with Huntington's disease, such as depression, psychosis, and chorea.[70]

Neural transplantation has been proposed as an alternative treatment for Huntington's disease. Because Huntington's disease and Parkinson's disease are both extrapyramidal movement disorders, accumulated data from neural transplant trials in Parkinson's disease can offer insights into similar therapeutic approaches to the treatment of Huntington's disease. Recently, Peschanski et al[79,80] outlined the rationale and accumulating evidence for proceeding with clinical trials of fetal neural transplantation as a treatment modality for Huntington's disease, much of which has been based on research with animal models.

Animal Models

Research has utilized injections of excitotoxins (glutamate analogs such as kainic acid, ibotenic acid, and quinolinic acid) into the striatum of adult rats. This produces anatomical and behavioral abnormalities similar to those seen in patients with Huntington's disease.[5] In adult rats, excitotoxins selectively destroy neuronal perikarya while leaving axons and terminals intact. This has resulted in strikingly similar neuropathological changes in the striatum of lesioned rats and the postmortem Huntington's disease striatum. More recently, a new neurotoxin, 3-nitropropionic acid (3-NP), has been introduced as an improved model of Huntington's disease.[4,9,10,14] 3-NP irreversibly inhibits the mitochondrial citric acid cycle and leads to depressed adenosine triphosphate levels and elevated lactate concentrations.[12,92] Chronic systemic injections of 3-NP in rats resulted in the evolution of deficits in spontaneous locomotor activity that resemble the progressive course of motor symptoms seen in Huntington's disease.[9,10] Because Huntington's disease has a progressive behavioral pathology, the 3-NP-induced behavioral symptoms more closely parallel those of the disease.[9,10]

Transplant Studies in Animals

A variety of studies have demonstrated that transplanted fetal striatal tissue readily survives and grows within the excitotoxin-lesioned striatum.[7,74] Morphological analysis has shown that the grafted tissue exhibits a patchy distribution of acetylcholinesterase-, metenkephalin-, and substance P-positive regions, which resemble those normally observed in the intact striatum.[7,50] The anatomical similarity is paralleled by a significant recovery of both acetylcholine and gamma-aminobutyric acid (GABA) within the previously depleted striatum.[7] GABA release is also partially restored in the globus pallidus and substantia nigra by striatal grafts.[27] Striatal transplants not only form synaptic contacts with the host, but are also innervated by afferent connections originating from the host substantia nigra and cortex, among others.[7]

These neuroanatomical and neurochemical results have generated substantial interest in the use of fetal striatal transplants to ameliorate behavioral deficits in animal models of Huntington's disease. The reversal of the behavioral abnormalities resulting from excitotoxic lesions has been demonstrated in several studies. In particular, fetal striatal grafts reversed the profound hyperkinesis observed in excitotoxin-lesioned rats.[4,9,10,14,24,49,89] Fetal striatal transplants also partially reversed impairments in a variety of learning and memory tasks.[23]

In primate models of Huntington's disease, Isacson and colleagues[52] described a profound drug-induced dyskinesia and hyperactivity resulting from intrastriatal injections of ibotenic acid into the primate striatum. As in the rodent studies, grafted fetal tissue was shown to survive, grow, and receive afferent innervation from the host. Moreover, a significant reduction in drug-induced dyskinesia, choreiform movements, and locomotor hyperactivity was reported.

Mechanisms of Striatal Graft Function

A number of possible mechanisms for the functional recovery following fetal striatal transplants have been postulated. One of the most frequently cited mechanisms is the development of anatomical connectivity between host and transplanted neurons.[7,74] Long axonal connections between graft and host neurons have not been demonstrated until up to 8-10 months posttransplantation, when it was demonstrated that tyrosine hydroxylase-containing neurons from the host innervated the transplanted striatal tissue.[100] Studies by Wictorin et al[100] have demonstrated both afferent and efferent connections between fetal grafts and host brain at 6-11 months posttransplantation.

However, it is unclear whether the recovery of behavioral deficits in animals seen as early as 3-5 weeks posttransplantation is specifically related to neuroanatomical integration between the transplant and host. Several rodent studies[10,83,87,90] dealing with transplant-induced behavioral changes have documented amelioration of lesion-induced deficits as early as 1 month posttransplantation. This relatively rapid recovery of locomotor function in the absence of well-formed structural connections between the graft and host brain suggests a two-stage recovery following intrastriatal transplantation: a rapid, transient neurochemically or neurotrophically mediated stage, followed by slower structural changes resulting in permanent recovery.[7,11,97]

Clinical Trials in Huntington's Disease

The application of fetal striatal transplant techniques to the treatment of Huntington's disease has become compelling for several reasons, including: 1) early successes with similar strategies in the treatment of Parkinson's disease; 2) the favorable behavioral and anatomical results from preclinical animal studies in models of Huntington's disease; and 3) the lack of adequate treatment for Huntington's disease, which is universally fatal. There are, however, many reasons why the use of human fetal tissue to treat Huntington's disease patients should be approached with caution. Several investigators[33,51,64] have argued that the complexity of the circuitry involved in the degeneration in Huntington's disease necessitates extensive experimentation and definition of optimal parameters before clinical trials are initiated. Freed[33] pointed out that even though the primate model may mimic the disease pathologically within the striatum, the behavioral similarity to Huntington's disease is apparent only after stimulation with dopamine-activating drugs, thereby limiting the ability of scientists to assess the efficacy of the transplants in primate models. Also, all animal models lack the progressive changes and multisystem involvement observed in Huntington's disease. However, the primate model of Huntington's disease facilitates the essential work of testing cell survival, connectivity, dosage, and functional effects on a drug-induced primate behavioral syndrome.[51] Whether such repair of neuronal circuitry will have substantial and sustained effect in patients with Huntington's disease can be tested only with clinical trials.

The first attempt to use fetal neural transplantation as a clinical procedure for Huntington's disease was performed collaboratively in Cuba and Poland in 1990,[96] followed months later by Madrazo et al.[69] Following the transplant of 13-week-old fetal tissue into a patient with Huntington's disease, Madrazo et al preliminarily reported no further neurological deterioration. In addition, some subjective signs of improvement were noted. However, abnormal movements frequently subside spontaneously in Huntington's disease despite continued disease progression. Madrazo et al have indicated that the patient was still improved at least 18 months later, and that subsequent patients have undergone the transplantation procedure. No further follow-up on this limited report is available.

The handling and dissection of tissue by the Madrazo group[69] was dissimilar to the procedures established by scientists who worked out the fundamental effects of striatal cell transplants in animal models. It should also be noted that the neurosurgical procedure employed by Madrazo et al is similar to that used for their patients with Parkinson's disease—making a cavity into the caudate, followed by placing the tissue into this cavity via a transventricular approach. Removing some of the already degenerated caudate nucleus could actually promote the progression of Huntington's disease. Furthermore, no recovery of function has been observed in a rodent model that had fetal striatal transplants placed into the lateral ventricles.[88] Animal research has shown that stereotactic placement of cells within the degenerated striatum appears to be the superior procedure for subsequent reduction of hyperkinetic behavior in rats. Therefore, clinical trials should employ stereotactic placement of transplanted tissue directly into the caudate nucleus and/or putamen.

There are a limited number of other research centers that have performed stereotactic implants of fetal striatal transplants in Huntington's disease patients. The only peer-reviewed publications at this time report preliminary findings.[69,82,96] Philpott et al[82] reported improved cognitive functioning 4-6 months posttransplantation in three patients with Huntington's disease. Most other investigators have been reluctant to begin Huntington's disease transplant programs, even though the animal literature has been supportive and early clinical studies of Parkinson's disease patients have shown that the transplantation technique is relatively safe. There are a number of issues that still need to be resolved. These include the determination, with human tissue, that: 1) suspension or solid tissue transplants provide survival of at least 80% of grafts; 2) uncontrolled graft overgrowth can be avoided; 3) the donor age that provides striatal graft survival is defined; and 4) fetal striatal dissection can be optimized to produce reliable human fetal graft survival and function.[16,40,79]

This latter issue has been the most significant obstacle in proceeding with clinical trials. The striatum consists of different compartments called striasomes and matrices. Grafts contain both striatal markers (p-zones) and cellular phenotypes of nonstriatal origin.[100] P-zones contain the primary afferent and efferent connections between the substantia nigra, cortex, and striatum, and can be demonstrated immunohistochemically by patches of acetylcholine and/or DARPP-32 (dopamine and cyclic adenosine monophosphate-regulated protein). Studies in rodents using grafts derived from rat and porcine embryonic tissue have suggested that a p-zone value of 25%-50% must be achieved in order to see consistent behavioral recovery.[16,72] Furthermore, only striatal GABA neurons (DARPP-32-positive neurons) are capable of making long axonal connections between the graft and striatal target areas. If the mechanism of graft-induced benefit is derived from such neuronal reconstruction, then a high p-zone value must be reliably produced in striatal grafts.[16,19,20,100]

Isacson and colleagues have shown that the lateral ganglionic eminence (LGE) contains most of the primordial striatum.[77] Transplants using this specific portion of the fetal rodent or porcine brain have resulted in grafts comprising mostly striatal tissue, upward of 80%. In humans, the primordial striatum is also derived from the LGE.[40,71] However, grafts derived from the human LGE have yet to reach the minimal p-zone criterion, possibly due to the extended duration of graft maturation and lack of expression of appropriate markers in human grafts early after transplantation.[16,71] Alternatively, dissection methods delineated in other species may not be appropriate for use in human grafts. In an attempt to increase the p-zone concentration of embryonic grafts, Freeman et al[39] eliminated the embryonic nucleus basalis by including only the lateral aspect of the LGE in the dissection. Analysis of grafts derived using this dissection technique with DARPP-32 showed p-zone values consistently above 40% of the graft volume, with some grafts containing p-zones of greater than 95% of the graft volume. These results suggest that lateral LGE grafts may be the most suitable tissue for transplantation in Huntington's disease patients.

Furthermore, all studies in rats from the 1980s and early 1990s that demonstrated behavioral changes after striatal grafting employed coarse striatal dissections that also included the medial ganglionic eminence and the body of the ventricular eminence.[16] Recently, improvement in paw-reaching has been noted following rodent allografts of LGE tissue.[72] The authors have also recently reported that grafts derived from the human fetal LGE can significantly reduce drug-induced rotation in a rodent model of Huntington's disease.[87]

Based on these preclinical results, the University of South Florida has begun a clinical trial of fetal lateral LGE transplants for the treatment of Huntington's disease. More clinical and laboratory data are likely to be forthcoming in the near future, which will permit a better assessment of this technique. At this time, fetal transplantation remains an experimental procedure.

References

1. Alexander GE, Crutcher MD, DeLong MR: Basal ganglia-thalamocortical circuits: parallel substrates for motor, oculomotor, "prefrontal" and "limbic" functions. **Prog Brain Res 85:**119-146, 1990
2. Annett LE, Torres EM, Ridley RM, et al: A comparison of the behavioural effects of embryonic nigral grafts in the caudate nucleus and in the putamen of marmosets with unilateral 6-OHDA lesions. **Exp Brain Res 103:**355-371, 1995
3. Bankiewicz KS, Whitwell HL, Sofroniew MV, et al: Survival of TH-positive cells and graft-induced host dopaminergic sprouting in patients with Parkinson's disease after intrastriatal grafting of fetal ventral mesencephalus. **Soc Neurosci Abst 19:**864, 1993 (Abstract)
4. Beal MF, Brouillet E, Jenkins BG, et al: Neurochemical and histologic characterization of striatal excitotoxic lesions produced by the mitochondrial toxin 3-nitropropionic acid. **J Neurosci 13:**4181-4192, 1993
5. Beal MF, Kowall NW, Ellison DW, et al: Replication of the neurochemical characteristics of Huntington's disease by quinolinic acid. **Nature 321:**168-171, 1986
6. Bernheimer H, Birkmayer W, Hornykiewicz O, et al: Brain dopamine and the syndromes of Parkinson and Huntington. Clinical, morphological and neurochemical correlations. **J Neurol Sci 20:**415-455, 1973
7. Björklund A, Lindvall O, Isacson O, et al: Mechanisms of action of intracerebral neural implants: studies on nigral and striatal grafts to the lesioned striatum. **Trends Neurosci 10:**509-516, 1987
8. Björklund A, Stenevi U, Schmidt RH, et al: Intracerebral grafting of neuronal cell suspensions I. Introduction and general methods of preparation. **Acta Physiol Scand Suppl 522:**1-7, 1983
9. Borlongan CV, Koutouzis TK, Sanberg PR: 3-nitropropionic acid animal model and Huntington's disease. **Neurosci Biobehav Rev 21:**289-294, 1997
10. Borlongan CV, Nishino H, Sanberg PR: Systemic, but not intraparenchymal administration of 3-nitropropionic acid mimics the neuropathology of Huntington's disease. **Neurosci Res 28:**185-189, 1997
11. Borlongan CV, Polgar S, Freeman TB, et al: Will fetal striatal transplants correct the akinetic end-stage of Huntington's disease? **Neurodegeneration 5:** 189-192, 1996
12. Bossi SR, Simpson JR, Isacson O: Age dependence of striatal neuronal death caused by mitochondrial dysfunction. **Neuroreport 4:**73-76, 1993
13. Breeze RE, Wells TH Jr, Freed CR: Implantation of fetal tissue for the management of Parkinson's disease: a technical note. **Neurosurgery 36:**1044-1048, 1995
14. Brouillet E, Jenkins BG, Hyman BT, et al: Age-dependent vulnerability of the striatum to the mitochondrial toxin 3-nitropropionic acid. **J Neurochem 60:**356-359, 1993
15. Brundin P, Björklund A: Survival, growth and function of dopaminergic neurons grafted to the brain. **Prog Brain Res 71:**293-308, 1987
16. Brundin P, Fricker RA, Nakao N: Paucity of p-zones in striatal grafts prohibit commencement of clinical trials in Huntington's disease. **Neuroscience 71:** 895-897, 1996
17. Brundin P, Strecker RE, Widner H, et al: Human fetal dopamine neurons grafted in a rat model of Parkinson's disease: immunological aspects, spontaneous and drug-induced behaviour, and dopamine release. **Exp Brain Res 70:**192-208, 1988
18. Brundin P, Widner H, Rehncrona S, et al: Influence of the size of the implantation instrument on the survival of dissociated fetal neural grafts. **Restor Neurol Neurosci 1:**155-156, 1989
19. Campbell K, Wictorin K, Björklund A: Neurotransmitter-related gene expression in intrastriatal striatal transplants—I. Phenotypical characterization of striatal and non-striatal graft regions. **Neuroscience 64:** 17-33, 1995
20. Campbell K, Wictorin K, Björklund A: Neurotransmitter-related gene expression in intrastriatal striatal transplants—II. Characterization of efferent projecting graft neurons. **Neuroscience 64:**35-47, 1995
21. Collier TJ, Gallagher MJ, Sladek CD: Cryopreservation and storage of embryonic rat mesencephalic dopamine neurons for one year: comparison to fresh tissue in culture and neural grafts. **Brain Res 623:** 249-256, 1993
22. Deacon T, Schumacher J, Dinsmore J, et al: Histological evidence of fetal pig neural cell survival after transplantation into a patient with Parkinson's disease. **Nat Med 3:**350-353, 1997
23. Deckel AW, Moran TH, Coyle JT, et al: Anatomical predictors of behavioral recovery following fetal striatal transplants. **Brain Res 365:**249-258, 1986
24. Deckel AW, Robinson RG, Coyle JT, et al: Reversal of long-term locomotor abnormalities in the kainic acid model of Huntington's disease by day 18 fetal striatal implants. **Eur J Pharmacol 93:**287-288, 1983
25. Defer GL, Geny C, Ricolfi F, et al: Long-term outcome of unilaterally transplanted parkinsonian patients. I. Clinical approach. **Brain 119:**41-50, 1996
26. Dunnett SB, Björklund A, Schmidt RH, et al: Intracerebral grafting of neuronal cell suspensions IV. Behavioural recovery in rats with unilateral 6-OHDA lesions following implantation of nigral cell suspensions in different forebrain sites. **Acta Physiol Scand Suppl 522:**29-37, 1983
27. Dunnett SB, Isacson O, Sirinathsinghji DJS, et al: Striatal grafts in the ibotenic acid-lesioned neostriatum: functional studies. **Prog Brain Res 78:**38-45, 1988
28. Folkerth RD, Durso R: Survival and proliferation of nonneural tissues, with obstruction of cerebral ventricles, in a parkinsonian patient treated with fetal allografts. **Neurology 46:**1219-1225, 1996
29. Freed CR, Breeze RE, Rosenberg NL, et al: Survival of implanted fetal dopamine cells and neurologic improvement 12 to 46 months after transplantation for Parkinson's disease. **N Engl J Med 327:**1549-1555, 1992
30. Freed CR, Breeze RE, Rosenberg NL, et al: Transplantation of human fetal dopamine cells for Parkinson's disease. Results at 1 year. **Arch Neurol 47:** 505-512, 1990
31. Freed CR, Breeze RE, Schnock SA, et al: Human fetal dopamine cells survive and develop processes after implantation into humans with Parkinson's disease. **Soc Neurosci Abst 20:**9, 1994 (Abstract)
32. Freed CR, Trojanowski JQ, Galvin JE, et al: Embryonic dopamine cells cultured as strands show long term survival without immunosuppression in a pa-

tient with advanced Parkinson's disease. **Soc Neurosci Abst 23:**1682, 1997 (Abstract)
33. Freed WJ: Neural transplantation: prospects for clinical use. **Cell Transplant 2:**13-31, 1993
34. Freeman TB: From transplants to gene therapy for Parkinson's disease. **Exp Neurol 144:**47-50, 1997
35. Freeman TB, Cosman E: New device for stereotactic transplantation of tissue into the human striatum. **Soc Neurosci Abst 19:**864, 1993 (Abstract)
36. Freeman TB, Kordower JH: Human cadaver embryonic substantia nigra grafts: effects of ontogeny, preoperative graft preparation and tissue storage, in Lindvall O, Björklund A, Widner H (eds): **Intracerebral Transplantation in Movement Disorders: Experimental Basis and Clinical Experience.** Amsterdam: Elsevier, 1991, pp 163-169
37. Freeman TB, Olanow CW: Fetal homotransplants in the treatment of Parkinson's disease. **Arch Neurol 48:**900-901, 1991 (Letter)
38. Freeman TB, Olanow CW, Hauser RA, et al: Bilateral fetal nigral transplantation into the postcommissural putamen in Parkinson's disease. **Ann Neurol 38:** 379-388, 1995
39. Freeman TB, Othberg AI, Jones SL, et al: Transplantation of the lateral aspect of the lateral ganglion eminence for Huntington's disease. **Soc Neurosci Abst 8:**1682, 1997
40. Freeman TB, Sanberg PR, Isacson O: Development of the human striatum: implications for fetal striatal transplantation in the treatment of Huntington's disease. **Cell Transplant 4:**539-545, 1995
41. Freeman TB, Sanberg PR, Nauert GM, et al: The influence of donor age on survival of solid and suspension intraparenchymal human embryonic nigral grafts. **Cell Transplant 4:**141-154, 1995
42. Freeman TB, Spence MS, Boss BD, et al: Development of dopaminergic neurons in the human substantia nigra. **Exp Neurol 113:**344-353, 1991
43. Freeman TB, Vawter D, Goetz CG, et al: Towards the use of surgical placebo-controlled trials. **Transplant Proc 29:**1925, 1997 (Abstract)
44. Hauser RA, Olanow CW, Snow BJ, et al: Fetal nigral transplantation in Parkinson's disease: the USF pilot program (12- to 24-month evaluation), in Freeman TB, Widner H (eds): **Cell Transplantation for Neurological Disorders: Toward Reconstruction of the Central Nervous System.** Totowa, NJ: Humana Press, 1998, pp 19-30
45. Hitchocock EH, Whitwell HL, Sofroniew MV, et al: Survival of TH-positive and neuromelanin-containing cells in patients with Parkinson's disease after intrastriatal grafting of fetal ventral mesencephalon. **Exp Neurol 129:**3, 1994 (Abstract)
46. Holt DA, Nauert GM, Othberg AI, et al: Infectious issues in fetal neural transplantation. **Cell Transplant 6:**553-556, 1997
47. The Huntington's Disease Collaborative Research Group: A novel gene containing a trinucleotide repeat that is expanded and unstable on Huntington's disease chromosomes. **Cell 72:**971-983, 1993
48. Iacono RP, Tang ZS, Mazziotta JC, et al: Bilateral fetal grafts for Parkinson's disease: 22 months' results. **Stereotact Funct Neurosurg 58:**84-87, 1992
49. Isacson O, Brundin P, Kelly PAT, et al: Functional neuronal replacement by grafted striatal neurones in the ibotenic acid-lesioned rat striatum. **Nature 311:** 458-460, 1984
50. Isacson O, Dawbarn D, Brundin P, et al: Neural grafting in a rat model of Huntington's disease: striosomal-like organization of striatal grafts as revealed by acetylcholinesterase histochemistry immunocytochemistry and receptor autoradiography. **Neurosci 22:**481-497, 1987
51. Isacson O, Hantraye P, Riche D, et al: The relationship between symptoms and functional anatomy in the chronic neurodegenerative diseases: from pharmacological replacement therapy in Huntington's disease, in Lindvall O, Björklund A, Widner H (eds): **Intracerebral Transplantation in Movement Disorders: Experimental Basis and Clinical Experience.** Amsterdam: Elsevier, 1991, pp 245-258
52. Isacson O, Riche D, Hantraye P, et al: A primate model of Huntington's disease: cross-species implantation of striatal precursor cells to the excitotoxically lesioned baboon caudate-putamen. **Exp Brain Res 75:**213-220, 1989
53. Kish SJ, Shannak K, Hornykiewicz O: Uneven pattern of dopamine loss in the striatum of patients with idiopathic Parkinson's disease. Pathophysiologic and clinical implications. **N Engl J Med 318:** 876-880, 1988
54. Kontur PJ, Leranth C, Redmond DE Jr, et al: Tyrosine hydroxylase immunoreactivity and monoamine and metabolite levels of cryopreserved human fetal ventral mesencephalon. **Exp Neurol 121:**172-180, 1993
55. Kopyov OV, Jacques D, Lieberman A, et al: Clinical study of fetal mesencephalic intracerebral transplants for the treatment of Parkinson's disease. **Cell Transplant 5:**327-337, 1996
56. Kordower JH, Freeman TB, Bakay RAE, et al: Treatment with fetal allografts. **Neurology 48:**1737-1738, 1997 (Letter)
57. Kordower JH, Freeman TB, Olanow CW: Neuropathology of fetal nigral grafts in patients with Parkinson's disease. **Mov Disord** (In press)
58. Kordower JH, Freeman TB, Snow BJ, et al: Neuropathological evidence of graft survival and striatal reinnervation after the transplantation of fetal mesencephalic tissue in a patient with Parkinson's disease. **N Engl J Med 332:**1118-1124, 1995
59. Kordower JH, Rosenstein JM, Collier TJ, et al: Functional fetal nigral grafts in a patient with Parkinson's disease: chemoanatomic, ultrastructural, and metabolic studies. **J Comp Neurol 370:**203-230, 1996
60. Kordower JH, Rosenstein JM, Collier TJ, et al: Functional fetal nigral grafts in a second patient with Parkinson's disease: a post-mortem analysis. **Soc Neurosci Abst 22:**318, 1996 (Abstract)
61. Kordower JH, Styren S, Clarke M, et al: Fetal grafting for Parkinson's disease: expression of immune markers in two patients with functional fetal nigral grafts. **Cell Transplant 6:**213-219, 1997
62. Kunzle H: Bilateral projections from precentral motor cortex to the putamen and other parts of the basal ganglia. An autoradiographic study in Maca fascicularis. **Brain Behav Evol 88:**195-209, 1975
63. Langston JW, Widner H, Goetz CG, et al: Core assessment program for intracerebral transplantations (CAPIT). **Mov Disord 7:**2-13, 1992
64. Lindvall O: Prospects of transplantation in human neurodegenerative diseases. **Trends Neurosci 14:** 376-384, 1991

65. Lindvall O, Brundin P, Widner H, et al: Grafts of fetal dopamine neurons survive and improve motor function in Parkinson's disease. **Science 247:**574-577, 1990
66. Lindvall O, Rehncrona S, Brundin P, et al: Human fetal dopamine neurons grafted into the striatum in two patients with severe Parkinson's disease. A detailed account of methodology and a 6-month follow-up. **Arch Neurol 46:**615-631, 1989
67. Lindvall O, Sawle G, Widner H, et al: Evidence for long-term survival and function of dopaminergic grafts in progressive Parkinson's disease. **Ann Neurol 35:**172-180, 1994
68. Lindvall O, Widner H, Rehncrona S, et al: Transplantation of fetal dopamine neurons in Parkinson's disease: one-year clinical and neurophysiological observations in two patients with putaminal implants. **Ann Neurol 31:**155-165, 1992
69. Madrazo I, Franco-Bourland RE, Castrejon H, et al: Fetal striatal homotransplantation for Huntington's disease: first two case reports. **Neurol Res 17:** 312-315, 1995
70. Marshall FJ, Shoulson I: Clinical features and treatment of Huntington's disease, in Watts RL, Koller WC (eds): **Movement Disorders: Neurologic Principles and Practice.** New York: McGraw-Hill, 1997, pp 491-502
71. Naimi S, Jeny R, Hantraye P, et al: Ontogeny of human striatal DARPP-32 neurons in fetuses and following xenografting to the adult rat brain. **Exp Neurol 137:**15-25, 1996
72. Nakao N, Grasbon-Frodl EM, Widner H, et al: DARPP-32-rich zones in grafts of lateral ganglionic eminence govern the extent of functional recovery in skilled paw reaching in an animal model of Huntington's disease. **Neuroscience 74:**959-970, 1996
73. Nauert GM, Freeman TB: Low-pressure aspiration abortion for obtaining embryonic and early gestational fetal tissue for research purposes. **Cell Transplant 3:**147-151, 1994
74. Norman AB, Lehman MN, Sanberg PR: Functional effects of fetal striatal transplants. **Brain Res Bull 22:** 163-172, 1989
75. Olanow CW, Freeman TB, Kordower JH: Transplantation strategies for Parkinson's disease, in Watts RL, Koller WC (eds): **Movement Disorders: Neurologic Principles and Practice.** New York, NY: McGraw-Hill, 1997, pp 221-236
76. Olanow CW, Kordower JH, Freeman TB: Fetal nigral transplantation as a therapy for Parkinson's disease. **Trends Neurosci 19:**102-109, 1996
77. Pakzaban P, Deacon TW, Burns LH, et al: Increased proportion of acetylcholinesterase-rich zones and improved morphological integration in host striatum of fetal grafts derived from the lateral but not the medial ganglionic eminence. **Exp Brain Res 97:** 13-22, 1993
78. Pate BD, Kawamata T, Yamada T, et al: Correlation of striatal fluorodopa uptake in the MPTP monkey with dopaminergic indices. **Ann Neurol 34:**331-338, 1993
79. Peschanski M, Césaro P, Hantraye P: Rationale for intrastriatal grafting of striatal neuroblasts in patients with Huntington's disease. **Neuroscience 68:** 273-285, 1995
80. Peschanski M, Césaro P, Hantraye P: What is needed versus what would be interesting to know before undertaking neural transplantation in patients with Huntington's disease. **Neuroscience 71:**899-900, 1996
81. Peschanski M, Defer G, N'Guyen JP, et al: Bilateral motor improvement and alteration of L-dopa effect in two patients with Parkinson's disease following intrastriatal transplantation of foetal ventral mesencephalon. **Brain 117:**487-499, 1994
82. Philpott LM, Kopyov OV, Lee AJ, et al: Neuropsychological functioning following fetal striatal transplantation in Huntington's chorea: three case presentations. **Cell Transplant 6:**203-212, 1997
83. Pundt LL, Kondoh T, Conrad JA, et al: Transplantation of human fetal striatum into a rodent model of Huntington's disease ameliorates locomotor deficits. **Neurosci Res 24:**415-420, 1996
84. Redmond DE Jr, Leranth C, Spencer DD, et al: Fetal neural graft survival. **Lancet 336:**820-822, 1990 (Letter)
85. Remy P, Samson Y, Hantraye P, et al: Clinical correlates of [^{18}F] fluorodopa uptake in five grafted parkinsonian patients. **Ann Neurol 38:**580-588, 1995
86. Robbins RJ, Torres-Aleman I, Leranth C, et al: Cryopreservation of human brain tissue. **Exp Neurol 107:**208-213, 1990
87. Sanberg PR, Borlongan CV, Koutouzis TK, et al: Human fetal striatal transplantation in an excitotoxic lesioned model of Huntington's disease. **Ann NY Acad Sci 831:**452-460, 1997
88. Sanberg PR, Giordano M, Henault MA, et al: Intraparenchymal striatal transplants required for maintenance of behavioral recovery in an animal model of Huntington's disease. **J Neural Transplant 1:** 23-31, 1989
89. Sanberg PR, Henault MA, Deckel AW: Locomotor hyperactivity: effects of multiple striatal transplants in an animal model of Huntington's disease. **Pharmacol Biochem Behav 25:**297-300, 1986
90. Sanberg PR, Koutouzis TK, Freeman TB, et al: Behavioral effects of fetal neural transplants: relevance to Huntington's disease. **Brain Res Bull 37:**493-496, 1993
91. Sawle GV, Bloomfield PM, Björklund A, et al: Transplantation of fetal dopamine neurons in Parkinson's disease: PET [^{18}F]-6-L-fluorodopa studies in two patients with putaminal implants. **Ann Neurol 31:** 166-173, 1992
92. Simpson JR, Isacson O: Mitochondrial impairment reduces the threshold for *in vivo* NMDA-mediated neuronal death in the striatum. **Exp Neurol 121:** 57-64, 1993
93. Snow BJ, Tooyama I, McGeer EG, et al: Human positron emission tomographic [^{18}F]-fluorodopa studies correlate with dopamine cell counts and levels. **Ann Neurol 34:**324-330, 1993
94. Snow BJ, Vingerhoets FJG, Hauser RA, et al: PET studies of bilateral fetal nigral transplantation for Parkinson's disease. **Mov Disord 11 (Suppl 1):**250, 1996
95. Spencer DD, Robbins RJ, Naftolin F, et al: Unilateral transplantation of human fetal mesencephalic tissue into the caudate nucleus of patients with Parkinson's disease. **N Engl J Med 327:**1541-1548, 1992
96. Sramka M, Rattaj M, Molina H, et al: Stereotactic technique and pathophysiological mechanisms of neurotransplantation in Huntington's chorea. **Ste-**

reotact Funct Neurosurg 58:79-83, 1992

97. Tulipan N, Huang S, Whetsell WO, et al: Neonatal striatal grafts prevent lethal syndrome produced by bilateral intrastriatal injection of kainic acid. **Brain Res 377:**163-167, 1986
98. Verney C, Zecevic N, Nikolic B, et al: Early evidence of catecholaminergic cell groups in 5- and 6-week-old human embryos using tyrosine hydroxylase and dopamine-ß-hydroxylase immunocytochemistry. **Neurosci Lett 131:**121-124, 1991
99. Wenning GK, Odin P, Morrish P, et al: Short- and long-term survival and function of unilateral intrastriatal dopaminergic grafts in Parkinson's disease. **Ann Neurol 42:**95-107, 1997
100. Wictorin K, Ouimet CC, Björklund A: Intrinsic organization and connectivity of intrastriatal transplants in rats as revealed by DARPP-32 immunohistochemistry: specificity of connections with host brain. **Eur J Neurosci 1:**690-701, 1989
101. Widner H, Tetrud J, Rehncrona S: Bilateral fetal mesencephalic grafting in two patients with parkinsonism induced by 1-methyl-4-phenyl-1,2,3,6-tetrahydropyridine (MPTP). **N Engl J Med 327:**1556-1563, 1992

PART D

Technical Advances in Surgery for Parkinson's Disease

CHAPTER 14

MAGNETIC RESONANCE IMAGING GUIDANCE IN SURGERY FOR PARKINSON'S DISEASE

RON L. ALTERMAN, MD, AND PATRICK KELLY, MD

Advances in stereotactic neurosurgery typically follow imaging breakthroughs. Whereas Horsley and Clarke introduced animal stereotaxis based on external cranial landmarks in 1908,[26] irregularities in human cranial morphology made clinical stereotaxis impractical until the advent of ventriculographic targeting 40 years later.[61] The introduction of axial computed tomography (CT) in the 1970s led to the reconfiguration of stereotactic frames, and computer planning systems capable of storing and manipulating increasingly complex imaging data were created. Today, magnetic resonance imaging (MRI) provides exquisite anatomical detail that heretofore was available only at postmortem examination. And, as we move into the era of high-resolution functional brain imaging, the noninvasive correlation of anatomy and pathophysiology may transform stereotaxis once again.

It is critical in this time of rapid technological advancement to have a detailed understanding of current and emerging imaging modalities. In this chapter, the current state of MRI guidance for Parkinson's disease surgery is discussed, concentrating on its comparative advantages and its limitations.

ALTERNATIVES TO MRI FOR STEREOTACTIC TARGETING

Ventriculography

Since 1947, when Spiegel et al[61] first used pneumoencephalography to relate anatomical targets to intracranial landmarks, ventriculography has been the mainstay of stereotactic imaging and the technique to which all others are compared. In 1955 Talairach[64] suggested that the deep brain structures were most consistently related to the anterior commissure (AC)-posterior commissure (PC) line. Human stereotactic atlases and targeting have henceforth been based on this easily constructed median, a convention that standardized stereotactic technique and facilitated the expansion of functional neurosurgery in the late 1950s and 1960s.

Ventriculography can be performed inexpensively with standard radiographic equipment. With good technique, the commissures are rapidly and accurately identified. In addition, if the proper facilities are established, biplanar x-rays can also be used for real-time feedback of probe position.

There are many factors, however, that make this method of targeting undesirable. Ventriculography is invasive and difficult to perform well. Radiographic technique must be perfect in order to eliminate distortion due to parallax.[36] Magnification must be factored into all measurements, increasing the risk of human error.[36] Intraoperative risk is increased, albeit minimally, by the need to cannulate the lateral ventricle. Intraventricular air or contrast medium can induce headaches, nausea, vomiting, or seizures.[17,18,36,38,66] Loss of cerebrospinal fluid can alter the position of brain structures.[66]

Even when performed by the most experienced and capable surgeons, there are numerous inaccuracies inherent to targeting based on ventriculography and stereotactic atlases. Ventriculography targets deep brain structures indirectly, relying on an inconstant relationship between these sites and the third ventricle.[3,7,20] The atlases from which target coordinates are derived are based on a small sample of brains and take little account of normal human variation.[59] Further error is introduced by tissue fixation for atlas preparation, which results in shrinkage.[50,59]

A number of authors have examined the inaccuracies of ventriculographic targeting. Amador et al[3] found that the movement of paraventricular structures in relation to increasing third ventricular width is not consistently proportional. Brierley and Beck[7] conducted an elegant examination of 53 human cerebral hemispheres, studying the relationship of the thalamic nuclei and globus pallidus to the PC. They discovered that the relationship of the PC to the thalamic nuclei was highly variable, raising questions about the accuracy of stereotactic targeting based on this landmark. Hardy et al[20] demonstrated that human third ventricular width, as seen on ventriculography, ranges from 2 to 13 mm, confirming the findings of previous studies. Further, they found that third ventricular width does correlate with the laterality of the thalamocapsular border, but the correlation is a loose one, serving only as an approximation as to where one should begin neurophysiological monitoring. Kawashima et al[33] demonstrated that even in individuals with identical third ventricular widths, the distance from the midline to the thalamocapsular border can vary by up to 5 mm, supporting a previous study by Kelly et al[37] which demonstrated that the electrophysiologically determined location of the ventral posterior thalamic nucleus could vary by as much as 6 mm from its location as predicted by ventriculography and a stereotactic atlas.

Potential targeting errors due to normal human variation are exacerbated by anatomical distortion due to ventriculography itself. Comparing ventriculographic and CT-derived measurements, Hariz et al[23,24] demonstrated that pneumoventriculography leads to widening and anterior displacement of the third ventricle. Huber and Rivoir[27] demonstrated significant distortion with air ventriculography and suggested that positive contrast was a better option, as it requires a smaller injection volume.

Given the inherent inaccuracies of indirectly targeting deep brain structures, and the complications and technical difficulties attendant upon ventriculography, it is surprising that Hanieh and Maloney[19] and Hassler et al[25] found most ventriculographically targeted lesions to be accurately placed at postmortem examination, and that prior generations of stereotactic neurosurgeons achieved such good results. In fact, ventriculography has proven so reliable that many stereotactic surgeons continue to use it in their contemporary practices despite the availability of MRI and CT.[29,34,35,60]

Computed Tomography

CT transformed stereotactic surgery by providing geometrically sound images of the brain noninvasively. This advance made direct targeting of visualized structures possible, permitting stereotactic procedures to be performed even in the presence of anatomically distorting pathology, such as mass lesions and ventriculomegaly. As a result, CT-compatible stereotactic systems were rapidly developed, CT-guided stereotactic biopsy became a routine neurosurgical procedure, and the groundwork for computer-assisted, image-guided stereotactic tumor resection was established.

The direct visualization of brain parenchyma and excellent gray/white matter differentiation on CT enhanced localization of the thalamocapsular and pallidocapsular borders; however, individual nuclear structures still could not be identified. Emerging computer technology was incorporated into CT-guided stereotaxy, in part to overcome this limitation. Digitized versions of human stereotactic atlases were developed that could be custom fit to the patient's anatomy in an attempt to improve targeting on axial CT images.[15,21,31,66]

Despite these advancements, the impact of CT on functional neurosurgery was not as great as had been hoped, primarily due to its inability to perform direct midsagittal imaging. Numerous techniques were proposed to address this problem, including the use of sagittal reconstructions of axial CT images, which poorly visualized the commissures[5,30]; attempts to identify consistent relationships between the AC-PC line and craniometric landmarks such as Reid's baseline[52,57]; mathematical calculations of the midcommissural point based on the coordinates of the anterior and posterior commissures imaged on separate axial slices[43,54]; the use of ventriculography to determine the AC-PC angle for axial CT imaging; and simple trial and error, angling the scanner in order to image both commissures on one slice.[51] None of these techniques proved ideal, and poor delineation of the commissures was cited as the most important source of error during CT-guided functional neurosurgery.[70,71]

Bucholz and colleagues[8] employed a phantom with points of varying size whose coordinates were known in order to analyze the sources of error in CT-guided stereotaxis. They discovered that the most important variables affecting accuracy were the user's ability to visualize the target, the size of the target, CT slice thickness, and interslice spacing. It is obvious from this study that the targeting demands of functional stereotactic procedures push the limits of CT guidance. Neither the commissures nor the targets are well visualized on CT, and both the targets and the margin for error are small.

Many surgeons abandoned ventriculography during the CT era, demonstrating acceptable results when performing neuroablative procedures with CT supported by neurophysiological techniques.[40,43,51,66] Others felt this was premature, citing the clear delineation of the AC-PC line as a critical factor in the proper performance of these procedures.[18,34,35,70,71] CT was incorporated into most surgeons' techniques; however, it was primarily used to delineate more accurately the thalamocapsular border during thalamotomy.[35] In all instances, neurophysiological confirmation of the functional anatomical target was advised.[4,5,9,18,30,31,34-37,40,43,51,52,54,57,66,70,71]

Magnetic Resonance Imaging

The advantages of MRI for performing functional neurosurgical procedures are obvious. MRI provides superior gray/white matter differentiation and visualization of some deep brain nuclei. Triplanar imaging permits ready identification of the commissures so that familiar ventriculographic targeting paradigms can be employed.[44,67] Newly developed pulse sequences, such as fast spin-echo inversion recovery (FSE/IR), visualize small structures such as the subthalamic nucleus, helping to expand the range of targets for surgical intervention.[55]

Image Distortion

The most important drawback to MRI is the potential for image distortion. It is interesting that many neurosurgeons who are comfortable with the myriad sources of error due to ventriculography cringe at the thought of using MRI alone for stereotactic targeting because of the potential for image distortion. Negating the overwhelming advantages of MRI, this factor alone has prevented the routine use of MRI as the sole means of anatomical stereotactic localization.

Magnetic field inhomogeneities and magnetic susceptibility artifacts can lead to small but important shifts in the apparent location of imaged structures.[58,63,65,68,69] A number of studies have been conducted to define the sources of image distortion so that they may be corrected. Sumanaweera et al[63] reviewed this topic in great detail. They defined gradient field nonlinearities and magnetic field inhomogeneities as the most important sources of error. Gradient field nonlinearities generate three types of distortion during two-dimensional (2-D) image acquisition (barrel, potato chip, and bow-tie effects), whereas only one form of distortion (barrel effect) occurs with three-dimensional (3-D) acquisitions. Barrel effects, as well as scanner-induced magnetic field inhomogeneities, are magnet-dependent and fairly constant, so they can be mathematically corrected. The authors therefore suggest the use of 3-D image sets performed on a well-calibrated magnet that is equipped with software to correct for the barrel effect.

In contrast to scanner-induced nonlinearities, the magnetic susceptibility effect, which occurs at the interface of tissues with markedly different magnetic susceptibilities (e.g., fat/water), is unique to the scanned subject and cannot be corrected.[63,65] Fortunately, such interfaces do not occur deep in the brain substance and should not affect subcortical targeting. In addition, Taren and co-workers[65] reported that FSE imaging techniques reduce magnetic susceptibility effects and provide excellent gray/white matter differentiation, making them ideal for performing functional neurosurgical procedures.

Walton et al[68,69] conducted a phantom-based analysis of MRI targeting, which revealed that distortion is spatially variant, occurring at the periphery of stereotactic space. This edge effect is not frame-related, as it occurred even with a specially constructed nonmetallic frame. Image distortion occurred in all planes and predominantly affected one coordinate in each plane. During axial imaging, anteroposterior (AP) coordinates were distorted near the frame base; during coronal imaging, large errors in depth occurred at the extremes of the AP axis; whereas sagittal imaging revealed distortions of depth at the extremes of laterality. Although image distortion was insignificant at the center of the stereotactic frame, image shifts at the periphery may result in misplaced stereotactic fiducials. Incorrectly registered fiducials result in poor targeting throughout the stereotactic image.

Cleverly, these authors noted that during coronal and axial imaging, the fiducials on the localizing panel that runs perpendicular to the other two (i.e., superior plate during coronal imaging, anterior plate during axial imaging) are the greatest source of error. By eliminating this "third plate" from fiducial registration, overall accuracy was greatly enhanced. For example, during axial imaging, elimination of the anterior plate fiducials reduced the absolute error along the y axis at extremes of z from 11 to 4 mm. The trade-off was a slight degradation in accuracy along the x axis. Elimination of the third plate should be employed only when the frame is perfectly orthogonal to the scanner, a situation that is dependent on the use of frame-to-scanner fixation devices employed with the various stereotactic systems.

As this discussion attests, the sources of MRI distortion have been well characterized and, for the most part, are correctable. In addition, we have learned from the ventriculography experience that clinical results can be surprising even with documented inaccuracies in targeting technique.

MRI-Guided Targeting for Functional Neurosurgical Procedures

In 1986, Lunsford et al[49] compared MRI- and CT-derived stereotactic coordinates in three patients, finding no significant difference between the two data sets. This prompted the successful performance of a thalamotomy guided solely by MRI, which was reported in 1988; Lunsford reported superior definition of the commissures with MRI, as compared to reformatted CT, and suggested that ventriculography was obsolete for stereotactic targeting.[48] This concept and the data upon which it was based were extended by a larger study published in 1992 by Kondziolka et al.[38] In this study MRI- and CT-derived coordinates were compared in

41 patients operated on at two separate centers. The authors found a maximum 2-mm difference in 2-D targeting between the modalities. They noted no accuracy degradation when targeting peripheral versus central sites, and no difference between a 0.5-tesla or 1.5-tesla scanner.

Gerdes et al[14] also compared MRI to CT, targeting four sites in each of four patients. They used the Brown-Roberts-Wells system and employed 4-mm thick axial CT slices and 5-mm axial MRI slices for targeting. They found a mean distance of 3.72 mm between the CT- and MRI-derived targets, prompting these authors to conclude that MRI should be used only in conjunction with CT and for larger lesions in non-eloquent brain. One might argue with these conclusions, pointing out that the targeting difference could be attributed in large part to the thick scan slices employed.

Recently, Favre et al (unpublished results, 1996) conducted a study in which they examined the necessity for microelectrode recording after pallidal targeting with MRI. Targeting was performed with sagittal T1-weighted sequences, as well as axial and coronal FSE/IR sequences. They discovered that the pallidal base, as determined by microelectrode recording, was within 1.5 mm of the MRI-derived location for this structure in all but one of their 48 patients (73 targets). They concluded that when employing their targeting paradigm, MRI sufficiently delineates the inferior border of the internal segment of the globus pallidus (GPi), obviating the need for microelectrode recording. They stress, however, that macroelectrode stimulation should still be performed for target confirmation.

COMPUTERS AND MRI GUIDANCE

The full potential of MRI guidance can be realized only when employed in concert with an advanced surgical planning system. These systems co-register different imaging modalities and different MRI pulse sequences in stereotactic space, allowing the neurosurgeon to capitalize on the particular advantages of each modality at different steps in the targeting process and to confirm final target coordinates on separate images. Digitized stereotactic atlases can be rapidly customized to a patient's anatomy, enhancing the accuracy of anatomical targeting.[22,32,35,46,53] CT-MRI fusion techniques have also been developed in order to address the problem of MRI distortion. By fitting a patient's MRI to his/her stereotactic CT, one can take advantage of the superior resolution of MRI and the geometric fidelity of CT. Kooy et al[39] have successfully adopted this technique for planning stereotactic radiosurgery. Finally, computers permit the rapid simulation of numerous trajectories to the target, reducing the likelihood of traversing the ventricle, which can lead to hemorrhage (see Chapter 16, "Interactive Computer-Assisted Image-Guided Technology as an Adjuvant to Neurosurgery for Movement Disorders").

MRI AND PALLIDOTOMY

In 1992, Laitinen and colleagues[41,42] resurrected pallidotomy as a viable treatment for medically refractory Parkinson's disease. Subsequent reports have supported their observations that lesions placed within the GPi relieve rigidity, dystonia, bradykinesia, and levodopa-induced dyskinesia in patients with moderate to severe Parkinson's disease.[6,11,28,29,46,47] While consistently good results have been reported for pallidotomy, a number of targeting strategies have been developed, demonstrating how personal bias and the particular strengths of an institution influence surgical technique.

Laitinen et al[41] use stereotactic CT and macroelectrode stimulation for targeting. Iacono et al[29] prefer proton density and T2-weighted MRI supported by ventriculography and macroelectrode stimulation. Baron et al[6] employ either MRI or CT, followed by microelectrode recording to delineate the borders of the GPi and macroelectrode stimulation. Lozano et al[46] perform initial targeting on "spoiled grass" MRIs, and a digitized version of the Schaltenbrand and Wahren atlas,[59] followed by microelectrode recording and microelectrode stimulation to localize the optic tract.

Although similar to the technique reported from the authors' institution by Dogali and colleagues,[10,11] the authors' pallidotomy technique has evolved over the last 3 years, reflecting ad-

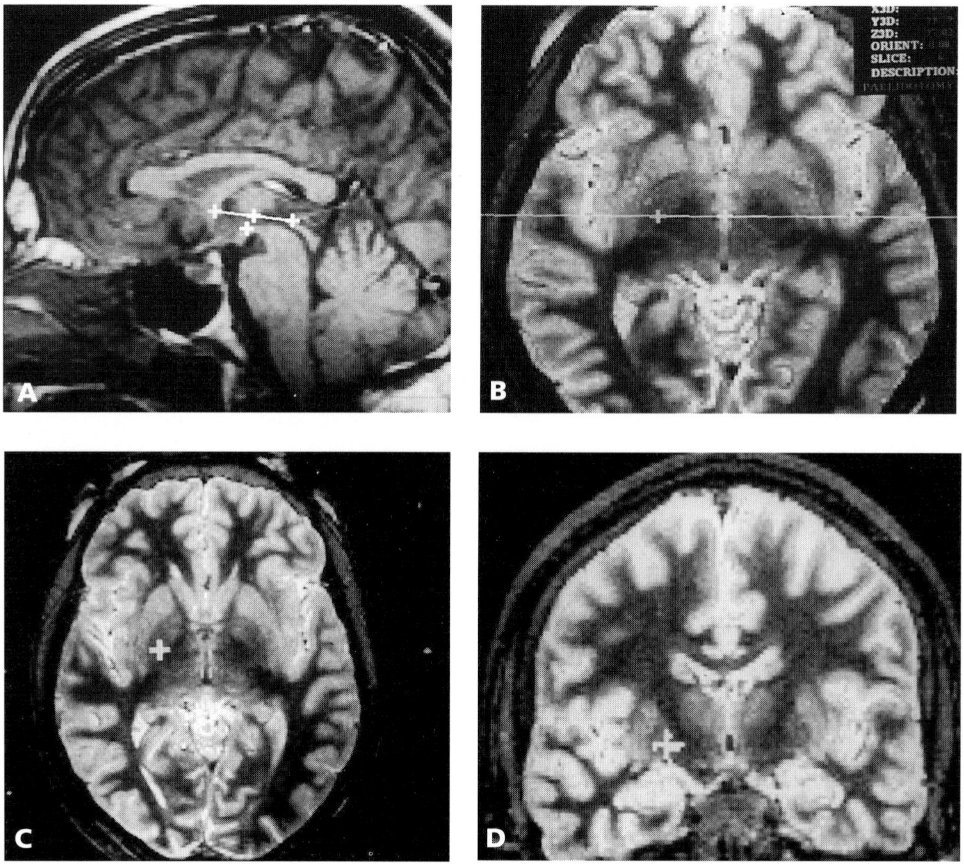

Figure 1: Computer-assisted, MRI-guided pallidal targeting. **A)** Midsagittal MRI demonstrating the commissures, the AC-PC line, midcommisural point, and a point 2 mm anterior and 4 mm ventral to the midcommissural point. **B)** Axial FSE/IR image 4 mm ventral to the intercommissural plane. The midpoint of the third ventricle and the posteroventral pallidal target are demonstrated. **C)** Axial FSE/IR image demonstrating the components of the lentiform nucleus and the pallidal target. **D)** Coronal FSE/IR image of the same target. See text for details of targeting procedure.

vances in computer and imaging technology as well as clinical experience.

The authors perform pallidotomy on awake patients who have been off medications for 12 hours. If tremor is significant in the "off" state, a short-acting benzodiazepine (such as lorazepam) can be given to suppress image-distorting tremor during MRI.

The Leksell G frame (Elekta Instruments, Atlanta, Georgia) is applied under local anesthesia and stereotactic MRI is performed with a 1.5-tesla magnet (Siemens Medical Systems, Iselin, New Jersey). The frame is applied so that the base ring is parallel to the orbitomeatal line, which the authors have found approximates the angle of the AC-PC line. T1-weighted axial, coronal, and sagittal images, as well as axial and coronal FSE/IR images, are obtained (3-mm slice thickness). The images are downloaded via Ethernet to the computer workstation (COMPASS International, Rochester, Minnesota), the fiducials are registered, and the pallidum is targeted as follows.

A T1-weighted midsagittal slice is employed for localizing the commissures, after which the computer draws the AC-PC line (Figure 1A). The computer is then directed to a locus 2 mm anterior to the midcommissural point and

TABLE 1

MICROELECTRODE RECORDING TRAJECTORIES PERFORMED DURING POSTEROVENTRAL PALLIDOTOMY*

Year	No. of Cases	Trajectories per Case: Mean ± SD	Trajectories per Case: Range
1992	10	3.6 ± 4.1	1-14
1993	21	3.1 ± 4.0	1-15
1994	21	1.5 ± 0.8	1-4
1995	43	2.0 ± 0.9	1-5
1996	37	1.8 ± 0.8	1-4
Totals	132	2.2 ± 2.1	1-15

*A total of 286 microelectrode recording trajectories were performed during 132 pallidotomies over a 5-year period. Experience and improved computer-assisted MRI targeting has led to a reduction in the average number of trajectories required for target localization. SD = standard deviation.

4 mm ventral to the AC-PC plane. The final target is then selected on the axial FSE/IR image that corresponds to the depth selected (Figure 1B). As already noted, FSE/IR beautifully demonstrates the basal ganglia (Figure 1B-D) and is resistant to distortion secondary to magnetic susceptibility. Final target laterality ranges from 18 to 23 mm lateral to the midline and is based on direct visualization of the internal pallidal segment on FSE/IR sequences.

Microelectrode recording is then used to "fine tune" the lesion. Microelectrode recording serves two critical functions: 1) confirmation of proper pallidal targeting; and 2) accurate definition of the ventral border of the GPi. Macroelectrode stimulation is employed to assess proximity to the internal capsule and optic tract. Details of the authors' microelectrode recording and macrostimulation techniques have been previously published.[62]

Employing this technique, the authors have achieved excellent therapeutic results with few complications when performing pallidotomy,[2,11] and have found that with experience and ever-improving MRI, the number of microelectrode recording trajectories required to perform pallidotomy has decreased dramatically. Table 1 demonstrates the number of microelectrode recording trajectories performed during pallidotomy for each of 5 years. In the last 3 years, 85% of pallidotomies were performed with one or two trajectories. On occasion, however, four trajectories may still be required to adequately target the GPi. Thus, while MRI may now be accurate enough to be the sole anatomical imaging modality employed for pallidal targeting, the authors believe that physiological confirmation of the target continues to be important for the safe performance of pallidotomy.

MRI AND THALAMOTOMY

The stereotactic principles that guided the development of the authors' pallidotomy technique are rooted in the extensive experience of the senior author (PK) with thalamotomy. Kall et al[31] first introduced the multicorrelative imaging technique for performing thalamotomy in 1992. Subsequently, Alterman et al[1] demonstrated that by employing this technique, MRI targeting for thalamotomy has become more accurate, requiring smaller targeting alterations based on semimicroelectrode recordings. This improved accuracy led those authors to conclude that ventriculography is no longer a required adjunct to MRI when performing thalamotomy but that neurophysiological confirmation of the target is still necessary.

The authors' thalamotomy technique differs from their pallidotomy protocol, accounting for differences in the anatomy and physiology of the respective targets. While FSE/IR sequences can clearly delineate the GPi, MRI with a 1.5-tesla magnet still cannot distinguish the thalamic subnuclei. Therefore, the authors are more dependent on neurophysiological techniques to target the ventral intermediate (VIM) and ventral oral posterior nuclei. Fortunately, the proximity of these nuclei to the ventral posterior thalamic nuclei, as well as their clearly delineated and corresponding topographies, permit us to accurately define target laterality whether treating upper- or lower-extremity tremor.

The AC-PC line is constructed on a midsagittal T1-weighted image, as in the pallidotomy protocol, after which the thalamic height is demonstrated on a parasagittal image toward the side to be operated. The computer then creates a Guiot-Talairach construct as previously described[31] (Figure 2). The VIM nucleus is selected

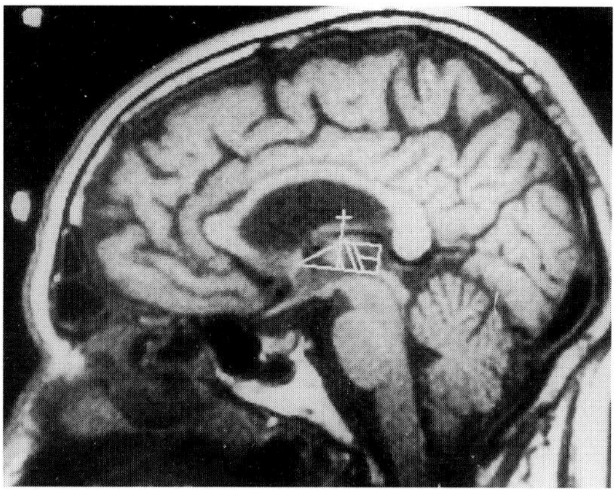

Figure 2: Computer-assisted, MRI-guided thalamic targeting. Midsagittal T1-weighted MRI demonstrating computerized Guiot-Talairach construct for targeting thalamic subnuclei. See text and prior publications[1,31] for details of targeting protocol.

interactively and the computer demonstrates an axial CT or MRI slice corresponding to the dorsoventral level selected. The thalamocapsular border is then identified interactively. Due to the possibility of MRI distortion, the authors have routinely performed positive contrast ventriculography in order to target the ventral posterior nucleus of the thalamus for semi-microelectrode recording. Target laterality is then determined by sensory field potentials exploiting the well-delineated topography of the ventral posterior thalamus. Once the appropriate laterality is determined, the electrode is moved anteriorly into the ventral lateral thalamus. Stimulation at low (5-Hz) and high (50-Hz) frequency is then performed in order to drive and suppress tremor, respectively. Stimulation also confirms the correct placement of the electrode in the ventral posterior thalamus by the absence of paresthesias. Employing this targeting paradigm, the senior author (PK) has reported excellent long-term amelioration of medically refractory hyperkinesia in patients with Parkinson's disease and essential tremor.[12,16]

Gamma Knife Pallidotomy and Thalamotomy

The Gamma Knife (Elekta Instruments) was originally conceived by Leksell for the performance of stereotactic neuroablative procedures without open surgery.[56] Neither ventriculography nor CT provided adequate anatomical targeting to perform neuroablation without neurophysiological localization, but ever-improving anatomical resolution with MRI has prompted limited trials of Gamma Knife lesioning procedures. In 1992, Lindquist et al[45] reported two cases of Gamma Knife thalamotomy. One patient developed hemiparesis and the second enjoyed only transient relief from tremor. Otsuki et al[53] reported a single case of Gamma Knife thalamotomy planned on MRI with a computerized atlas overlay. Tremor was relieved in this patient, without recurrence for more than 1 year. Rand et al[56] reported improvement in four of seven parkinsonian patients who received Gamma Knife thalamotomy for tremor and four of eight patients undergoing pallidotomy for rigidity and bradykinesia. Friedman et al[13] reported improvement in parkinsonism in only one of four patients undergoing Gamma Knife pallidotomy, leading them to abandon this approach.

In addition to relying solely on MRI for targeting, radiosurgical approaches have the disadvantage of a delay in their clinical effects. Patients must wait weeks to months to notice any positive changes. As a consequence, the clinical effects of the lesion cannot be assured at the time of the procedure, and the possibility of detecting potential complications via stimulation is denied. Taken together, the data from these small series that report inferior results when compared to larger series of "open" pallidotomy and thalamotomy suggest that functional neuroablative procedures should still be performed with neurophysiological support, necessitating the use of implanted electrodes.

Conclusions

There is little question that MRI is now superior to CT or ventriculography for anatomically localizing deep brain targets. Legitimate concerns about image distortion are being adequately addressed and the sources of distortion systematically eliminated. Computer planning systems enhance the capabilities of MRI, permitting rapid correlation of target coordinates on multiple MRI pulse sequences as well as other imaging modalities. In addition, safe trajectories to the target can be planned prior to incision.

The study by Favre et al (unpublished data, 1996) as well as the cumulative experience with Gamma Knife pallidotomy and thalamotomy for Parkinson's disease suggest that while high-resolution, thin-slice MRIs with distortion-resistant sequences provide highly accurate anatomical targeting, some form of neurophysiological localization is still required for the efficacious performance of neuroablative procedures. The authors and others[6,46] continue to employ microelectrode recording for physiological localization during pallidotomy, although this is controversial. The authors believe that microelectrode recording provides superior delineation of the ventral pallidal border, minimizing the likelihood of optic tract injury when lesioning the critical transition zone from the GPi to the ansa lenticularis. Current MRI technology does not yet distinguish thalamic subnuclei; thus, neurophysiological confirmation is still advised when lesioning or chronically stimulating the ventral lateral thalamic nucleus. Further advances in anatomical MRI as well as the introduction of functional imaging, whether with MRI, magnetoencephalography, high-resolution positron emission tomography, or some other modality, may well lead to a time when invasive neurophysiological techniques are obsolete. On the other hand, if chronic, high-frequency deep brain stimulation proves superior to neuroablation for treating movement disorders, functional imaging may not have an appreciable impact on current targeting technique. For now, computer-assisted MRI-guided targeting with thin-slice FSE/IR sequences, and neurophysiological confirmation provide the most consistent, and therefore the safest, means of localizing a deep brain target for surgical intervention.

REFERENCES

1. Alterman RL, Kall BA, Cohen H, et al: Stereotactic ventrolateral thalamotomy: is ventriculography necessary? **Neurosurgery 37:**717-722, 1995
2. Alterman RL, Kelly PJ, Beric A, et al: Selection criteria for unilateral posteroventral pallidotomy. **Acta Neurochir Suppl 68:**18-23, 1997
3. Amador LV, Blundell JE, Warren W: Description of coordinates of the deep structures; in Schaltenbrand G, Bailey P (eds): **Introduction to Stereotaxis With an Atlas of the Human Brain.** Stuttgart: Thieme, 1959, Vol 1, pp 16-28
4. Asakura T, Uetsuhara K, Kanemaru R, et al: An applicability study on a CT-guided stereotactic technique for functional neurosurgery. **Appl Neurophysiol 48:**73-76, 1985
5. Aziz T, Torrens M: CT-guided thalamotomy in the treatment of movement disorders. **Br J Neurosurg 3:** 333-336, 1989
6. Baron MS, Vitek JL, Bakay RAE, et al: Treatment of advanced Parkinson's disease by posterior GPi pallidotomy: 1-year results of a pilot study. **Ann Neurol 40:**355-366, 1996
7. Brierley JB, Beck E: The significance in human stereotactic brain surgery of individual variation in the diencephalon and globus pallidus. **J Neurol Neurosurg Psychiatry 22:**287-298, 1959
8. Bucholz RD, Ho HW, Rubin JP: Variables affecting the accuracy of stereotactic localization using computerized tomography. **J Neurosurg 79:**667-673, 1993
9. Burchiel KJ, Ojemann GA, Bolender N: Localization of stereotaxic centers by computerized tomographic scanning. Technical note. **J Neurosurg 53:**861-863, 1980
10. Dogali M, Beric A, Sterio D, et al: Anatomic and physiological considerations in pallidotomy for Parkinson's disease. **Stereotact Funct Neurosurg 62:** 53-60, 1994
11. Dogali M, Fazzini E, Kolodny E, et al: Stereotactic ventral pallidotomy for Parkinson's disease. **Neurology 45:**753-761, 1995
12. Fox MW, Ahlskog JE, Kelly PJ: Stereotactic ventrolateralis thalamotomy for medically refractory tremor in post-levodopa era Parkinson's disease patients. **J Neurosurg 75:**723-730, 1991
13. Friedman JH, Epstein M, Sanes JN, et al: Gamma Knife pallidotomy in advanced Parkinson's disease. **Ann Neurol 39:**535-538, 1996
14. Gerdes JS, Hitchon PW, Neerangun W, et al: Computed tomography versus magnetic resonance imaging in stereotactic localization. **Stereotact Funct Neurosurg 63:**124-129, 1994
15. Giorgi C, Gartibotto G, Garozzo S, et al: Three-dimensional processing of a stereotactic brain atlas. **Appl Neurophysiol 45:**419-425, 1982
16. Goldman MS, Ahlskog JE, Kelly PJ: The symptomatic and functional outcome of stereotactic thalamotomy for medically intractable essential tremor. **J Neurosurg 76:**924-928, 1992
17. Gonsette RE, Liesenborghs L: Iohexol: a new nonionic contrast medium for myelography and cisternography with markedly reduced neurotoxicity. **Invest Radiol 20 (Suppl 1):**S32-S35, 1985
18. Hadley MN, Shetter AG, Amos MR: Use of the Brown-Roberts-Wells stereotactic frame for functional neurosurgery. **Appl Neurophysiol 48:**61-68, 1985
19. Hanieh A, Maloney AFJ: Localization of stereotaxic lesions in the treatment of parkinsonism: a clinicopathological comparison. **J Neurosurg 31:**393-399, 1969
20. Hardy TL, Bertrand G, Thompson CJ: Position of the medial internal capsular border in relation to third-ventricular width. **Appl Neurophysiol 42:**234-247, 1979

21. Hardy TL, Koch J, Lassiter A: Computer graphics with computerized tomography for functional neurosurgery. **Appl Neurophysiol 46:**217-226, 1983
22. Hardy TL, Smith JR, Brynildson LRD, et al: Magnetic resonance imaging and anatomic atlas mapping for thalamotomy. **Stereotact Funct Neurosurg 58:**30-32, 1992
23. Hariz MI, Bergenheim AT: A comparative study on ventriculographic and computerized tomography-guided determinations of brain targets in functional stereotaxis. **J Neurosurg 73:**565-571, 1990
24. Hariz MI, Bergenheim AT, Fodstad H: Air-ventriculography provokes an anterior displacement of the third ventricle during functional stereotactic procedures. **Acta Neurochir 123:**147-152, 1993
25. Hassler R, Mundinger F, Reichert T: Correlations between clinical and autoptic findings in stereotaxic operations of parkinsonism. **Confin Neurol 26:** 282-290, 1965
26. Horsley V, Clarke RH: The structure and functions of the cerebellum examined by a new method. **Brain 31:** 45-124, 1908
27. Huber P, Rivoir R: The influence of intraventricular pressure on the size and shape of the anterior part of the third ventricle. **Neuroradiology 5:**33-36, 1973
28. Iacono RP, Lonser RR: Reversal of Parkinson's akinesia by pallidotomy. **Lancet 343:**418-419, 1994
29. Iacono RP, Shima F, Lonser RR, et al: The results, indications, and physiology of posteroventral pallidotomy for patients with Parkinson's disease. **Neurosurgery 36:**1118-1127, 1995
30. Jeanmonod D, Thomas DGT: Application of CT-directed stereotaxy in the determination of functional neurosurgical targets in the diencephalon and cerebral hemisphere. **Br J Neurosurg 3:**337-342, 1989
31. Kall BA, Goerss SJ, Kelly PJ: A new multimodality correlative imaging technique for VOP/VIM (VL) thalamotomy procedures. **Stereotact Funct Neurosurg 58:**45-51, 1992
32. Kall BA, Kelly PJ, Goerss SJ, et al: Methodology and clinical experience with computed tomography and a computer-resident stereotactic atlas. **Neurosurgery 17:**400-407, 1985
33. Kawashima Y, Chen HJ, Takahashi A, et al: Application of magnetic resonance imaging in functional sterotactic thalamotomy for the evaluation of individual variations in the thalamus. **Stereotact Funct Neurosurg 58:**33-38, 1992
34. Kelly PJ: Comment on Lunsford LD: Magnetic resonance imaging stereotactic thalamotomy: report of a case with comparison to computed tomography. **Neurosurgery 23:**367, 1988
35. Kelly PJ: Contemporary stereotactic ventralis lateral thalamotomy in the treatment of parkinsonian tremor and other movement disorders, in Heilbrun MP (ed): **Stereotactic Neurosurgery**. Baltimore, Md: Williams & Wilkins, 1988, pp 133-148
36. Kelly PJ: Principles of stereotactic surgery, in Youmans JR (ed): **Neurological Surgery.** 3rd ed. Philadelphia, Pa: WB Saunders, 1990, pp 4183-4226
37. Kelly PJ, Derome P, Guiot G: Thalamic spatial variability and the surgical results on lesions placed with neurophysiologic control. **Surg Neurol 9:**307-315, 1978
38. Kondziolka D, Dempsey PK, Lunsford LD, et al: A comparison between magnetic resonance imaging and computed tomography for stereotactic coordinate determination. **Neurosurgery 30:**402-407, 1992
39. Kooy HM, van Herk M, Barnes PD, et al: Image fusion for stereotactic radiotherapy and radiosurgery treatment planning. **Int J Radiat Oncol Biol Phys 28:** 1229-1234, 1994
40. Laitinen LV: CT-guided ablative stereotaxis without ventriculography. **Appl Neurophysiol 48:**18-21, 1985
41. Laitinen LV, Bergenheim AT, Hariz MI: Leksell's posteroventral pallidotomy in the treatment of Parkinson's disease. **J Neurosurg 76:**53-61, 1992
42. Laitinen LV, Bergenheim AT, Hariz MI: Ventroposterolateral pallidotomy can abolish all parkinsonian symptoms. **Stereotact Funct Neurosurg 58:**14-21, 1992
43. Laitinen LV, Liliequist B, Fagerlund M, et al: An adapter for computed tomography-guided stereotaxis. **Surg Neurol 23:**559-566, 1985
44. Leksell L, Leksell D, Schwebel J: Stereotaxis and nuclear magnetic resonance. **J Neurol Neurosurg Psychiatry 48:**14-18, 1985
45. Lindquist C, Steiner L, Hindmarsh T: Gamma Knife thalamotomy for tremor: report of two cases, in Steiner L (ed): **Radiosurgery: Baseline and Trends.** New York, NY: Raven Press: 1992, pp 237-243
46. Lozano A, Hutchison W, Kiss Z, et al: Methods for microelectrode-guided posteroventral pallidotomy. **J Neurosurg 84:**194-202, 1996
47. Lozano AM, Lang AE, Galvez-Jimenez N, et al: Effect of GPi pallidotomy on motor function in Parkinson's disease. **Lancet 346:**1383-1387, 1995
48. Lunsford LD: Magnetic resonance imaging stereotactic thalamotomy: report of a case with comparison to computed tomography. **Neurosurgery 23:** 363-367, 1988
49. Lunsford LD, Martinez AJ, Latchaw RE: Stereotaxic surgery with a magnetic resonance- and computerized tomography-compatible system. **J Neurosurg 64:** 872-878, 1986
50. Mark VH, Yakovlev PI: A note on problems and methods in the preparation of a human stereotactic atlas. Including a report of measurements of the posteromedial portion of the ventral nucleus of the thalamus. **Anat Rec 121:**745-752, 1955
51. McKean JDS, Allen PBR, Filipow LJ, et al: CT guided functional stereotaxic surgery. **Acta Neurochir 87:** 8-13, 1987
52. Ohye C, Kawashima Y, Hirato M, et al: Stereotactic CT scan applied to stereotactic thalamotomy and biopsy. **Acta Neurochir 71:**55-68, 1984
53. Otsuki T, Jokura H, Takahashi K, et al: Stereotactic γ -thalamotomy with a computerized brain atlas: technical case report. **Neurosurgery 35:**764-768, 1994
54. Page RD, Miles JB: Validation of CT targeting for functional stereotaxis with postoperative magnetic resonance imaging. **Br J Neurosurg 8:**461-467, 1994
55. Pollak P, Benabid AL, Limousin P, et al: Subthalamic nucleus stimulation alleviates akinesia and rigidity in parkinsonian patients. **Adv Neurol 69:**591-594, 1996
56. Rand RW, Jacques DB, Melbye RW, et al: Gamma Knife thalamotomy and pallidotomy in patients with movement disorders: preliminary results. **Stereotact Funct Neurosurg 61 (Suppl 1):**65-92, 1993
57. Rosenfeld JV, Barnett GH, Palmer J: Computed tomography guided stereotactic thalamotomy using the Brown-Roberts-Wells system for nonparkinson-

ian movement disorders. Technical note. **Stereotact Funct Neurosurg 56:**184-192, 1991
58. Schad L, Lott S, Schmitt F, et al: Correction of spatial distortion in MR imaging: a prerequisite for accurate stereotaxy. **J Comput Assist Surg 11:**499-505, 1987
59. Schaltenbrand G, Wahren W: **Guide to the Atlas for Stereotaxy of the Human Brain.** Stuttgart: Georg Thieme, 1977, pp 1-26
60. Siegfried J, Lippitz B: Bilateral chronic electrostimulation of ventroposterolateral pallidum: a new therapeutic approach for alleviating all parkinsonian symptoms. **Neurosurgery 35:**1126-1130, 1994
61. Spiegel EA, Wycis HT, Marks M, et al: Stereotaxic apparatus for operations on the human brain. **Science 106:**349-350, 1947
62. Sterio D, Berić A, Dogali M, et al: Neurophysiological properties of pallidal neurons in Parkinson's disease. **Ann Neurol 35:**586-591, 1994
63. Sumanaweera TS, Adler JR Jr, Napel S, et al: Characterization of spatial distortion in magnetic resonance imaging and its implications for stereotactic surgery. **Neurosurgery 35:**696-704, 1994
64. Talairach J: **VI Congreso Latin-Americano de Neurocirugia, Montevideo,** pp 865-925, 1955
65. Taren JA, Ross DA, Gebarski SS: Stereotactic localization using fast spin-echo imaging in functional disorders. **Acta Neurochir Suppl 58:**59-60, 1993
66. Tasker RR, Dostrovsky JO, Dolan EJ: Computerized tomography (CT) is just as accurate as ventriculography for functional stereotactic thalamotomy. **Stereotact Funct Neurosurg 57:**157-166, 1991
67. Villemure JG, Marchand E, Peters T, et al: Magnetic resonance imaging stereotaxy: recognition and utilization of the commissures. **Appl Neurophysiol 50:**57-62, 1987
68. Walton L, Hampshire A, Forster DMC, et al: Stereotactic localization using magnetic resonance imaging. **Stereotact Funct Neurosurg 64 (Suppl 1):**155-163, 1995
69. Walton L, Hampshire A, Forster DMC, Kemeny AA: A phantom study to assess the accuracy of stereotactic localization using T1-weighted magnetic resonance imaging with the Leksell stereotactic system. **Neurosurgery 38:**170-178, 1996
70. Whittle IR, O'Sullivan MG, Ironside JW, et al: Accuracy of ventrolateral thalamic nucleus localization using unreformatted CT scans and the B-R-W system. Experimental studies and clinical findings during functional neurosurgery. **Acta Neurochir Suppl 58:**61-64, 1993
71. Whittle IR, O'Sullivan MG, Ironside JW, et al: An experimental study to evaluate the accuracy of diencephalic and pallidal target localization using the Brown-Roberts-Wells stereotactic system and unreformatted axial GE8800 CT scanning. **Br J Neurosurg 8:**63-72, 1994

CHAPTER 15

Intraoperative Electrophysiological Recording Techniques

Donald J. Weisz, PhD, and Bo-Yi Yang, PhD

The goal of this chapter is to describe the electrophysiological techniques that can be used to assist in the localization of the subthalamic nucleus (STN) and the internal segment of the globus pallidus (GPi) during stereotactic surgery in patients with Parkinson's disease. These techniques, which include extracellular single-cell recording, electrical stimulation, and recording of visual evoked responses, can provide verification of electrode placement that is based on magnetic resonance imaging (MRI).[4,7,22] By using a combination of these techniques, the accuracy of lesion location and the placement of electrodes for chronic deep brain stimulation or ablative procedures can be improved, and damage to the optic tract, internal capsule, and other nearby structures can be minimized.

Intraoperative electrophysiological techniques relative to localization of the ventral intermediate (VIM) nucleus of the thalamus are reviewed in Chapter 8, "Thalamotomy for Movement Disorders: Indications, Techniques, and Results."

General Microelectrode Recording Procedures

Rationale

For purposes of localization of a targeted brain structure, single-cell recording techniques can assist the surgical team in two different ways. First, these recordings can differentiate areas that have a high density of cell bodies from areas that have few or no cell bodies. As discussed below, this information can be useful in defining the dorsal and ventral boundaries of the GPi and the anterior, anteroventral, and lateral boundaries of the STN. Second, in many cases, recordings from single cells in a particular area can be differentiated from recordings in adjacent areas on the basis of firing rates and firing patterns. For example, the dominant cell type in the GPi typically exhibits a high-frequency and rather continuous discharge that is different from the firing patterns of cells in the surrounding areas, such as the external segment of the globus pallidus (GPe).[5] In addition, the waveform of an extracellular single-cell recording (also called a spike) can at times be used to differentiate areas of the brain, because spikes from one area may possess characteristics (e.g., width or shape) that spikes from adjacent areas do not possess.

General Approach

In the operating room, it is important to extract information about the firing rates, firing patterns, and waveform topographies of the spikes as rapidly as possible in order to avoid needless delay in the surgical procedure. The authors use a combination of hardware and software to provide: 1) an audio signal of the microelectrode recordings; 2) a continuous display of the firing rate of a recorded cell; 3) a continuous display of the firing patterns; and 4) the waveform topography of the individual spikes.

Microelectrode Construction

Single-cell responses are recorded extracellularly using high-impedance tungsten microelectrodes with tip diameters of approximately 0.25 μm. At the time of manufacture, the impedance of the electrodes used by the authors is 1-2 MΩ, but this is reduced to approximately 250-350 kΩ by electrolytic plating of the electrode tip with chloroplatinic acid. (The impedance of the microelectrodes used in various centers varies from 0.2 kΩ to over 1.0 MΩ.) The shaft of the electrode is insulated with Epoxylite, except at the tip. The end of the electrode opposite the tip is stripped of Epoxylite, bent to assure good electrical contact, and inserted into a 25-gauge insulated stainless steel tube. At the junction between the electrode and the tube, a 3.0-mm epoxy seal anchors the microelectrode to the tube, and a male gold pin is crimped onto the opposite end of the tube. This entire assembly is then placed into a guide cannula (19-gauge stainless steel tube). During storage, the electrode is pulled back into the guide cannula to protect the tip. A piece of Silastic tubing is placed over the gold pin and the end of the guide cannula to prevent the electrode from moving within the cannula. The microelectrodes and all connecting leads are then packaged for gas sterilization prior to use.

Two leads, constructed from shielded coaxial cable, are connected to the microelectrode at the time of recording. One lead is connected to the gold pin at the end of the microelectrode and serves as the active lead. The second lead is attached to the guide tube via an alligator clip and serves as the reference. A lead from an electrocoagulation pad on the patient is used to ground the patient. The three leads are connected to the first stage of a differential preamplifier, which is placed as close to the patient as possible in order to minimize noise.

Placement of the Microelectrode

At the time of surgery, a guiding cannula with a stylette is placed 20 mm above the STN and 25 mm above the GPi localized stereotactically, as described in Chapter 11, "Chronic Deep Brain Stimulation: Indications and Techniques." The stylette is withdrawn and the microelectrode assembly is inserted into the guide cannula. When properly positioned in the guide cannula, the tip of the microelectrode extends 10 mm beyond the end of the guide cannula. Therefore, microelectrode mapping begins approximately 10 mm above the STN target or at least 15 mm above the GPi target. At this time, the electrode impedance is verified. Electrodes are replaced if the impedance is <200 kΩ or >400 kΩ.

Processing of Microelectrode Recordings

The microelectrode is advanced in approximately 0.1-mm increments and at each advance the recordings are analyzed. Electrode impedance is frequently checked to verify that it has not changed significantly during the surgery.

The microelectrode recordings are differentially amplified with a gain of 5000, and filtered using a bandwidth of 300-10,000 Hz. The output of the amplifier is sent to: 1) two storage oscilloscopes; 2) an audio amplifier; 3) a window discriminator; 4) an analog-to-digital converter that is connected to a personal computer; and 5) a digital tape drive (for archival storage).

Two oscilloscopes are used for simultaneous display of the recordings. The shape of each spike's waveform is viewed on a fast time base on one oscilloscope (5 msec sweep duration), and the firing pattern is viewed on a slower time base on another oscilloscope (1.0 sec sweep duration).

An audio system, which includes an amplifier, custom-made noise clipping filter, and speakers, permits real-time audio monitoring of the recorded signals by the surgeon and the neurophysiologist. The audio signal is a very useful indicator of the changes in background activity level that occur when an electrode tip moves from an area of densely packed cells to an area of no or sparse cells. In addition, the audio signal of isolated cells provides a fast initial assessment of the firing rate and firing pattern. For example, the audio signal of a cell that exhibits bursts of spikes interspersed with pauses has a different sound from the audio signal of a cell that has sustained activity with no pauses.

For a quantitative evaluation of firing rate, the authors use a commercially available window discriminator (Frederick Haer & Co., Brunswick, Maine) and a custom-made frequency counter with a light-emitting diode (LED) display. The window discriminator can be set to trigger on the rising or falling phase of a spike. Each time the discriminator detects a response, it sends a digital pulse to the counting device, which provides a second-to-second measure of the firing rate on the LED display.

The firing rate information is useful if it is certain that the recording samples are from only one cell. To verify a single-cell recording, the authors display the analog signal on an oscilloscope (0.1-0.5 msec/div) in which the sweep is triggered on the initial deflection of the waveform. If the recordings include two or more cells, the traces will normally exhibit two or more patterns in which the amplitudes and/or spike widths are different. If the traces have virtually the same shape and size, a single-cell recording is likely, although not certain. More sophisticated methods exist for a more definitive determination of the number of cells in a recording (e.g., analysis based on comparison of signals obtained from two or more closely spaced electrodes), but these methods may prolong the surgery and probably are not necessary in the operating room.

The authors also extract information about firing patterns and rates using a commercial software package. For this analysis, single-cell recordings are digitized and the digitized values are sent to a personal computer. Commercial products that can be used to analyze single-cell recordings are available, such as CED Spike 2 (Cambridge Electronic Design Ltd., Cambridge, England) and DataWave (DataWave Technologies, Longmont, Colorado). The authors use the software for both on-line and off-line analysis of archived data.

Relevant data from the microelectrode recordings and electrical stimulation are entered for all electrode tracks on a wall chart, upon which is drawn an outline of the patient's brain around the target site.[13] The outline is traced immediately prior to surgery from an MRI of the patient. This wall chart is invaluable in interpreting the electrophysiological data prior to making a determination of final lesion or implantation coordinates.

Electromyographic Recordings

Electromyography (EMG), recorded from surface electrodes and/or limb movements and recorded by an accelerometer, is monitored by many groups who perform stereotactic surgery in patients with Parkinson's disease. Although these recordings are made primarily for research reasons, they also have clinical value. In both the STN[23] and the GPi,[5,19] the firing of approximately 20% of the cells can be modulated by movement. Typically, each cell responds selectively to movements of a particular limb or joint. The stereotactic coordinates of responsive cells may be used to select a target area in the GPi[11] or STN. The simultaneous display of the microelectrode and movement recordings makes it easier to determine if a relationship exists between the firing pattern and the movements.

EMG is recorded from a pair of surface electrodes placed over each target muscle. Accelerometers are commonly attached to the wrists or fingers of the patients. EMG and the accelerometer outputs are amplified, bandpass filtered, displayed on an oscilloscope and computer monitor, and saved to tape.

How Many Electrode Penetrations Are Needed?

The number of electrode penetrations used to record neuronal activity varies a great deal from center to center. Favre et al[6] found that only 14 of 28 centers in their survey used microelectrode recordings during pallidotomy, whereas 26 of 28 used electrical stimulation (either with a microelectrode or a macroelectrode) to localize motor pathways and the optic tract. In the centers that used microelectrode recordings, there was a wide range in the number of tracks that were mapped (1-8 tracks, median 3). These statistics indicate that surgical centers vary in their use of recording and stimulation techniques during pallidotomy and that at present there is no consensus regarding the optimal technique for target localization.

At one end of the continuum are the centers where microelectrode recordings are used to define the boundaries of the GPi. At a minimum, three electrode tracks are needed: one to map the dorsal-ventral plane at the target site, one to establish either a medial or a lateral boundary, and one track to establish either an anterior or posterior boundary. In actual practice, four tracks are normally needed to define the boundaries of the GPi using microelectrode recordings. In addition, at some centers the sensorimotor region of the GPi is defined by careful microelectrode mapping before selecting coordinates for the lesion.[2] At the other end of the continuum, of course, are the centers where microelectrode recordings are not used, and lesion or electrode placement is based on stereotactic coordinates and electrical stimulation using macroelectrodes.

Therefore, the answer to the question of how many electrode tracks need to be mapped during pallidotomy depends largely on the goals of the surgical staff. Eventually the clinical outcomes of the various approaches will be used to make a more intelligent decision regarding the best approach to deep brain stimulation or ablative procedures.

The goal of microelectrode recording during the implantation of chronic stimulating electrodes (e.g., in the VIM, GPi, or STN) is essentially the same as the goal of recording during pallidotomy; that is, the recordings can be used to define the boundaries of the target site. There is one major difference, however, that may reduce the number of microelectrode tracks needed prior to implantation of a chronic stimulating electrode. The difference is that, during surgery for deep brain stimulation, an MRI can be obtained following tentative placement of the stimulating electrode, and the final location can be adjusted based on the results of that MRI. There is a greater safety margin for deep brain stimulaton than there is for pallidotomy, and it is probably not necessary to define all of the boundaries of the target structure prior to initial implantation.

Currently, the authors make microelectrode recordings during surgery for implantation of an STN stimulating electrode until it is clear that recordings from the STN and the substantia nigra have been obtained. The approximate depth and thickness of the STN at the target coordinates are noted, and from these measures, the stimulating electrode is placed. Stimulation coupled with neurological examination will confirm clinical accuracy. By using this approach, the authors believe that the number of electrode tracks can be kept to a minimum without sacrificing accuracy in placement.

Localizing the Subthalamic Nucleus

Single-Cell Recordings From the Subthalamic Nucleus

The authors use a combination of MRI-guided stereotactic procedures, electrophysiological recordings, and electrical stimulation to localize the STN during surgery to implant chronic stimulating electrodes.[12,15,16,24] MRI guidance is used initially to lower the tip of a recording microelectrode to a point 10 mm above the target in the STN. Figure 1 shows a diagrammatic representation of the STN and adjacent structures. After waiting 2-3 minutes for the brain to stabilize its position relative to the recording electrode, the tip is slowly advanced in 0.1-mm increments until cell body spikes are seen and heard in the recordings. The electrode tip at the time of the initial recordings should be located in either the thalamus or the

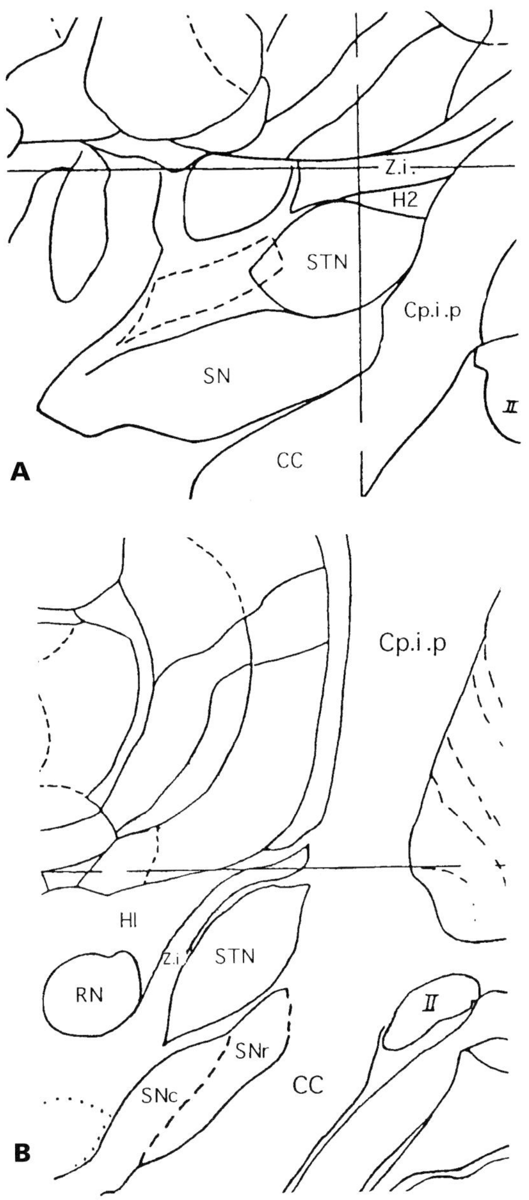

Figure 1: Drawings of parasagittal **(A)** and coronal **(B)** views of the STN and surrounding areas. (Reproduced from Schaltenbrand and Bailey[17] with permission.) Abbreviations of key structures: CC = crus cerebri; Cp.i.p = internal capsule, posterior limb; H_1 and H_2 = tegmental fields; II = optic nerve; RN = red nucleus; SN = substantia nigra; Z.i = zona incerta.

internal capsule. If the tip is in the thalamus, recordings will typically exhibit multiple and single cell activity over 4-6 mm of electrode travel. The authors' experience is that thalamic recordings are notable for their heterogeneity; that is, cells with different waveforms, different firing rates, and different firing patterns will be seen. If the electrode tip is in the internal capsule, the recordings consist primarily of small-amplitude activity in which individual signals have very narrow waveforms (spike width <0.2 msec). These recordings produce an audio signal that is characterized by a weak, high-frequency hiss.

If the microelectrode tip was originally located in a fiber bundle, the appearance of the first spikes is usually preceded by an increase in background activity, which indicates that the electrode tip is passing from a fiber bundle to an area of cell bodies. Recordings immediately dorsal to the STN frequently reveal single cells that are separated from other cells, demonstrated by very brief periods in which background activity is low. It is unlikely that a high density of cell body responses will be seen in the area immediately above the STN, which includes the tegmental field H_2 and the zona incerta.

As the microelectrode enters the STN, there is a sudden increase in the number of spikes being recorded. Cells in the primate STN are densely packed and tonically active.[23] It is important to note the exact depth at which the STN is entered. If possible, single cells should be isolated in order to obtain additional information about the neuronal firing patterns and rates. It is the authors' experience that these cells can be slightly more difficult to isolate than cells in surrounding areas because of the higher cell density of the STN.

Extracellular single-cell recordings of STN cells can exhibit at least two different waveforms, a biphasic one in which the initial deflection is usually positive and a monophasic negative-going waveform.[9] For the negative-going waveform, the duration of the extracellularly recorded potentials in the STN is usually between 0.5 and 0.8 msec. If biphasic waveforms are seen, the spike width could be slightly broader. These two types of waveforms are probably a function of differential distances between the tip of the microelectrode and the cell body, rather than representative of different neuronal populations.[9] Using microelectrodes of 200-400 kΩ

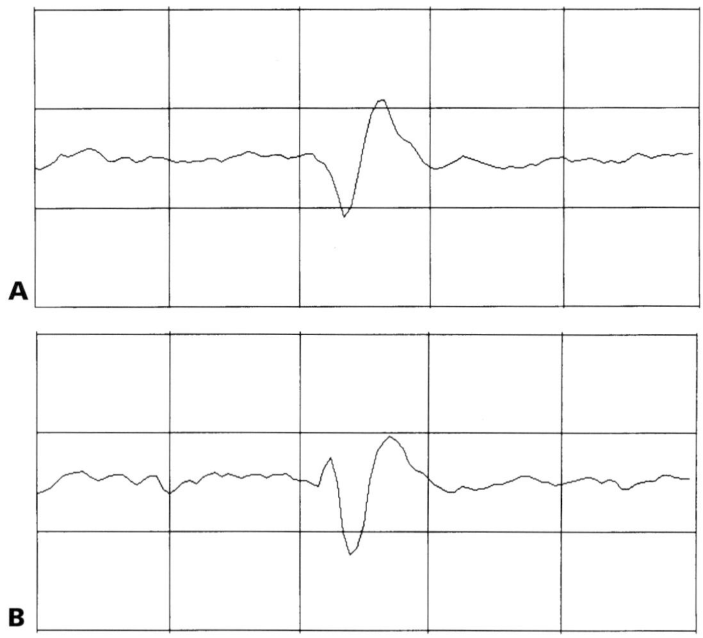

Figure 2: Examples of two types of spike morphologies seen in STN recordings. **A)** The dominant shape is a spike that has an initial negative deflection followed by a positive component. The width of the spike is typically 0.5-0.8 msec. **B)** Infrequently, STN spikes may have a brief initial positive component followed by negative and positive deflections. This spike is slightly wider than the more dominant type. The two spike morphologies are probably from the same cell type. The different shapes are probably due to differences in the physical relationship between the recording tip and STN cell bodies[9] (x axis = 5 msec).

impedance, the authors have seen both types of waveforms (Figure 2), although, by far, more negative-going spikes are seen.

Spontaneous firing rates of STN cells in primates are in the range of 10-40 spikes/sec, although Bergman et al[3] found that treatment with 1-methyl-4-phenyl-1,2,3,6-tetrahydropyridine (MPTP) resulted in an increase in the mean firing rates of monkey STN cells from 19 ± 10 spikes/sec to 26 ± 15 spikes/sec. In addition, Bergman et al found that approximately 16% of STN cells showed 4-8-Hz oscillatory firing patterns and another 10% showed oscillatory patterns at higher frequencies. Furthermore, MPTP treatment increased the percentage of oscillatory neurons that exhibited a 4-8-Hz pattern. In recordings from the authors' patients, almost all STN cells have shown an irregular firing pattern with periods of bursts and pauses (Figure 3). The authors are currently analyzing these cells for any oscillatory patterns. The cell density (high), pattern of activity (bursts of spikes and irregular firing patterns), firing rate (10-50 spikes/sec), and spike morphology (spike width 0.5-0.8 msec) are the main criteria for STN localization.

As the microelectrode is slowly advanced through the STN, the recordings will continue to reflect the presence of high-density, tonically active neurons. When the ventral border of the STN is passed (usually 3-4 mm from its dorsal border), one of two types of recordings should be seen. If the electrode has passed through the rostral or caudolateral regions of the STN, the background activity will abruptly revert to a low-amplitude, soft hiss that is characteristic of fiber bundles—in this case, the crus cerebri. Further advancement with the microelectrode will lead to continued silence, indicative of a rostral or caudolateral trajectory through the STN. It is important to note the exact depth at which the electrode leaves the STN. Subtracting the dorsal coordinate of the STN from its ventral coordinate will provide an estimate of the thickness of the STN at that electrode track. Because the STN is thicker in its center, a thickness of <2.0 mm indicates that the electrode has passed near the margins of the STN.

If the electrode passes through the medial part of the STN in the caudal portion, there may be a very brief quiet period when the tip exits the STN; however, very shortly, cell bodies will be encountered that have firing patterns different from those in the STN. These cells are probably

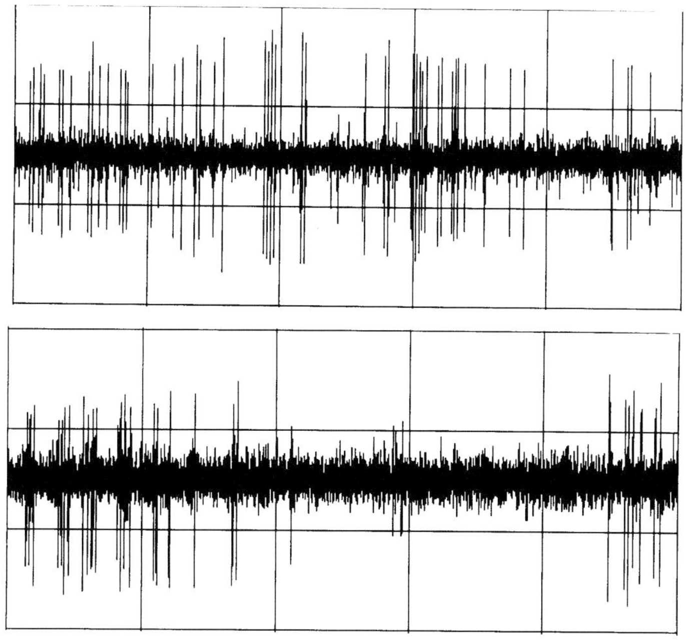

Figure 3: Representative samples of the firing patterns of two STN cells (x axis = 1.0 sec).

in the pars reticulata of the substantia nigra (SNr). Although it is possible that a recording could be made from a cell in the pars compacta of the substantia nigra (SNc), it is unlikely in Parkinson's disease patients because the disease process destroys a high percentage of SNc cells.

Cells in the SNr and SNc can be easily discriminated on the basis of electrophysiological recordings. Single-cell responses from SNr cells in primates have firing rates of 15-150 spikes/sec, with a median rate of approximately 70 spikes/sec[8,14,18] and spike widths of approximately 0.6-1.0 msec in duration.[18] In recordings from the authors' patients, the firing patterns of SNr cells have resembled those of cells in the GPi; that is, they tend to fire more or less continuously with no long pauses[8,14,18] (Figure 4). Cells in the SNc have firing rates of <8 spikes/sec, with long duration spike widths (>2.0 msec). Ventral to the SNr and SNc lies the crus cerebri, which lacks cell bodies.

Typically, two or three passes with the microelectrode are made before deciding on the target coordinates for placement of the chronic stimulating electrode. The chronic stimulating electrode (Medtronics, Minneapolis, Minnesota) has four contacts (see Figure 4 in Chapter 11, "Chronic Deep Brain Stimulation: Indications and Techniques"). The most distal contact is lowered to the target. Test stimulation is always performed at this time to determine the effect of the stimulation on Parkinson's disease symptoms and if the stimulation has any unwanted effects (e.g., paresthesias). Low-frequency stimulation (e.g., 2 Hz) that elicits motor responses or paresthesias at a low voltage (<3 V) indicates a placement that is too close to the internal capsule. On the other hand, high-frequency stimulation (e.g., 100 Hz) at the correct target can inhibit an ongoing tremor. Intermediate rates of stimulation (e.g., 50 Hz) can enhance tremor activity.[6]

Recordings That Indicate an Off-Target Electrode Track

Electrophysiological recordings can be useful not only in determining the accuracy of MRI-based stereotactic coordinates, but also in providing information regarding the direction in which an error may have been made. Unfortu-

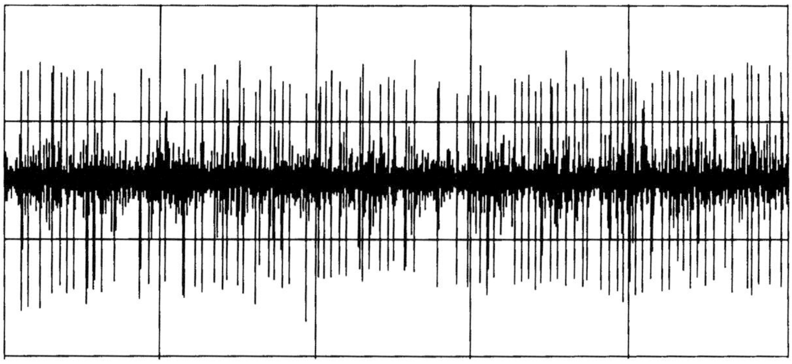

Figure 4: Representative sample of the firing pattern of an SNr cell. One second of activity is shown (x axis = 1.0 sec).

nately, the placement of a misdirected STN electrode may be difficult to determine because the STN is surrounded on most sides either by white matter or by areas of low cell density. The internal capsule lies anterior and lateral to the STN, and the cerebellothalamic track and the cell-poor region of the tegmental field H lie medial to the STN. Therefore, if recordings at the target depth are notable for the scarcity of cell body spikes, it may be difficult to determine in which direction an error was made. If no clear cell body spikes are recorded in the first 10-15 mm of travel, it is likely that the electrode track is too far lateral, but it is also possible that it is too far anterior. If the recordings indicate a fiber bundle location, electrical stimulation (2 or 50 Hz) may be delivered through the microelectrode in an effort to elicit somatic sensations or motor responses. If the electrode track misses the STN in a posterior direction, then a different pattern of recordings is seen. When the electrode tip is at the target depth of the STN but too far posterior, very few cell body spikes are recorded because this area has a much lower cell density than does the STN. Posterior and ventral to the STN lies the substantia nigra, which is much larger than the STN. Therefore, if activity is recorded that appears to be from the SNr but activity fails to be recorded on the electrode track that looks to be in the STN, it is assumed that the electrode is posterior to the STN.

Localizing the Posteroventral Globus Pallidus

Neuronal Recordings From the Globus Pallidus

The major risk of a posteroventral pallidotomy is damage to either the internal capsule or the optic tract. Therefore, electrophysiological recording and stimulation techniques are focused on identifying these structures. In addition, electrophysiological recordings can be helpful in determining the optimal coordinates for lesions of the posteroventral globus pallidus, by identifying the dorsal and ventral borders of the GPi and by determining the location of the sensorimotor region of the GPi. Figure 5 is a diagrammatic representation of the GPi and adjacent structures.

The target for the lesion varies somewhat from one surgical group to another, but is usually 1-3 mm anterior to the midpoint of the anterior commissure (AC)-posterior commissure (PC) line, 18-23 mm lateral and 4-7 mm below the AC-PC line.[6] Using MRI guidance, a recording microelectrode is lowered to a point approximately 20-30 mm above the target at an angle of approximately 65° (±15°) from the horizontal axis of the stereotactic frame. Baron et al[2]

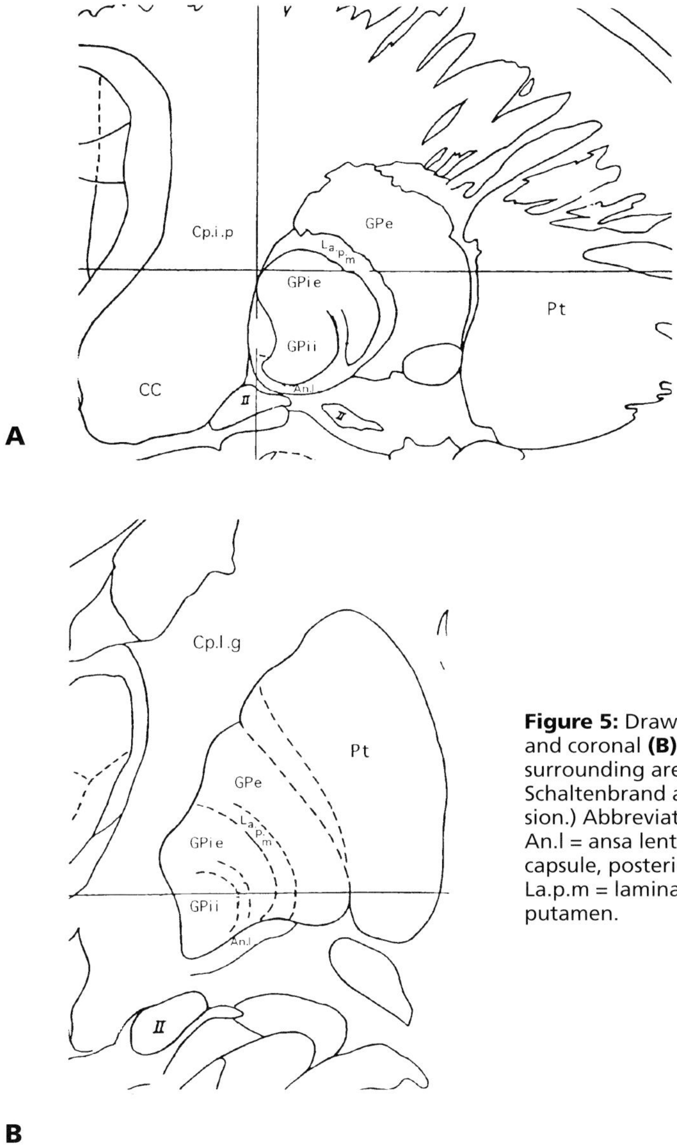

Figure 5: Drawings of parasagittal **(A)** and coronal **(B)** views of the GPi and surrounding areas. (Reproduced from Schaltenbrand and Bailey[17] with permission.) Abbreviations of key structures: An.l = ansa lenticularis; Cp.i.p = internal capsule, posterior limb; II = optic nerve; La.p.m = lamina pallidi medialis; Pt = putamen.

recommend that electrophysiological recordings should begin above the globus pallidus in order to accurately define the dorsal and ventral borders of the GPe and GPi. If recordings begin from above the GPe, the recordings will contain either no cell body spikes, indicating that the electrode tip is in white matter, or low-frequency activity, indicating that the tip is probably in the putamen.[1] Two types of neuronal recordings are generally seen from electrodes in the putamen. The first and dominant type of recording (from a type I neuron) has a very low firing rate (<1 spike/sec) and a narrow spike width, whereas the second (from a type II neuron) has a firing rate of 2-5 spikes/sec and a much broader spike width.[1]

After waiting 2-3 minutes for the brain to stabilize its position relative to the recording electrode, the tip is slowly advanced until high-frequency spikes are seen and heard from the

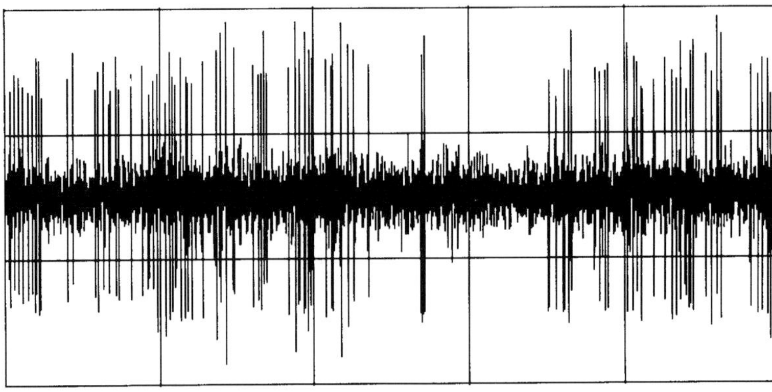

Figure 6: Representative sample of the firing pattern of a GPe cell (x axis = 1.0 sec).

recordings. As with the STN, it is important to note the depth at which the GPe is entered and exited. Cells in the GPe normally exhibit one of two patterns of firing, neither of which is regular.[5,13,19] One pattern consists of rapid bursts of activity lasting for ≥500 msec that are separated by very low rates of discharge or silence that can last for more than 0.5 sec (Figure 6). The mean overall firing rate for these cells in monkeys[5] and humans[13,19] is approximately 50 spikes/sec. The second pattern consists of very slow firing interspersed with an occasional short burst of spikes. These patterns have been seen in GPe recordings in both humans and monkeys but not in GPi recordings.[5,13,19]

As the electrode tip moves from the GPe to the GPi, there may be a brief period of silence and reduced background activity, indicating that the tip is probably in the internal medullary lamina. Increased background activity, and high-frequency discharges are typically recorded as the electrode enters the GPi. Unlike GPe cells, GPi cells exhibit continuous discharges without periods of silence.[5,13,19] Firing rates of GPi cells range from approximately 10 spikes/sec to over 100 spikes/sec. Although these cells fire more or less continuously, their firing patterns usually exhibit irregular fluctuations in rate (Figure 7). The depth of this transition also needs to be noted. The absolute thickness of the GPe and the GPi, as well as the ratio of the thicknesses of these two areas, can assist in the determination of electrode location along the anterior-posterior and medial-lateral axes.[11,20]

In some cases, spikes exhibiting a regular firing pattern of 10-40 spikes/sec may be recorded. Cells showing this rate have been called border cells[5,13,19] and can be found in areas of transition in the globus pallidus (e.g., the internal or external medullary lamina). They can be discriminated from GPi and GPe cells by their more regular firing patterns.

As the microelectrode exits the GPi, background activity abruptly decreases, indicating that the tip is passing the ventral margin of the GPi into the ansa lenticularis. In properly targeted tracks, this transition occurs approximately 1-2 mm before the optic tract is encountered. Taha et al[20] found that the thickness of the transition zone between the GPi and ansa lenticularis was not constant, but instead varied from 0.4 to 2.0 mm. The variability in the thickness of this zone could be due, for example, to an irregular border between the two areas. Because of the importance of defining this coordinate, Taha et al[20] developed a computer analysis that improved identification of the coordinates for this transition. It is possible that this type of analysis will improve the accuracy of pallidal lesions and the placement of chronic stimulating electrodes.

At the point where the background activity decreases, many surgical groups begin to deliver electrical stimulation through the microelectrode in an attempt to activate the optic tract. Microstimulation through an electrode in the optic tract should evoke visual sensations (e.g., seeing lights or stars) at currents of <20 μA.[13] The elicitation of visual sensations may be facil-

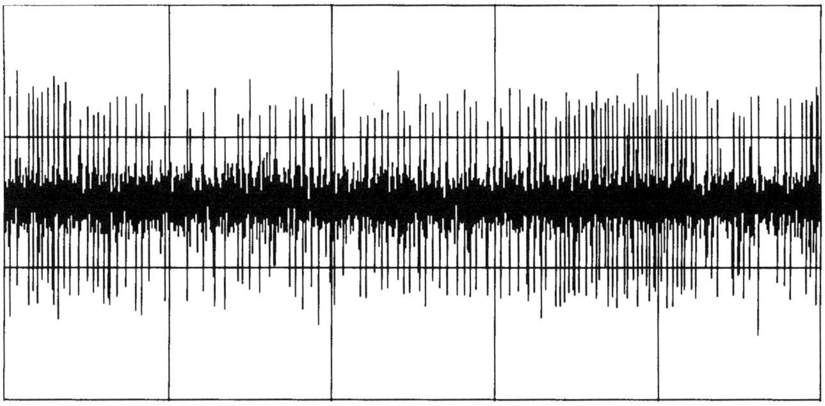

Figure 7: Representative sample of the firing pattern of a GPi cell (x axis = 1.0 sec).

itated by reducing the room lighting. If current levels of >20 μA are required to obtain a positive response, then the microelectrode is probably near but not in the optic tract.[13] It is very useful to determine the threshold current necessary to elicit visual sensations at various distances below the GPi before deciding on the lesion site. Lozano et al[13] make their lesions 3-4 mm away from areas at which electrical stimulation elicits visual or motor responses.

Visual Evoked Responses

If electrical stimulation fails to elicit visual sensations in a patient, some groups will attempt to record visual evoked responses (VERs) from an electrode that is located in or near the optic tract.[13,21,25] The same active reference and ground connections that were used for the single-cell recordings can be used for recording VERs. These leads are fed into a differential amplifier (gain 5000, bandwidth filter 10-1000 Hz), and recordings are made in response to a flashing light that is computer-controlled. Generally the responses to 20-50 stimuli are averaged, although if the electrode is in the optic tract, single flashes can elicit VERs that will be seen on oscilloscope traces and heard if the signal is sent to an audio amplifier.[13] If the recording electrode is in or very near the optic tract, repeatable VERs can be seen at approximately 30-60 msec.[13,21,25]

Recordings That Indicate an Off-Target Electrode Track

Medial and posterior to the globus pallidus lies the internal capsule, and recordings that exhibit no cell body spikes and only low-amplitude background activity throughout the targeted area are most likely in the internal capsule. When an electrode is thought to be in the internal capsule, electrical stimulation through the microelectrode can be delivered in an effort to elicit sensory or motor responses. Sensory responses can take the form of mild paresthesias, whereas motor responses can consist of tetanic contractions.[13] Microstimulation does not always elicit responses even when the electrode tip is in the optic tract or internal capsule, probably because the high impedance of the microelectrode may limit the amount of current that can be delivered. Therefore, most groups perform additional stimulation tests using a macroelectrode after the microelectrode has been withdrawn. The stimulation parameters are usually similar to those used for microstimulation. Low-frequency (2-Hz) stimulation at up to 3 V is commonly delivered.[10]

Lateral and anterior to the globus pallidus is the putamen. Recordings from cells in this area are easily discriminated from those in the globus pallidus because putamenal cells fire at very low rates.

SUMMARY

This chapter contains a brief description of electrophysiological recording techniques that are used during stereotactic surgery of the GPi and STN in patients with Parkinson's disease. These techniques include microelectrode recordings of single cells, microelectrode recordings of VERs, and electrical stimulation. At the present time there is no consensus regarding the use of microrecording in performing stereotactic functional procedures for movement disorders. Some centers would not consider doing a pallidotomy without microelectrode recordings and microstimulation, while at other centers microelectrode recording is considered to be unnecessary.[6] Controlled studies assessing which combination of recording and stimulation techniques leads to the best outcomes are needed to bring insights into this expanding field.

REFERENCES

1. Alexander GE, DeLong MR: Microstimulation of the primate neostriatum. II. Somatotopic organization of striatal microexcitable zones and their relation to neuronal response properties. **J Neurophysiol 53:** 1417-1430, 1985
2. Baron MS, Vitek JL, Bakay RAE, et al: Treatment of advanced Parkinson's disease by posterior GPi pallidotomy: 1-year results of a pilot study. **Ann Neurol 40:**355-366, 1996
3. Bergman H, Wichmann T, Karmon B, et al: The primate subthalamic nucleus. II. Neuronal activity in the MPTP model of Parkinsonism. **J Neurophysiol 72:**507-520, 1994
4. Cohen DS, Lustgarten JH, Miller E, et al: Effects of coregistration of MR to CT images on MR stereotactic accuracy. **J Neurosurg 82:**772-779, 1995
5. DeLong MR: Activity of pallidal neurons during movement. **J Neurophysiol 34:**414-427, 1971
6. Favre J, Taha JM, Nguyen TT, et al: Pallidotomy: a survey of current practice in North America. **Neurosurgery 39:**883-892, 1996
7. Gerdes JS, Hitchon PW, Neerangun W, et al: Computed tomography versus magnetic resonance imaging in stereotactic localization. **Stereotact Funct Neurosurg 63:**124-129, 1994.
8. Hikosaka O, Wurtz RH: Visual and oculomotor functions of monkey substantia nigra pars reticulata. I. Relation of visual and auditory responses to saccades. **J Neurophysiol 49:**1230-1253, 1983
9. Hollerman JR, Grace AA: Subthalamic nucleus cell firing in the 6-OHDA-treated rat: basal activity and response to haloperidol. **Brain Res 590:**291-299, 1992
10. Iacono RP, Shima F, Lonser RR, et al: The results, indications, and physiology of posteroventral pallidotomy for patients with Parkinson's disease. **Neurosurgery 36:**1118-1127, 1995
11. Kelly PJ: Pallidotomy in Parkinson's disease. **Neurosurgery 36:**1154-1157, 1995
12. Limousin P, Pollak P, Benazzouz A, et al: Effect on parkinsonian signs and symptoms of bilateral subthalamic nucleus stimulation. **Lancet 345:**91-95, 1995
13. Lozano A, Hutchinson W, Kiss Z, et al: Methods for microelectrode-guided posteroventral pallidotomy. **J Neurosurg 84:**194-202, 1996
14. Magariños-Ascone C, Buño W, García-Austt E: Activity in monkey substantia nigra neurons related to a simple learned movement. **Exp Brain Res 88:**283-291, 1992
15. Pollak P, Benabid AL, Gross C, et al: Effets de la stimulation du noyau sous-thalamique dans la maladie de Parkinson. **Rev Neurol 149:**175-176, 1993
16. Pollak P, Benabid AL, Limousin P, et al: Subthalamic nucleus stimulation alleviates akinesia and rigidity in parkinsonian patients. **Adv Neurol 69:**591-594, 1996
17. Schaltenbrand G, Bailey P: **Introduction to Stereotaxis with an Atlas of the Human Brain.** Stuttgart: Georg Thieme Verlag, 1959
18. Schultz W: Activity of pars reticulata neurons of monkey substantia nigra in relation to motor, sensory, and complex events. **J Neurophysiol 55:**660-677, 1986
19. Sterio D, Berić A, Dogali M, et al: Neurophysiological properties of pallidal neurons in Parkinson's disease. **Ann Neurol 35:**586-591, 1994
20. Taha JM, Favre J, Baumann TK, et al: Functional anatomy of the pallidal base in Parkinson's disease. **Neurosurgery 39:**1164-1168, 1996
21. Tobimatsu S, Shima F, Ishido K, et al: Visual evoked potentials in the vicinity of the optic tract during stereotactic pallidotomy. **Electroencephalogr Clin Neurophysiol 104:**274-279, 1997
22. Walton L, Hampshire A, Forster DMC, et al: Stereotactic localization using magnetic resonance imaging. **Stereotact Funct Neurosurg 64 (Suppl 1):**155-163, 1995
23. Wichmann T, Bergman H, DeLong MR: The primate subthalamic nucleus. I. Functional properties in intact animals. **J Neurophysiol 72:**494-506, 1994
24. Wichmann T, Bergman H, DeLong MR: The primate subthalamic nucleus. III. Changes in motor behavior and neuronal activity in the internal pallidum induced by subthalamic inactivation in the MPTP model of parkinsonism. **J Neurophysiol 72:**521-530, 1994
25. Yokoyama T, Sugiyama K, Nishizawa S, et al: Visual evoked potential guidance for posteroventral pallidotomy in Parkinson's disease. **Neurol Med Chir 37:** 257-264, 1997

CHAPTER 16

Interactive Computer-Assisted Image-Guided Technology as an Adjuvant to Neurosurgery for Movement Disorders

Isabelle M. Germano, MD, and M. Peter Heilbrun, MD

Stereotaxy was conceived by Horsley and Clarke[11] at the beginning of the 20th century, to overcome the difficulty of localizing intracranial structures based on skull landmarks in humans. The use of the stereotactic frame to increase the precision of surgery for functional disorders of the central nervous system was first demonstrated by Spiegel et al[24] in 1947 using a stereotactic reference frame that provided rigid skull fixation by means of screws and that established a stereotactic coordinate system for mechanically directing a probe or other surgical instrument to a defined intracranial point. Stereotactic calculations to place the probe at a specific intracranial location were performed by manual measurement of the relationship of the targets to ventricular landmarks visualized on two-dimensional (2-D) x-ray images. In the 1970s, computers were first used to perform the calculations of the stereotactic coordinates. Investigators at the Montreal Neurological Institute[2] in 1974 used computers to display probe tracts on brain maps. In the 1980s, several teams designed software that implemented stereotaxy by providing preoperative visualization of the planned surgical path.[9,13,16,21]

With the price of computers decreasing, coupled with their increased performance and speed, computer use is rapidly expanding in most neurosurgical practices. In the 1990s, there has been an explosion of computer-assisted image-guided technology, also known as "frameless stereotaxy," to use for intracranial and spinal procedures.[1,4,7,8,10,12,14,19,20,23] An advantage of this technology is the avoidance of a rigid frame, which is uncomfortable for the patient and intrusive intraoperatively for the surgeon.[9] These systems are easy to use for neurosurgical planning. Preoperatively the neurosurgeon can correlate corresponding points in various three-planar and three-dimensional (3-D) images and examine different trajectories on reconstructed oblique images.

In this chapter, the use of the frameless StealthStation system (Sofamor Danek, Memphis, Tennessee) interfaced with the frame-based Cosman-Roberts-Wells (CRW) stereotactic system (Radionics, Burlington, Massachusetts) is described, as well as the advantages of the use of this technology for neurosurgical treatment of movement disorders.

Frameless Systems and Accuracy

Frameless stereotaxy relies on accurately registering physical space with image space. In other words, the patient's anatomy as seen on preoperative images is "superimposed" on the physical anatomy of the patient. This process is called registration. After registration is completed, the position of a surgical instrument used for a particular procedure can be seen projected in real-time on the patient's preoperative images, which are displayed on the computer screen. Fundamentally, the mode of operation of frameless systems currently available is similar and based on three pieces of equipment: 1) a computed tomography (CT) or magnetic resonance imaging (MRI) scanner for acquisition of preoperative images; 2) a digitizer for the registration process; and 3) a high-capacity computer workstation. Several digitizing technologies have been adapted to be used with these systems, including articulated mechanical arms and sonic, electromagnetic, and optical digitizers.[10,12,20,21,23,25]

Although a review of the existing frameless technology is beyond the scope of this chapter, it should be emphasized that there have been several reports on the degree of accuracy that these systems can achieve.[1,7,15] In frame-based stereotaxy, accuracy is determined for the most part by the mechanical characteristics of the stereotactic system and the imaging characteristics, including MRI distortion and the thickness of the images used for localization. In frameless stereotaxy, in addition to the above-mentioned factors, the registration process itself can be a source of inaccuracy. Each of these factors is additive in a vector sum and can ultimately result in a more significant error than an error of each step by itself. Furthermore, there is a difference between bench accuracy and accuracy when the system is used clinically. The term "application accuracy" was therefore introduced in 1994.[18] Application accuracy refers to the accuracy of a stereotactic device when used in the clinical setting.

Stereotactic frames have provided extreme levels of application accuracy for surgical localization. To supplant the technology of stereotactic frames, equivalent levels of localization accuracy should be provided by frameless systems of interactive image-guided neurosurgery. Recent literature suggests that frameless systems can be as accurate as frame-based systems. For example, the accuracy of the StealthStation system under optimal conditions in the laboratory compares favorably with that of four commonly used conventional stereotaxy systems: the Brown-Roberts-Wells and CRW systems (Radionics), the Leksell system (Elekta Instruments, Atlanta, Georgia), and the Kelly-Goerss system (Stereotactic Medical Systems, Rochester, Minnesota).[3,17]

Although several groups have been working to gain higher accuracy with frameless systems in the clinical setting,[17] the author's (IMG) clinical experience using frameless technology for over 150 intracranial cases supports the evidence that frameless techniques cannot be used alone when the desired degree of accuracy is within 1 mm, such as in deep brain stimulation or ablative procedures.

Interface Between Frame and Frameless Systems

Stereotactic localization of nuclei of the basal ganglia, which are the target for ablative and restorative procedures, is fundamental in the surgical treatment of movement disorders. At the present time, most frame-based systems provide an accuracy that is satisfactory for the high precision required for this type of surgery. While frame-based systems provide accurate localization of the desired target, other factors are essential in functional neurosurgery, namely, the choice of a trajectory that avoids blood vessels, sulci, eloquent structures, and the ventricular cavity. These systems allow the surgeon to perform preplanning, simulation, and optimization of the surgical procedure and show the safest approach to the target. Furthermore, real-time visualization of the recording electrode inserted in the brain allows easier readjustment of its location if needed, as defined by microelectrophysiology recordings.

These advantages of frameless technology (including interactive image-guided computer assistance) are very appealing, especially if it can be superimposed with the high degree of accuracy seen with frame-based stereotaxy. The concept of interfacing frame-based with frameless equipment has been explored for use in other stereotactic procedures,[6,26] and has contributed to interfacing of frame-based and frameless equipment for use in the neurosurgical treatment of movement disorders. A description of an interface developed by the authors to integrate the CRW system with the StealthStation follows.

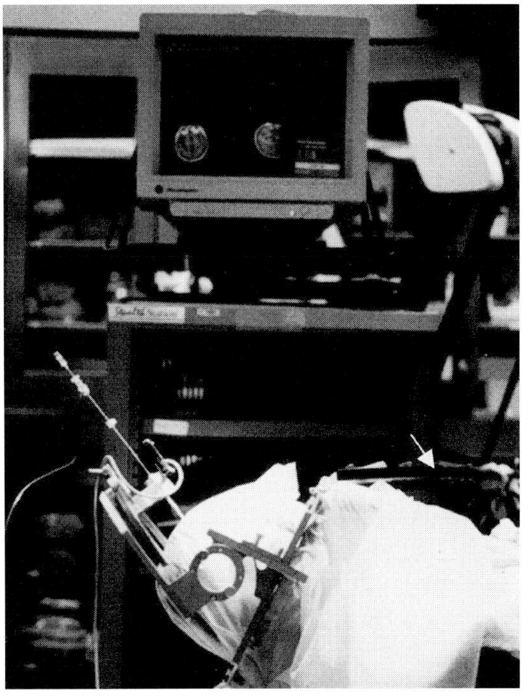

Figure1: Intraoperative photograph showing the patient positioned on the operating room table with the hardware interface for frame-based (CRW) and frameless (StealthStation) technology. The *arrow* indicates the reference arc for the frameless system. See text for details.

Hardware Interface

Image acquisition via MRI or CT is performed, as described elsewhere,[5] during the morning of surgery after applying the CRW frame and the self-adhesive markers in a conventional fashion. Intraoperatively, the patient is positioned supine on the operating table. The CRW system is secured to the table using a CRW-Mayfield adapter, which is modified to allow simultaneous attachment with the post holding the frameless reference arc. The reference arc is positioned approximately 20 cm in front of the CRW ring. Care must be taken to position the lateral post supporting the frameless reference arc at least 20 cm away from the CRW ring to allow placement of the CRW arc (Figure 1).

Software Interface

The frameless registration process is first completed in the conventional fashion, as described elsewhere.[4] Then, the CRW system coordinates are computer-generated after clicking on the nine CRW rods shown in the axial image displayed on the computer screen. For CT scans, the rods are clicked off in a counterclockwise direction, starting from the widest rod. For MRIs, the rods are marked in a clockwise direction, starting from the most anterior rod on the right-hand side. After entering the positions of all nine rods, the CRW coordinates are automatically displayed on the computer screen. After a surgical plan is determined (see below), the arc setting, i.e., the arc angles, is computer-calculated (Figure 2).

Functional Software and Surgical Planning

The next step in the integration of the frame-based and frameless systems includes the addition in the software of a digitized stereotactic atlas and several functions to optimize selection of the target. For determination of the ventral intermediate (VIM) nucleus of the thalamus and the internal segment of the globus pallidus (GPi), an axial image showing both the anterior commissure (AC) and the posterior commis-

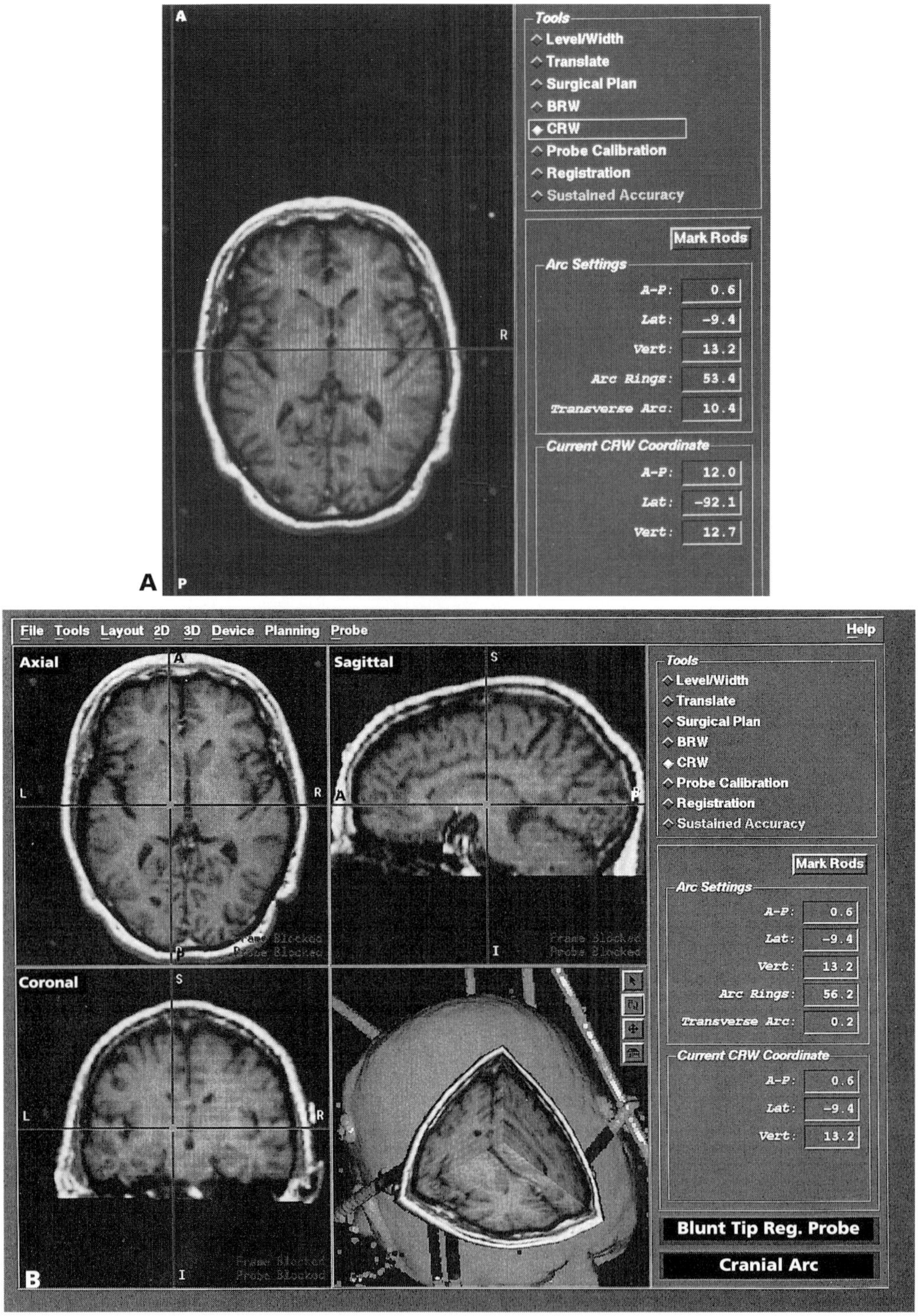

Figure 2:. Intraoperative photographs of the computer screen displayed while interfacing frame-based and frameless techniques. **A)** The CRW coordinates are obtained after entering the position of the CRW rods into the computer, i.e., by clicking on each rod in the axial image displayed on the screen. **B)** The target is then selected by clicking on the desired anatomical structure, in this case the VIM. The computer-generated anteroposterior (AP), lateral, and vertical CRW coordinates of the target ("Current CRW Coordinate") and the AP ("Arc Rings") and lateral ("Transverse Arc") angle of the CRW arc are displayed in the dialog box on the screen ("Arc Settings").

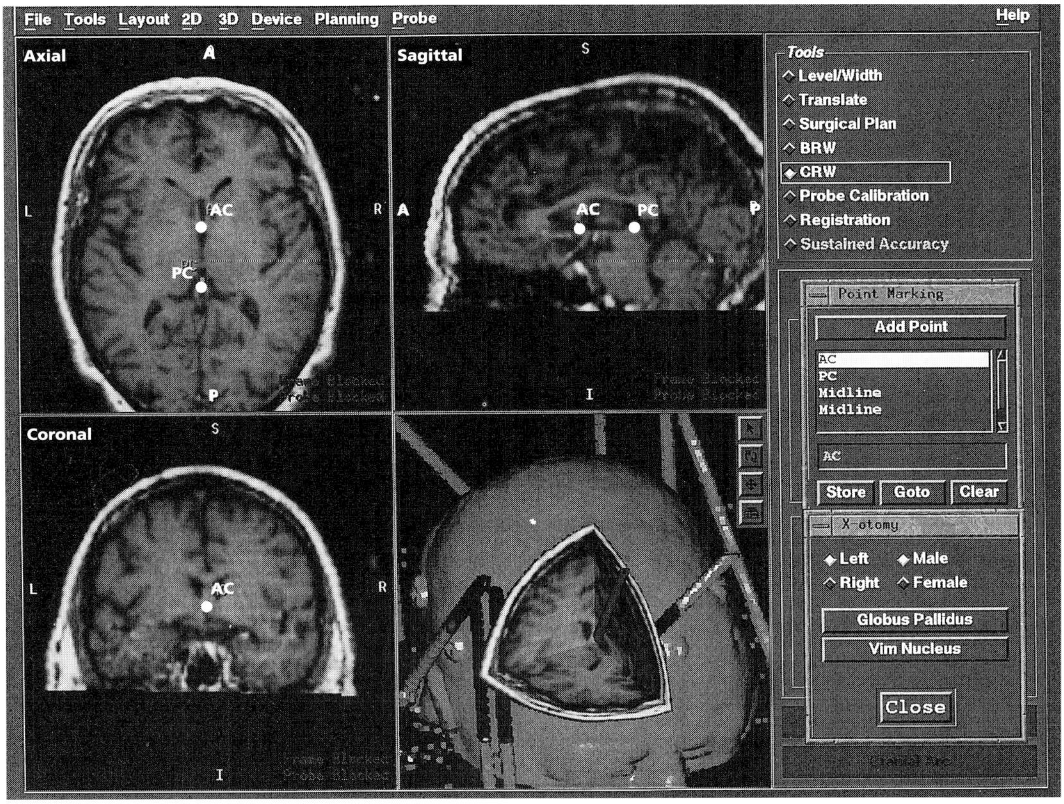

Figure 3: Intraoperative photograph of the computer screen displayed while marking the AC and PC on the axial slice showing the midcommissural point. Three midline points are also selected. Selection of the appropriate fields in the "X-otomy box" results in the calculation of the CRW coordinates for the VIM or GPi (as shown in Table 1). The calculated point is seen on the screen as crosshairs.

sure (PC) should be selected by the surgeon. These two points are marked on the computer by clicking on each. Furthermore, three midline points are selected and entered (Figure 3). At this point, the computer calculates the CRW coordinates based on standard stereotactic locations of the VIM and GPi (Table 1).

A digitized copy of the Schaltenbrand and Wahren stereotactic brain atlas[22] is superimposed onto the axial images, choosing the appropriate window from the menu, and then formatted by the surgeon to fit the patient's anatomy by matching the length of the AC-PC line and the size of the ventricle (Figure 4). The

TABLE 1

COMPUTED CALCULATIONS FOR LOCALIZATION OF THE VIM AND THE GPI

	Coordinates		
Nucleus	Anteroposterior	Lateral	Vertical
VIM	(0.25 × length of AC-PC line) anterior to PC	(0.55 × length of AC-PC line) lateral to AC-PC line	(0.05 × length of AC-PC line) below AC-PC line
GPi	2 mm anterior to midcommissural point	21 mm lateral to AC-PC line	4 mm inferior to AC-PC line

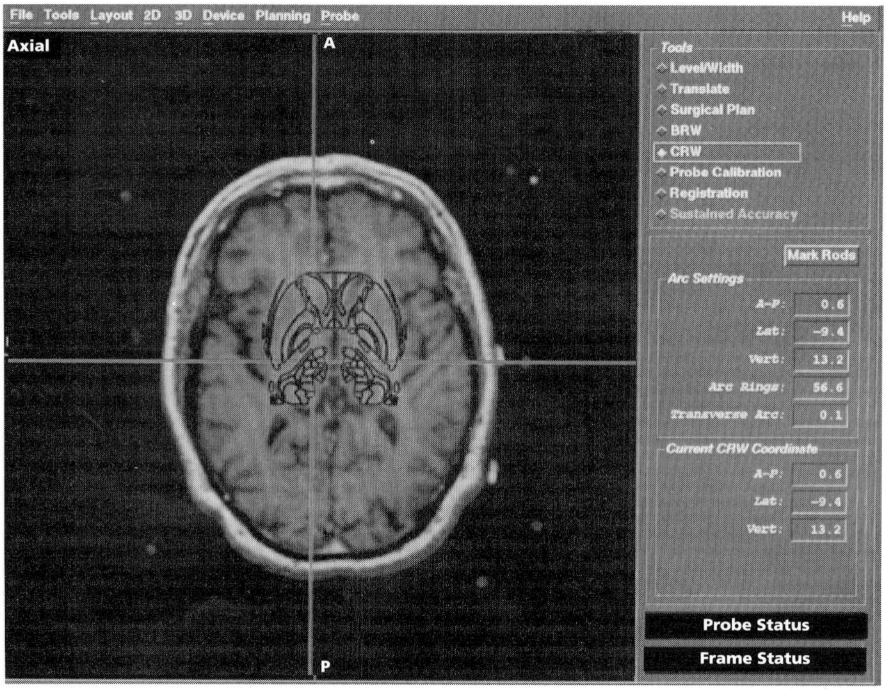

Figure 4: Intraoperative photograph of the computer screen showing the Schaltenbrand and Wahren atlas reformatted to fit the patient's anatomy. This is accomplished by matching the length of the AC-PC line and the size of the ventricles. The atlas can be modified in all three dimensions.

atlas can be modified in all three dimensions. At this point, the computer-selected target for the VIM or the GPi can be seen in relationship to the outlines of the basal ganglia structures in the atlas. Typically, the location of the target is optimized based on anatomical landmarks and/or atlas-based physiology.

After the target is selected, an entry point is chosen and the planned trajectory is optimized using computer images (Figure 5). The authors choose an entry point anterior to the coronal suture and verify that the trajectory does not involve sulci or the ventricular cavity, to decrease the risk of hemorrhage and brain shift, respectively. Once a surgical plan is formulated by choosing the entry point and the target, the computer displays a trajectory of the planned path. This can be visualized not only on the three-planar and 3-D images but also on other images reconstructed by the computer. Trajectory views, i.e., images reconstructed in the two planes orthogonal to the electrode are very helpful in conceptualizing the real-time trajectory of the probe. Similarly, the "probe's eye view," i.e., an image reconstructed in the same angle as the probe's trajectory, allows visualization of the tissue to be traversed by the electrode to reach the target. The "planned pathway" option allows the surgeon to scroll through images from the entry point to the target in a sequential fashion. Based on feedback regarding this "virtual surgery," the trajectory can be modified until satisfactory. In the authors' experience, the preoperative planning is a very important step because it not only allows optimization of the placement of deep brain electrodes or ablative lesions, but also reduces morbidity risks. Based on the neurosurgeon's view of the calculated functional targets, the software allows direct targeting or the use of customized formulas.

Advantages, Disadvantages, and Future Directions

Surgical navigation systems provide a real-time virtual linkage between digitized neuroradiological images and anatomical structures,

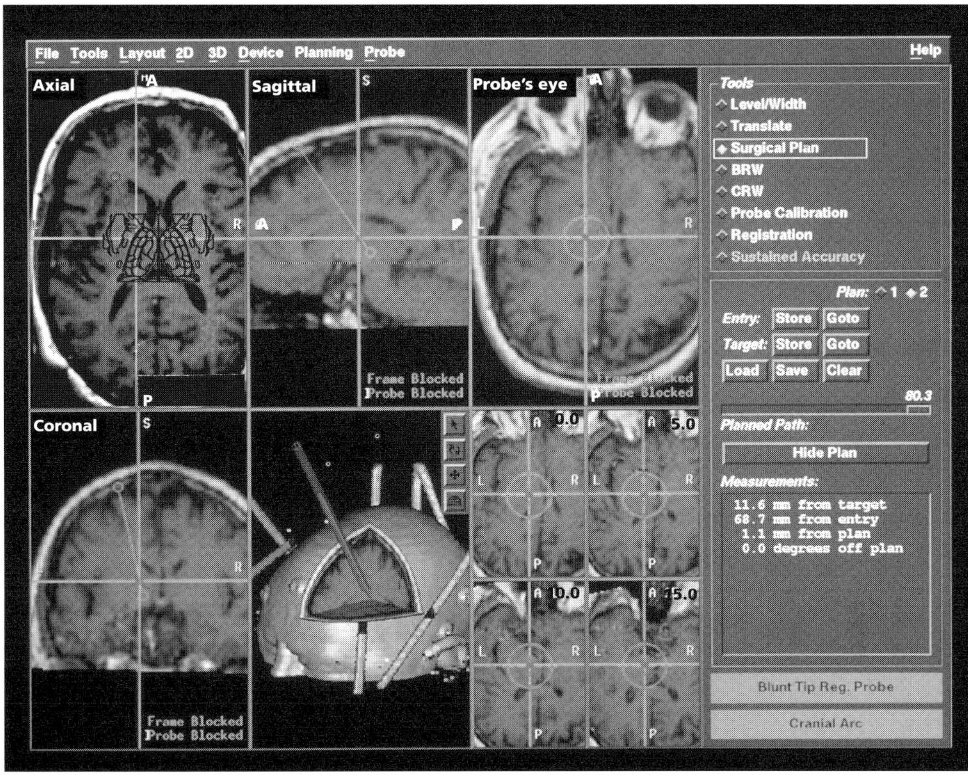

Figure 5: Intraoperative photograph of the computer screen showing the real-time position of the recording electrode (crosshairs) prior to beginning the electrophysiological microrecording. The distance from the chosen target is indicated in the dialog box ("Measurement"): 11.6 mm. The trajectory is seen as a lighter line between two circles on the 2-D images and as a hollow cylinder on the 3-D image. "Trajectory view 1" is an image reconstructed in a plane orthogonal to the electrode. The "look ahead" view *(lower right)* shows the location of the electrode tip at the present time (0.0) and its "virtual location" 5 (5.0), 10 (10.0), and 15 (15.0) mm further along the same trajectory.

thus allowing an accurate 3-D orientation by real-time graphic-anatomical interaction. At Mount Sinai Medical Center, the CRW-StealthStation systems interface has been used in seven patients undergoing implantation of deep brain electrodes in the GPi, the VIM nucleus, and the subthalamic nucleus for treatment of movement disorders. Furthermore, it has been used for diagnostic brain needle biopsies of lesions with a maximum longitudinal diameter of <1.5 cm.[5] This system has been found to be advantageous for several reasons. First, a presurgical plan can be prepared with an optimal trajectory designed to avoid sulci and the ventricular cavity. This is best done using the planned pathway option, which allows the surgeon to scroll through the three-planar images and view the proposed trajectory. The probe's eye view shows the reconstructed image in a plane orthogonal to the probe, allowing excellent visualization of the proposed trajectory. Additionally, "performing" the planned surgery on the computer before its execution is a valuable training experience for residents. Second, intraoperatively, the recording electrode can be seen in real-time on the computer images, which provides an excellent correlation between the electrophysiological recording and the patient's anatomy. In the authors' experience, this expedites the placement of the permanent electrode by reducing the number of passes. In the authors' series of patients, no morbidity has been related to the use of this system.

A disadvantage of using the frameless system is that it adds 15 minutes to the procedure, to register the frameless equipment. In the authors' experience, this is not a significant drawback, as the interface has been shown to expedite and facilitate the placement of the permanent electrode. Thus, the authors believe that the overall surgical time is decreased.

Future directions in this field include the implementation of storing a library of cases managed at various institutions, based on the final placement of the electrode in each patient and easily accessible during presurgical planning. Further advances in frameless technology may result in its sole use for functional surgical procedures.

Conclusion

The authors' clinical and bench experience with the StealthStation system shows that it is a very accurate frameless device. At the present time, however, the authors prefer to rely on a frame-based system to perform ablative and restorative intracranial procedures for movement disorders. Nonetheless, preliminary clinical experience shows that computer-assisted image-guided technology is a valuable adjunct to frame-based systems for neurosurgical treatment of movement disorders.

References

1. Barnett GH, Kormos DW, Steiner CP, et al: Use of a frameless, armless stereotactic wand for brain tumor localization with two-dimensional and three-dimensional neuroimaging. **Neurosurgery 33:**674–678, 1993
2. Bertrand G, Olivier A, Thompson CJ: Computer display of stereotaxic brain maps and probe tracts. **Acta Neurochir Suppl 21:**235-243, 1974
3. Galloway RL Jr, Maciunas RJ, Latimer JW: The accuracies of four stereotactic frame systems: an independent assessment. **Biomed Instrum Technol 25:** 457-460, 1991
4. Germano IM: The NeuroStation system for image-guided, frameless stereotaxy. **Neurosurgery 37:** 348-350, 1995
5. Germano IM, Queenan JV: Clinical experience with intracranial brain needle biopsy using frameless surgical navigation. **Comput Aided Surg** (In press)
6. Goerss SJ, Kelly PJ, Kall B, et al: A stereotactic magnetic field digitizer. **Stereotact Funct Neurosurg 63:** 89-92, 1994
7. Golfinos JG, Fitzpatrick BC, Smith LR, et al: Clinical use of a frameless stereotactic arm: results of 325 cases. **J Neurosurg 83:**197–205, 1995
8. Guthrie BL, Adler JR Jr: Computer-assisted preoperative planning, interactive surgery, and frameless stereotaxy. **Clin Neurosurg 38:**112–131, 1992
9. Heilbrun MP: Computed tomography-guided stereotactic systems. **Clin Neurosurg 31:**564-581, 1984
10. Heilbrun MP, McDonald P, Wiker C, et al: Stereotactic localization and guidance using a machine vision technique. **Stereotact Funct Neurosurg 58:**94-98, 1992
11. Horsley V, Clarke RH: The structure and functions of the cerebellum examined by a new method. **Brain 31:** 45-124, 1908
12. Horstmann GA, Reinhardt HF: Ranging accuracy test of the sonic microstereometric system. **Neurosurgery 34:**754–755, 1994
13. Kall BA, Kelly PJ, Goerss SJ: Comprehensive computer-assisted data collection treatment planning and interactive surgery. **Med Imag SPIE 767:**509-514, 1987
14. Kato A, Yoshimine T, Hayakawa T, et al: A frameless, armless navigational system for computer-assisted neurosurgery. Technical note. **J Neurosurg 74:** 845-849, 1991
15. Kaus M, Steinmeier R, Sporer T, et al: Technical accuracy of a neuronavigation system measured with a high-precision mechanical micromanipulator. **Neurosurgery 41:**1431–1437, 1997
16. Kelly PJ , Kall BA, Goerss S, et al: Present and future developments of stereotactic technology. **Appl Neurophysiol 48:**1-6, 1985
17. Maciunas RJ, Fitzpatrick JM, Galloway RL, et al: Beyond stereotaxy: Extreme levels of application accuracy are provided by implantable fiducial markers for interactive image-guided neurosurgery, in Maciunas RJ (ed): **Interactive Image-Guided Neurosurgery.** Park Ridge, Ill: American Association of Neurological Surgeons, 1993, pp 259-270
18. Maciunas RJ, Galloway RL Jr, Latimer JW: The application accuracy of stereotactic frames. **Neurosurgery 35:**682–695, 1994
19. Olivier A, Germano IM, Cukiert A: Frameless stereotaxy for surgery of the epilepsies: preliminary experience. Technical note. **J Neurosurg 81:**629-633, 1994
20. Reinhardt HF, Horstmann GA, Gratzl O: Sonic stereometry in microsurgical procedures for deep-seated brain tumors and vascular malformations. **Neurosurgery 32:**51-57, 1993
21. Roberts DW, Strohbehn JW, Hatch JF, et al: A frameless stereotaxic integration of computerized tomographic imaging and the operative microscope. **J Neurosurg 65:**545-549, 1986
22. Schaltenbrand G, Wahren W: **Atlas for Stereotaxy of the Human Brain.** New York, NY: Thieme, 1977
23. Smith KR, Frank KJ, Bucholz RD: The NeuroStation—a highly accurate minimally invasive solution to frameless stereotactic neurosurgery. **Comput Med Imaging Graph 18:**247-256, 1994
24. Spiegel EA, Wycis HT, Marks M, et al: Sterotaxic apparatus for operations on the human brain. **Science 106:**349-350, 1947
25. Watanabe E, Watanabe T, Manaka S. Three-dimensional digitizer (Neuronavigator): new equipment for computed tomography-guided stereotaxic surgery. **Surg Neurol 27:**543-547, 1987
26. Zamorano L, Nolte L, Kodi M, et al: Modification of stereotactic frame guidance arcs using optical encoder verniers, in Maciunas RJ (ed): **Interactive Image-Guided Neurosurgery.** Park Ridge, Ill: American Association of Neurological Surgeons, 1993, pp 97-103

PART E

Treatment of Hyperkinesias: Surgical Techniques

CHAPTER 17

Operative Treatment of Hemifacial Spasm

Peter J. Jannetta, MD, and Mark R. McLaughlin, MD

History

The first clinical-pathological correlation of vascular compression in hemifacial spasm was reported in 1875, when Schultze[31] described aneurysmal compression of the seventh cranial nerve on postmortem examination in a patient with a history of hemifacial spasm. The first intraoperative observations of arterial ectasia compressing the seventh and eighth nerve complex were described by Campbell and Keedy[5] and subsequently by Gardner.[11,12] Gardner found vascular compression of the seventh cranial nerve in 8 of 19 operations for hemifacial spasm. However, he did not use magnification technique nor did he inspect the dorsal root exit zone, and he treated all patients with "neurolysis" (mild nerve trauma).[11-13] Scoville,[32] in 1969, again without magnification, reported the successful treatment of hemifacial spasm by moving a distal arterial loop in the cerebellopontine angle away from the seventh cranial nerve. Although he did not look at the dorsal root exit zone, it is presumed that he unknowingly freed the more proximal seventh cranial nerve from compression of a mildly traumatized facial nerve.

Diagnosis

There are two subtypes of hemifacial spasm. Typical hemifacial spasm is characterized by the onset of intermittent, unilateral spontaneous contraction of one of the orbicularis oculi muscles. These spasms progress in a rostral-to-caudal fashion and gradually encompass the cheek and buccal muscles, ultimately involving the platysma. Atypical hemifacial spasm, which was found in approximately 8% of the authors' patients, is characterized by intermittent spasms that begin within the buccal muscles and ascend in a caudal-to-rostral fashion to involve the facial musculature, ultimately affecting the frontalis muscle.[2] In the late stages of either type, all of the muscles of facial expression may be involved.

Patients with long-standing hemifacial spasm usually have "tonus phenomenon," which is characterized by sustained facial musculature contractions with grimacing, eye closure, and some pulling of the corner of the mouth. These episodes can persist for many seconds to several minutes before relaxation. Frequently there is a positional component to the spasm, and it is usually present while the patient is sleeping. Diagnosis can be made easily by clinical history and observation.

Differential Diagnosis

Other diseases that may mimic some of the aspects of hemifacial spasm include essential blepharospasm, facial myokymia, "habit" spasm, focal cortical seizures involving the facial muscles, synkinesis due to aberrant nerve regeneration after facial nerve injury, tardive dyskinesia, and Meige's syndrome.[4,35,36] Essential blepharospasm can be easily ruled out, as this condition is characterized by involuntary, bilateral repetitive and symmetrical blinking of the eyes.[14] Patients with aberrant nerve regeneration after seventh cranial nerve injury usually have a history of trauma.[35] Facial myokymia is a continuous facial spasm without remission, and often is associated with an intrinsic brain-stem lesion demonstrated on magnetic resonance imaging.[6] Meige's syndrome is characterized by oromandibular dystonia and blepharospasm.[33] Habit spasms usually have a volitional component and involve muscles not innervated by the seventh cranial nerve.[8] The remaining conditions in the differential diagnosis are excluded by a thorough history and physical examination.

Medical Management

Medical therapy for hemifacial spasm is either ineffective or provides the patient with only temporary relief. Nearly unanimously in the patients in the authors' series, carbamazepine, phenytoin, baclofen, and clonazepam were found to be useless.[2] Other treatments have included psychotherapy, electrical stimulation, massage, and radiotherapy with a linear accelerator, all of which have provided minimal or no benefit.[35] Some patients have had improvement with the use of haloperidol and baclofen, although these reports have been in small series and have had short follow-up.[3,30]

Botulinum toxin injection for hemifacial spasm has been reported to be successful in several series.[7,23,25] The duration of relief, however, averages only 12-18 weeks, and thus requires three to four courses of injections per year until it becomes ineffective.[2,23] In addition, this therapy substitutes muscle hypoactivity for hyperactivity and has potential complications.[7,25] Furthermore, there are no reports of hemifacial spasm remission with botulinum toxin therapy.[2]

Given the relative ineffectiveness of medical therapy, including only transient relief with a high complication rate from botulinum toxin therapy, the authors recommend microvascular decompression for all patients medically able to undergo a 2-hour procedure under anesthesia.

Operative Technique: Retromastoid Craniectomy and Microvascular Decompression

Patient Positioning

It has often been said that the most important part of a surgical procedure is performed before the skin incision is made. Proper patient positioning for this operation is critical to maximize surgical exposure and minimize the risks for complications. The patient is placed in a reverse position on the operating room table such that the patient's head is at the foot of the bed. This allows the surgeon the most comfortable position while operating under the microscope by providing adequate foot room. Anesthesia for the procedure cannot include paralytics, as intraoperative electromyography (EMG) is utilized to aid the surgeon in determining which vessel is the cause of the hemifacial spasm. This point must be emphasized to the anesthesia team prior to induction so that adequate EMG can be performed.[27] After induction and intubation, a three-point pin fixation device is applied, and the patient is turned to the lateral park bench position with the affected side up. Appropriate pressure points are padded, and the patient is secured to the table as shown in Figure 1. The head is held with one of the surgeon's arms supporting the neck and the other holding the pin fixation system, and the neck is placed on the stretch. The head is flexed slightly, and the vertex is tilted approximately 10° toward the floor. By placing the vertex 10° toward the floor, the sev-

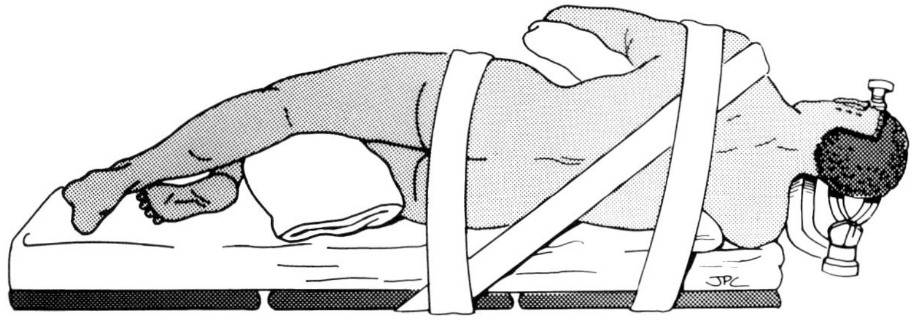

Figure 1: Proper patient positioning for microvascular decompression of the seventh cranial nerve. The head is slightly flexed and tilted 10°, with the vertex down. An axillary roll prevents brachial plexus injury, and the patient is secured so that the table can be rotated toward or away from the surgeon during the microdissection without risking patient movement.

enth and eighth cranial nerve complex is rotated into a more accessible position and the caudal aspect of the seventh nerve is exposed once the microsurgical exposure is obtained. The head is locked into place, and the proper position verified by the surgeon. A 3 × 5-cm patch of hair is shaved behind the ear, and the area is prepped. A linear incision line is drawn approximately 0.5 cm posterior and parallel to the hairline. The inferior aspect of the incision should extend down to slightly below the level of the mastoid tip (Figure 2). The area is then draped.

The incision, 2.5-5 cm long (shorter in Asians and in long-necked patients, slightly longer in muscular, short-necked patients), is made and dissection is performed down to the periosteum. Occasionally an occipital artery branch may require suture ligation. However, the majority of vessels can be cauterized using a bipolar forceps and divided easily. The muscle dissection is carried down to the occipital bone, carefully following the skull contour as it gradually falls away from the surgical field. The dissection must be low and lateral, and should extend superiorly to the junction of the sigmoid and transverse sinuses. The digastric groove is identified, and the mastoid emissary vein, which is usually located at the top of the digastric groove, is occluded with bone wax. This dissection is slightly lower and more lateral than the typical dissection for a microvascular decompression of the trigeminal nerve. To assure adequate exposure, periosteal dissection should be extended to approximately 0.5 cm lateral to the digastric groove, over the mastoid eminence. An angled cerebellar retractor is utilized for retraction.

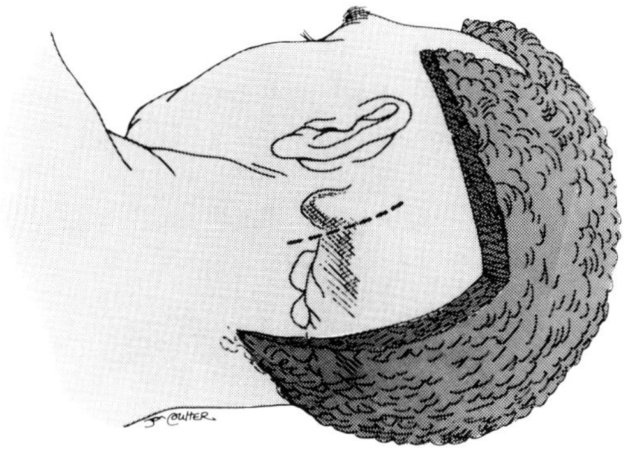

Figure 2: A linear incision line is drawn approximately 0.5 cm posterior and parallel to the hairline with the inferior aspect extending slightly below the level of the mastoid tip. The length of the incision varies from 2 to 5 cm depending on the body habitus of the patient.

Prior to craniectomy, the operative site must be completely dry. The craniectomy is then performed using an osteotome or high-speed drill and enlarged using Leksell and Raney rongeurs. The edge of the sigmoid sinus must be identified and clearly exposed. The finished craniectomy is shaped in a generally triangular fashion with the apex pointing toward the mastoid tip, as shown in Figure 3. Mastoid air cells and bone edges are then waxed thoroughly.

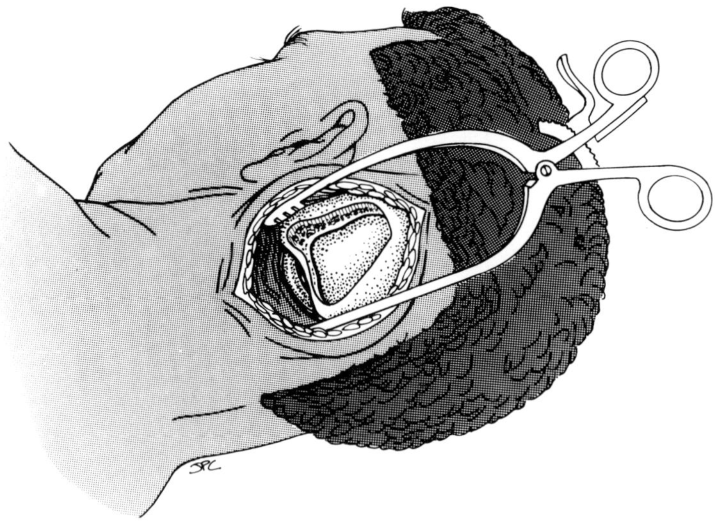

Figure 3: A triangular craniectomy is made with the apex pointing toward the mastoid tip. The edge of the sigmoid sinus must be clearly exposed. Mastoid air cells are waxed thoroughly "on the way in and (again) on the way out."

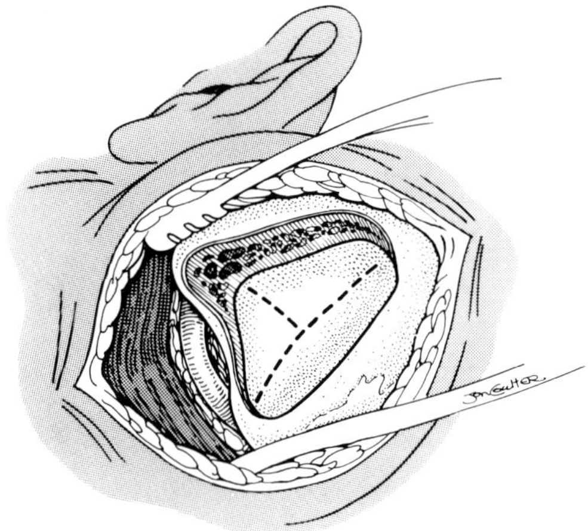

Figure 4: The dura is opened in a T-shaped fashion to optimize exposure of the low and lateral corner of the craniectomy. An alternative curvilinear durotomy can be made adjacent to the sigmoid sinus.

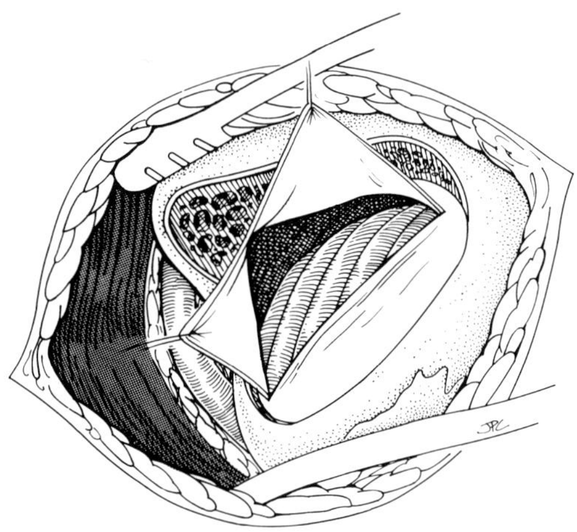

Figure 5: The dural leaflets are tacked back to the periosteum to expose the inferolateral cerebellum.

The dural opening is then made in either a curvilinear or a T-shaped fashion so as to maximize exposure to the lowest and most lateral point of the dura (Figure 4). The authors do not utilize lumbar drainage or the administration of mannitol prior to opening the dura. In the vast majority of cases, simple cerebrospinal fluid (CSF) drainage from the dural opening is adequate to obtain exposure. Occasionally in a young person, the cerebellum may herniate outward after the durotomy. In these cases a rubber dam-covered cottonoid patty is placed over the entire cerebellar surface exposed after the dural opening. Gentle, even pressure on the cottonoid with either a forceps or the surgeon's finger can easily prevent a cerebellar contusion. The surgeon must then simply "walk" the rubber dam-covered cottonoid caudally, gently elevating the cerebellum until the cistern can be identified and drained.

After the dural opening, the operating microscope is brought into the field. Once CSF drainage is accomplished, the cerebellum will fall away rapidly (Figure 5). The cottonoid patty should then be advanced inferiorly to expose the subarachnoid cistern over the ninth and tenth

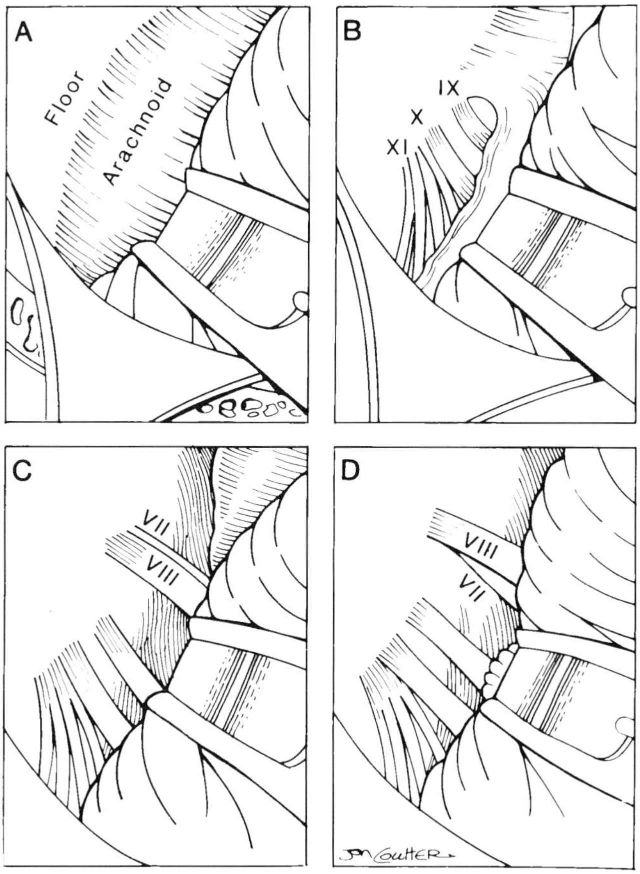

Figure 6: Microsurgical view of the floor of the posterior fossa **(A)** and the progressive changes in the angulation of the microscope and the adjustment of the retractor blade. The arachnoid over the ninth and tenth cranial nerves is opened first **(B)**. The microscope and retractor blade are then directed rostrally to elevate the flocculus and expose the seventh and eighth nerve complex **(C** and **D)**.

cranial nerves. It is critical to make an approach well inferior to the seventh and eighth nerve complex to avoid damage to the cochlear nerve. The arachnoid cistern over the ninth and tenth nerve complex is opened using sharp dissection. The arachnoid is then widely opened, first over cranial nerves IX and X, and then over cranial nerves VII and VIII. The operating microscope is then angled superiorly, and the seventh and eighth nerve complex should come into view (Figure 6). The majority of the cerebellar retraction is obtained by adequate CSF drainage. The cerebellum is gently elevated, and the choroid plexus and lateral recess of the fourth ventricle are visualized. The facial nerve exits the brain stem in a diagonal fashion, appearing somewhat like a flag pole coming off a building. The intraoperative area of the seventh cranial nerve often is obscured by the vascular pathology and occasionally by the flocculus or choroid plexus. The retractor blade is slowly and carefully advanced. Ultimately, the tip should gently elevate the flocculus and choroid plexus from the ninth and tenth nerve complex. Sharp dissection of the flocculus off the ninth and tenth nerve complex is critical to visualizing the dorsal root exit zone of seven.

The offending pathology is most commonly

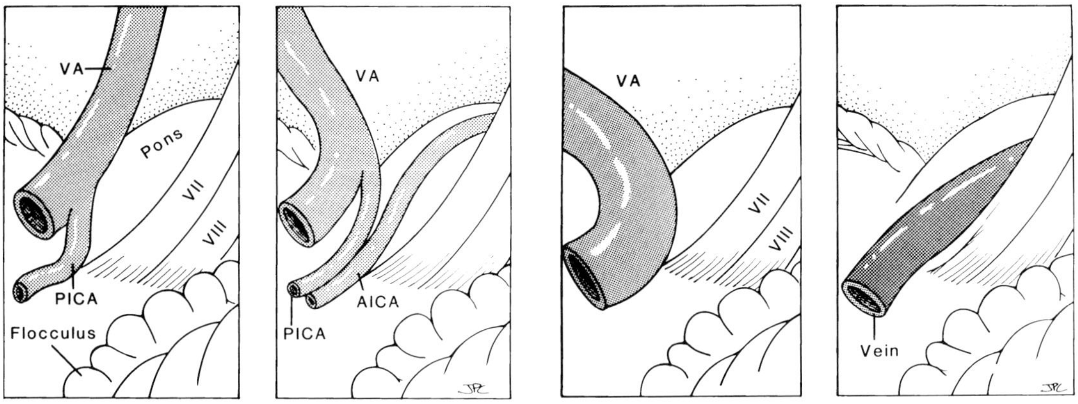

Figure 7: The four most commonly observed vascular relationships in typical hemifacial spasm. Note the cross-compression is at the anterior-caudal portion of the nerve. VA = vertebral artery.

the posterior inferior cerebellar artery (PICA) with the anterior inferior cerebellar artery (AICA) second in frequency (Figure 7). The vertebral artery can also be the causative agent. Not infrequently, two or three of these arteries will be compressing a nerve. Venous compression was also noted in approximately 20% of patients in the authors' most recent series (Table 1). Arteries and veins often can be seen compressing, abutting, or coursing through the seventh and eighth cranial nerve complex between the brain stem and the porus acusticus; however, these vessels are *not* the cause of hemifacial spasm. Most importantly, the surgeon must decompress the facial nerve at and proximal to the nerve root exit zone, including the intrapontine portion of the seventh cranial nerve all the way down to the pontomedullary junction. The vascular arterial loop must be dissected away from and lifted off this area. A small implant of nonabsorbable, soft felt material must be interposed between the vessel and the nerve. Arachnoid bands must be completely removed using sharp dissection to fully mobilize the offending vessel. Once the vessel is mobilized, one or more soft plastic implants are placed. The sizes and shapes of the implants vary depending on the vessel anatomy and configuration. When the offending vessel is mobilized and lifted off the dorsal root exit zone, abnormal facial EMG responses (lateral spread) should disappear instantaneously. If this lateral spread does not disappear, the surgeon must vigilantly look for other vessels causing compression.[26] Venous compression is relieved by coagulation and division of the abnormal veins. Division of the veins is necessary, as recanalization can occur in veins that are merely coagulated. Atypical hemifacial spasm is caused by a blood vessel rostral or posterior to the facial nerve (Figure 8). Therefore, the rostral side of the nerve should be exposed. Veins are coagulated and divided. The AICA running between the seventh and eighth cranial nerves must be elevated off the brain stem and padded very gently to avoid tearing away perforating arterial branches to the brain.

TABLE 1

Operative Findings in 648 Consecutive First Operations for Hemifacial Spasm

Offending Vessel	Percentage of Cases
PICA	68%
AICA	35%
Vertebral artery	24%
Vein	20%
Vein only	3%
Other	21%

Once adequate decompression has been verified, several Valsalva maneuvers are performed to verify hemostasis. The area is then gently irrigated with warm saline, and the retractor blade

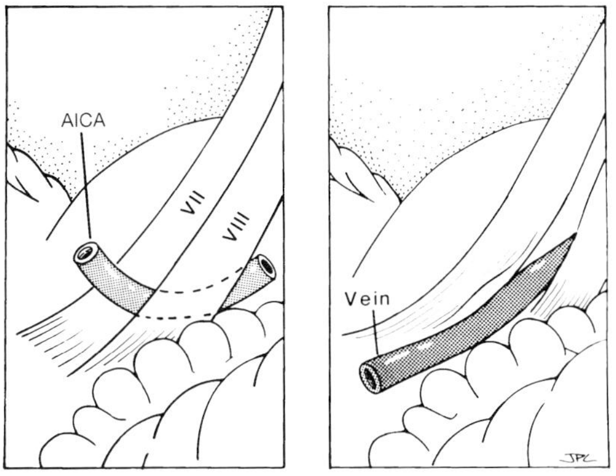

Figure 8: The two most commonly observed vascular relationships in atypical hemifacial spasm. The vascular compression is at the rostral-posterior aspect of the facial nerve root exit zone and is more difficult to treat than typical hemifacial spasm.

is removed. The cerebellar surface is inspected and then the dura is closed in a watertight fashion using running, nonabsorbable 4-0 sutures. Mastoid air cells are thoroughly waxed a second time, and a small piece of absorbable cellulose is placed over the durotomy. A cranioplasty is performed. Muscle and fascial layers are approximated and the skin is closed. A dry dressing is applied.

Postoperative care is similar to other intracranial procedures. Special attention is focused on minimizing nausea and emesis. Blood pressure is monitored carefully, and hypertension is aggressively treated. The patient is observed overnight in the intensive care unit. Diet is advanced as tolerated, and analgesics are administered *ad libidum*. Patients are mobilized on postoperative Day 1 and are usually ready for discharge at 72 hours.

Surgical Pearls

Operative angle and exposure are critical in minimizing complications. Every millimeter more caudal and lateral that a surgeon can achieve decreases cerebellar retraction. Proper head positioning maximizes the surgeon's view of the seventh and eighth cranial nerve complex. By tilting the vertex of the head 10° toward the floor, the seventh and eighth nerve complex is rotated to expose vascular pathology at the caudal portion of the seventh cranial nerve. The incision line should be drawn prior to draping such that external landmarks can aid the surgeon in properly placing the incision. An incision placed improperly by as little as 0.5 cm can decrease the exposure and require further cerebellar retraction. The dural opening should maximize the entire craniectomy.

TABLE 2

OUTCOMES

1 Month	
Excellent	86%
Partial relief	5%
Failure	9%
10 Years	
Excellent	84%
Partial relief	7%
Failure	9%

Results

Short- and Long-Term Outcome

In the authors' most recent communication, 86% of the patients had an excellent result (defined as ≥98% absence of the spasm) and 5% had partial relief (defined as spasms diminished by ≥75%) at 1 month follow-up. At 1 month, 9% of patients did not have significant relief of their spasm. This high early success rate continued at long-term follow-up: 84% of the patients at 10 years had an excellent result (Table 2). The majority of the failures occurred within 2 years of the first operation and were not affected by patient age, duration of symptoms, side, or history of Bell's palsy. There were 12 patients who had no improvement of their spasm within the first postoperative week. Eleven of these patients underwent early repeat microvascular decompression, and 10 of them ultimately obtained long-term excellent results.[2] For this reason, if no improvement is seen within the first week after surgery, re-exploration is recommended. If, however, the slightest improvement is detected after

TABLE 3

COMPLICATIONS IN 782 OPERATIONS IN A TOTAL OF 703 PATIENTS

Complication	Percentage of Cases
Transient facial weakness	3.2%
Complete ipsilateral hearing loss	2.7%
CSF leak	2.4%
Mild permanent facial weakness	1.8%
Severe permanent facial weakness	1.5%
Wound infection	1.2%
Pseudomeningocele	0.5%
Bacterial meningitis	0.5%
Cerebellar hematoma	0.5%
Brain stem infarct	0.3%
Operative death	0.1%
Other (meningitis, pseudomeningocele)	<1.0%

surgery, a close course of follow-up is recommended, as the majority of these patients will experience continued improvement. High success rates with microvascular decompression have been confirmed in other series as well.[1,7,9,10,15-22,24,28,29,34]

Complications

In the authors' most recent analysis,[2] approximately 3% of the patients developed a transient delayed facial weakness, which improved completely, while 1.5% of the patients experienced some form of severe facial weakness. Ipsilateral deafness occurred in 2.7% of the authors' entire series, with a very low incidence in recent years. The figure is somewhat higher than the complication rate with microvascular decompression for trigeminal neuralgia, and is thought to be related to the anatomical relationship between the seventh and eighth cranial nerves. There was a 2.4% incidence of CSF leak treated by closed drainage, and a 1.2% incidence of wound infection. One patient (a repeat operation) in the series of 782 operations died postoperatively. Cerebellar hematoma, brain stem infarct, and pseudomeningocele were rare complications (Table 3).

Complication Avoidance

The incidence of hearing loss is minimized by careful attention to surgical technique in conjunction with the use of brain stem auditory evoked potentials. The neurophysiologist and neurosurgeon must work closely together during the critical part of decompression, and any prolonged delay or decrease in amplitude must be considered a threat to the cochlear nerve.[26,27] There appears to be a variable sensitivity among patients to cerebellar retraction and vascular manipulation. Some patients are extremely sensitive, and even the smallest cerebellar retraction causes significant changes in brain stem evoked response. Occasionally, the surgeon must intermittently remove the retractor to allow the brain stem auditory evoked potentials to recover prior to proceeding with decompression.

Facial weakness can be minimized by carefully forming a proper implant. The authors prefer the use of shredded Teflon felt to Ivalon sponge implants, because the sponge implant is hard and irregular. CSF leak can be minimized by meticulously waxing the mastoid air cells. In addition, a small piece of cellulose foam placed over the waxed cells can prevent melting of the bone wax secondary to heat from the methylmethacrylate cranioplasty. A watertight closure of the wound is essential to prevent any CSF leakage from the wound. The incidence of cerebellar hematoma can be minimized by utilizing low and lateral exposure on both the craniectomy and the dural opening. The authors have recently used a wire mesh cranioplasty.

CONCLUSIONS

Microvascular decompression for hemifacial spasm is safe and highly effective.[1,7,9,10,15-22,24,28,29,34] Long-term results demonstrate an excellent outcome in 84% of patients in the authors' series after 10 years. With rare exceptions, microvascular decompression should be considered the treatment of choice in patients with hemifacial spasm.

References

1. Auger RG, Piepgras DG, Laws ER Jr: Hemifacial spasm: results of microvascular decompression of the facial nerve in 54 patients. **Mayo Clin Proc 61:** 640-644, 1986
2. Barker FG II, Jannetta PJ, Bissonette DJ, et al: Microvascular decompression for hemifacial spasm. **J Neurosurg 82:**201-210, 1995
3. Benos J: Zur medikamentösen. Therapie des Hemifacialspasmus. **Nervenarzt 43:**650-652, 1972
4. Blair RL, Berry H: Spontaneous facial movement. **J Otolaryngol 10:**459-462, 1981
5. Campbell E, Keedy C: Hemifacial spasm: a note on the etiology in two cases. **J Neurosurg 4:**342-347, 1947
6. Cherington M, Sadler KM, Ryan DW: Facial myokymia. **Surg Neurol 11:**478-480, 1979
7. Dutton JJ, Buckley EG: Long-term results and complications of botulinum A toxin in the treatment of blepharospasm. **Ophthalmology 95:**1529-1534, 1988
8. Ehni G, Woltman HW: Hemifacial spasm. Review of one hundred and six cases. **Arch Neurol Neurosurg Psychiatry 53:**205-211, 1945
9. Fukushima T: Microvascular decompression for hemifacial spasm: results in 2890 cases, in Carter LP, Spetzler RF, Hamilton MG (eds): **Neurovascular Surgery.** New York, NY: McGraw Hill, 1995, pp 1133-1146
10. Fukushima T: [Posterior cranial fossa neurovascular decompression (Jannetta method) for trigeminal neuralgia and hemifacial spasm.] **No Shinkei Geka 10:**1257-1261, 1982 (Jpn)
11. Gardner WJ: Concerning the mechanism of trigeminal neuralgia and hemifacial spasm. **J Neurosurg 19:** 947-957, 1962
12. Gardner WJ: Five-year cure of hemifacial spasm. Report of a case. **Cleveland Clin Q 27:**219-221, 1960
13. Gardner WJ, Sava GA: Hemifacial spasm—a reversible pathophysiologic state. **J Neurosurg 19:** 240-247, 1962
14. Grandas F, Elston J, Quinn N, et al: Blepharospasm: a review of 264 patients. **J Neurol Neurosurg Psychiatry 51:**767-772, 1988
15. Huang CI, Chen IH, Lee LS: Microvascular decompression for hemifacial spasm: analyses of operative findings and results in 310 patients. **Neurosurgery 30:**53-57, 1992
16. Iwakuma T, Matsumoto A, Nakamura N: Hemifacial spasm: comparison of three different operative procedures in 110 patients. **J Neurosurg 57:**753-756, 1982
17. Jannetta PJ: Microsurgical exploration and decompression of the facial nerve in hemifacial spasm. **Curr Top Surg Res 2:**217-220, 1970
18. Jannetta PJ: Microvascular decompression of the facial nerve for hemifacial spasm, in Wilson CB (ed): **Neurosurgical Procedures: Personal Approaches to Classic Operations.** Baltimore, Md: Williams & Wilkins, 1992, pp 154-162
19. Jannetta PJ: Neurovascular compression in cranial nerve and systemic disease. **Ann Surg 192:**518-525, 1980
20. Jannetta PJ: Neurovascular compression of the facial nerve in hemifacial spasm: relief by microsurgical technique, in Merei FT (ed): **Reconstructive Surgery of Brain Arteries.** Budapest: Publishing House of the Hungarian Academy of Sciences, 1974, pp 193-199
21. Jannetta PJ, Abbasy M, Maroon JC, et al: Etiology and definitive microsurgical treatment of hemifacial spasm. Operative techniques and results in 47 patients. **J Neurosurg 47:**321-328, 1977
22. Kondo A, Ishikawa J, Yamasahi T, et al: [Microvascular decompression of cranial nerves, particularly of the 7th cranial nerve.] **Neurol Med Chir 20:**739-751, 1980 (Jpn)
23. Kraft SP, Lang AE: Cranial dystonia, blepharospasm and hemifacial spasm: clinical features and treatment, including the use of botulinum toxin. **Can Med Assoc J 139:**837-844, 1988
24. Loeser JD, Chen J: Hemifacial spasm: treatment by microsurgical facial nerve decompression. **Neurosurgery 13:**141-146, 1983
25. Mauriello JA, Aljian J: Natural history of treatment of facial dyskinesias with botulinum toxin: a study of 50 consecutive patients over seven years. **Br J Ophthalmol 75:**737-739, 1991
26. Møller AR: Cranial nerve dysfunction syndromes: pathophysiology of microvascular compression, in Barrow DL (ed): **Surgery of the Cranial Nerves of the Posterior Fossa.** Park Ridge, Ill: American Association of Neurological Surgeons, 1993, pp 105-129
27. Møller AR: Intraoperative neurophysiologic monitoring of cranial nerves, in Barrow DL (ed): **Surgery of the Cranial Nerves of the Posterior Fossa.** Park Ridge, Ill: American Association of Neurological Surgeons, 1993, pp 175-199
28. Piatt JH Jr, Wilkins RH: Treatment of tic douloureux and hemifacial spasm by posterior fossa exploration: therapeutic implications of various neurovascular relationships. **Neurosurgery 14:**462-471, 1984
29. Rhoton AL Jr: Microsurgical neurovascular decompression for trigeminal neuralgia and hemifacial spasm. **J Fla Med Assoc 65:**425-428, 1978
30. Sandyk R, Gillman MA: Baclofen in hemifacial spasm. **Int J Neurosci 33:**261-264, 1987
31. Schultze F: Linksseitiger facialiskrampf in folge eines aneurysma der arteria vertebralis sinistra. **Virchows Arch Pathol Anat 65:**385-391, 1875
32. Scoville WB: Hearing loss following exploration of cerebellopontine angle in treatment of hemifacial spasm. **J Neurosurg 31:**47-49, 1969
33. Tolosa E, Martí MJ: Blepharospasm-oromandibular dystonia syndrome (Meige's syndrome): clinical aspects. **Adv Neurol 49:**73-84, 1988
34. Wilkins RH: Facial nerve decompression for hemifacial spasm, in Apuzzo MLJ (ed): **Brain Surgery: Complication Avoidance and Management.** New York, NY: Churchill Livingstone, 1993, Vol 2, pp 2115-2143
35. Wilkins RH: Hemifacial spasm: a review. **Surg Neurol 36:**251-277, 1991
36. Wilkins RH: Hemifacial spasm and other facial nerve dysfunction syndromes, in Barrow DL (ed): **Surgery of the Cranial Nerves of the Posterior Fossa.** Park Ridge, Ill: American Association of Neurological Surgeons, 1993, pp 221-232

CHAPTER 18

Surgical Treatment of Spasmodic Torticollis: Selective Peripheral Denervation Revisited

Claude M. Bertrand, CC, MD, FRCS(C), and Reina Benabou, MD, PhD

The main purpose of this chapter is to review and analyze the data obtained during the past 20 years, since selective denervation was first introduced as a complement to thalamotomy. Since 1978, selective peripheral denervation has become the only surgical procedure used for the treatment of spasmodic torticollis at the author's (CMB) institution. It is also currently performed in other centers in the United States (Department of Neurosurgery, University of Florida, Jacksonville, Florida, and Mayo Clinic, Rochester, Minnesota) and Europe (Department of Neurosurgery, Universität Ulm, Germany). The use of electromyography (EMG), stimulation, nerve blocks, and especially direct observation of the results of intraoperative stimulation have considerably increased our knowledge of the distribution and functions of the various branches of the cervical nerves.

It is generally accepted that spasmodic torticollis is an adult-onset focal dystonia involving the cervical region, which usually appears within the third to fifth decade of life and is characterized by involuntary abnormal movements and/or postures of the head and neck. Usually it is a limited dystonic manifestation;[46] however, in rare cases, it may be the first focal symptomatology of an evolving generalized dystonia.[13,60]

Until the early 20th century, spasmodic torticollis was commonly considered and treated as a psychogenic disease.[20,28] This concept has changed throughout the years, in view of frequent personal or familial history of essential tremor in these patients.[24] Familial spasmodic torticollis has also been reported.[33] More recently, the role of heredity has been well established, with the important discovery by Ozelius et al[50] of a human gene for torsion dystonia. However, psychological factors, such as anxiety and reactive depression, may play a modulatory role in the intensity of the symptoms. An emotional shock may even act as a precipitating factor for some patients. The surgeon should take into account the fact that there might be conversion symptoms resembling spasmodic torticollis, mainly in cases in which a secondary reward is involved. The distinction between psychogenic and organic spasmodic torticollis should be made through careful clinical examination of the abnormal movements, and the dystonic muscle pattern should be reproducible and visualized during EMG. If there is persisting doubt, the physician may request a psychological evaluation.

Pathophysiology

In general, dyskinesias are probably a manifestation of basal ganglia dysfunction,[45,53,55,62,64] but the underlying pathological condition that induces a focal, adult-onset dystonia such as spasmodic torticollis is still unknown, except in rare cases of spasmodic torticollis with a definite lesion within the basal structures of the brain.[37,38,54]

Tarlov[61] described pathological findings in humans, such as bilateral cavitation of the putamen and substantia innominata in a patient with retrocollis. Bilateral loss of ganglion cells in the caudate, putamen, and globus pallidus was found in a patient with spasmodic torticollis and choreoathetosis.

Poirier et al[56] summarized reports of unilateral stereotatic lesions of the periaqueductal gray matter and immediately adjacent structures in monkeys that caused marked and sustained torticollis. They added that bilateral thalamic lesions involving the ventral lateral and intralaminar thalamic nuclei almost completely abolish dystonic postures, and suggested that the striatopallidal system, which is connected to the latter thalamic structures, may contribute to the appearance of dystonic movements and postures.

It is very likely that vestibular dysfunction also plays an important role in the pathophysiology of spasmodic torticollis: vestibular lesions have been described as the cause of permanent postural derangement of head position since early on. Batten,[4] in 1903, described two patients with unilateral cerebellar lesions and contralateral head rotation and flexion, but concluded that lesions of the cerebellum can only produce the rotated posture through their compressive effects on neighboring structures (eighth cranial nerve or brain stem), because ablation of one cerebellar hemisphere did not produce the same effects on head posture. Cushing[25] observed the posture in patients with an acoustic nerve tumor and remarked that on the side of the tumor, "the mastoid is usually drawn towards the shoulder." Magnus[43] performed labyrinth extirpations in monkeys and described head rotation to the affected side, so that the occiput was rotated and flexed to the side from which the labyrinth was removed. Brain[18] published a series of five patients with different tumors of the pons and midbrain and contralateral rotation of the head. Based on both his own findings and those of previous authors, Brain concluded that "the rotated posture of the head was the result of interference with a tonic reflex in which the extensor muscles of the neck, under the influence of impulses from the labyrinths, are maintained in a state of tonus adequate to resist the effect of gravity on the head." To support this idea, Brain also described another of his patients with bilateral eighth nerve tumors in whom posture of the head was normal. This concept was also taken into consideration by Svien and Cody,[59] who in 1969 performed iontophoresis to suppress labyrinthine activity (as treatment for spasmodic torticollis), but the long-term results were not satisfactory. Tarlov[59] reproduced different abnormal neck postures in experimental animals with focal brain stem lesions involving the vestibular nuclei, with different postural effects in different primate species. Clinical studies also suggest primary involvement of the vestibular system in spasmodic torticollis.[21,22]

Conservative Management

Without a doubt, botulinum toxin injection therapy is a major step forward in the conservative treatment of spasmodic torticollis.[34,39] It provides marked improvement of the symptoms for about 3-4 months in most cases, but among these cases, there are some patients who become progressively resistant to the treatment due to the production of specific antibodies. In a few cases, there is no response at all. In some other patients, it may become difficult to pursue the treatment indefinitely.

Initial medical treatment still includes anticholinergic drugs such as trihexyphenidyl and biperiden, and tranquilizers, such as diazepam and clonazepam.[29,42,47] These can offer some relief, particularly in high doses, although this may cause undesirable side effects. Recently, Marino et al[44] and Benabou et al[5] reported a study on flunitrazepam, a benzodiazepine derivative, which had a specific therapeutic effect in a group of dystonic patients, including patients with spasmodic torticollis. It provided moderate to very good improvement of the dystonic symptomatology and of quality of life.

Long-term therapies, such as physiotherapy and biofeedback, may offer some relief in mild cases of spasmodic torticollis.[41]

Other Surgical Techniques

Of all of the surgical techniques developed for the treatment of spasmodic torticollis, only selective peripheral denervation and two others seem to still be used: bilateral cervical rhizotomy and microvascular lysis of the accessory nerve.

Bilateral Cervical Rhizotomy

Cervical rhizotomy was first designed by Cushing and McKenzie as a unilateral approach to denervate the posterior cervical group of muscles.[48,57] This was done by sectioning the anterior roots of C1, C2, C3, and part of C4. It became a bilateral procedure, mostly under the influence of Dandy,[26] in the hope that a more radical procedure would improve results; however, the fact that the antagonists to the abnormal movements were being denervated was ignored. It was the procedure most frequently used for the relief of spasmodic torticollis until the 1970s, in spite of side effects such as weakness of the neck and frequent swallowing problems.[2,32,35,52] In fact, the concept of bilaterality became so ingrained in the neurological community that, in the early stages of selective denervation, it was constantly brought up as an objection. One can hardly defend its use now that it has been firmly established that the anterior divisions of C1 and C2 innervate the muscles in the throat responsible for swallowing and that they have nothing to do with the posterior cervical musculature. In addition, denervation of the posterior primary divisions of C4 and C5 is essential to obtain proper denervation of the posterior cervical group, and preservation of the antagonists is very important for recuperation of normal movements after surgery.

Microvascular Lysis of the Spinal Accessory Nerve Roots

The only other procedure that is still mentioned in the literature is microvascular lysis of the accessory nerve roots, a restricted approach that nevertheless requires a laminectomy. It was probably inspired by decompression of the facial nerve for facial tics.[1]

After their initial report[31] in 1981, Freckmann and associates[30] in 1986 stated that "the notion that neurovascular contacts of the spinal accessory nerve can be of relevance, as in other cranial nerve dysfunction syndromes, like hemifacial spasms, cannot be considered valid in our experience." In the six patients who required selective peripheral denervation after spinal accessory nerve decompression, all muscle groups, including the sternocleidomastoid, remained very active.

The fact remains that there are a few reports of relief of spasmodic torticollis following spinal accessory nerve decompression.[51,58] The report by Jho and Jannetta[40] is the more recent. They described 20 patients who underwent microvascular decompression for spasmodic torticollis. After a 5-year follow-up, 13 patients (65%) were cured, 4 (20%) were improved, 1 (5%) still had moderate spasms, and 2 (10%) were unchanged.

The results of this procedure are usually delayed for many months before they become apparent.

Selective Peripheral Denervation

It was in the hope of avoiding the sequelae of bilateral rhizotomy that, following the lead of Cooper[23] in 1964, then Hassler and Dieckmann[36] in 1970, the author (CMB) started using thalamotomy for rotatory torticollis.[14,17] Although the results were excellent, in some cases they were very inconsistent, which is why it was decided to combine thalamotomy with selective periph-

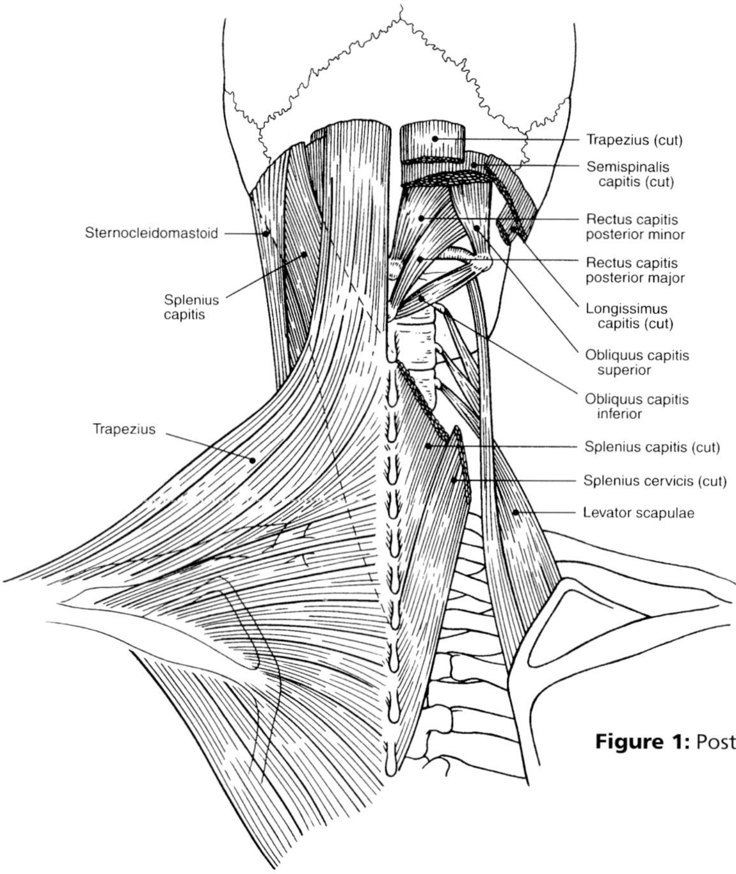

Figure 1: Posterior view of the cervical muscles.

eral denervation following EMG and nerve blocks.[8,10,12] It became evident that peripheral denervation could suppress abnormal movements. As a result of this, selective denervation has been the only procedure used for spasmodic torticollis at the author's (CMB) institution since 1978. However, unilateral thalamotomy is still indicated for generalized dystonia unresponsive to medication. Even then, if there is a strong cervical component, selective denervation should be done first and may suffice to improve the patient's posture.

The success of selective peripheral denervation is due to the fact that only the muscles involved in the abnormal movement of the head are denervated. Therefore, it is essential to make the right choice of muscles. For that, one has to determine which form of abnormal movement one is dealing with and then relate it to the specific muscles.

A videotape of the patient at rest and while performing voluntary movements with the head is required. This allows repeated analysis of the abnormal movements. It is also a basis for analysis of the results after surgery. When the patient lives far from the medical center, a control video is requested 3 months postoperatively.

There are essentially three pure forms of spasmodic torticollis: rotatory torticollis, laterocollis, and retrocollis. Figure 1 and Table 1 provide a review of all of the muscles that may be involved in each particular form of spasmodic torticollis and their specific innervation. Muscles such as the sternocleidomastoid, splenius capitis, and levator scapulae can be palpated, and sometimes one can even see them because they may become quite hypertrophic. Muscles are classified as agonists or synergists, depending on the importance of their contribution and the frequency of their involvement in a particular form of spasmodic torticollis. The agonists are almost always involved. The synergists, on the other hand, may or may not be involved, depending on the pattern and severity of each case; nevertheless, they

TABLE 1

MUSCLES FREQUENTLY INVOLVED IN DIFFERENT TYPES OF SPASMODIC TORTICOLLIS AND THEIR INNERVATION*

Rotatory Spasmodic Torticollis		
CL	*Sternocleidomastoid* (A)	Cranial nerve XI and VR of C2 and C3
IL	*Splenius capitis* (A)	PR of C2-6
IL	*Splenius cervicis* (A)	PR of C4-8
IL	*Rectus capitis posterior major* (S)	PR of C1
IL	*Obliquus capitis inferior* (S)	PR of C1-2
CL	*Obliquus capitis superior* (S)+	PR of C1
CL	*Semispinalis capitis* (S)	PR of C1-6
CL	*Semispinalis cervicis* (S)	PR of C4-8
IL	*Longissimus capitis* (S)	PR of C3-8
Laterocollis		
IL	*Splenius capitis* (A)	PR of C2-6
IL	*Levator scapulae* (A)‡	VR of C3-4
IL	*Obliquus capitis superior* (S)§	PR of C1
IL	*Trapezius* (S)‡	Cranial nerve XI and VR of C3-4
IL	*Sternocleidomastoid* (S)	Cranial nerve XI and VR of C2-3
Retrocollis		
BL	*Splenius capitis* (A)	PR of C2-6
BL	*Splenius cervicis* (S)	PR of C4-8
BL	*Semispinalis capitis* (A)	PR of C1-6
BL	*Semispinalis cervicis* (S)	PR of C4-8
BL	*Longissimus capitis* (A)	PR of C3-8
BL	*Rectus capitis posterior major and minor* (A)	PR of C1
BL	*Obliquus capitis inferior* (S)	PR of C1-2
BL	*Obliquus capitis superior* (S)	PR of C1

* A = main agonist; BL = bilateral; CL = contralateral; IL = ipsilateral; PR = posterior rami; S = synergist; VR = ventral rami.
+ Combined with slight inclination, contralateral to the rotation, and extension.
‡ When the shoulder is fixed.
§ Combined with slight extension and rotation to the opposite side.

should always be investigated as well. There are also combined forms of spasmodic torticollis: rotatory plus laterocollis, rotatory plus retrocollis, retrocollis plus laterocollis, and so on. In these cases, each of the abnormal movements should be defined and related to specific muscles. Each case of spasmodic torticollis corresponds to a particular pattern that should be investigated as a separate entity.

Electromyographic Recording

Once one has an idea of the muscles that could be involved in a particular form of spasmodic torticollis, through the analysis of individual movements or postures and through palpation, the next step is to confirm the choice of muscles using EMG to identify which muscles are hyperactive and which ones are inhibited.

As a standard procedure,[16] four muscles are recorded simultaneously: both sternocleidomastoid and both splenius capitis muscles. Two monopolar needles (electrodes) are placed 5 mm apart in each muscle. To confirm that the electrodes are placed accurately in the proper muscles, the patient is asked to perform head rotation toward each side, as well as extension. The recording is performed with the patient at rest (usually in a sitting position) and while performing voluntary movements of the head, such as rotation, inclination, extension, and flexion. The recording at rest shows which muscles are hyperactive during the involuntary movements, i.e., the ones responsible for the abnormal posture. They may produce varying degrees of strong discharges. During the performance of repetitive voluntary movements, the recording also shows the abnormally inhibited muscles, which should not be denervated because they will be important for the recovery of normal movements postoperatively. It may be necessary to repeat the recording because of variation in the discharge of some muscles.

If necessary, the examination may be complemented by recording some other muscles, such as the levator scapulae, the oblique, or the rectus muscles. In the case of more deeply located muscles, a longer bipolar concentric electrode is very helpful.

Blocks

Even in typical cases, a temporary block with 1% lidocaine without epinephrine is useful to outline the relative action of individual muscles.[8,12] The sternocleidomastoid and the levator scapulae are the muscles most frequently blocked. This can also give an idea of possible functional deficits after denervation of muscles, such as the trapezius or the oblique muscles.

Blocks can be performed under EMG control, and the injection is done at the point where the electric stimulation produces maximum contraction of the muscle to be blocked. Frequent aspirations should be done to ensure that the needle is not in a blood vessel. An injection of 5-10 ml is sufficient for one muscle. Even if the blocks are incomplete, they help predict what can be expected after surgical denervation of a particular muscle. In more complex cases, many blocks are performed at different times; each block lasts around 30 minutes. If the first block is satisfactory by itself, denervation may be limited to that muscle, with the understanding that a more extensive procedure may be required later on.

In cases of lateroretrocollis, it is necessary to discover whether the contralateral posterior cervical group of muscles is involved. This may require a greater amount of lidocaine (10-15 ml). Care should be taken not to inject into the cervical posterior venous plexus.

Temporary blocks have recently been found helpful in clarifying the role of some muscles in cases of lateroretrocollis. When denervation of the posterior cervical muscles was not enough to improve the abnormal lateral inclination of the head, a selective block of the ipsilateral levator scapulae provided good improvement of the residual lateral tilting, without deficits such as weakness of the shoulder. Block of the trapezius muscle, on the other hand, usually led to marked impairment of movements of the shoulder. This finding, together with EMG recordings that showed significant hyperactivity of the levator scapulae, established that this muscle is one of the main agonists for laterocollis. Its denervation can be contemplated without the risk of a postoperative sagging shoulder. In some cases in which the head is simultaneously tilted and pulled slightly forward, EMG demonstrates synergistic activity from the ipsilateral sternocleidomastoid (cleidal portion). A selective temporary block of this muscle provides relief of this abnormal posture. The blocks are not used when there is any previous history of allergy to local anesthetics.

Selection Criteria

Selective peripheral denervation has been a successful surgical treatment for spasmodic torticollis since 1978. Over 400 patients have undergone selective denervation for spasmodic torticollis through these years at the author's (CMB) institution. They were evaluated with standard pre- and postoperative clinical and electrophysiological protocols. From these data, the following premises have been established as the best indications for this surgical treatment:[6,16]

1. Previous conservative medical treatments, mainly BOTOX (botulinum toxin) injections, no longer provide satisfactory relief, they cause significant side effects, or they are becoming too difficult to pursue indefinitely.
2. The clinical picture should be stable for at least 1 year, preferably evolving for 3 years. Before this period of stabilization, spasmodic torticollis may still change its pattern, i.e., other muscles may become active because the final pattern is still evolving.

3. The dystonic symptomatology must be restricted to or at least prevalent in the cervical region.
4. Dystonic features elsewhere may indicate that we are dealing with a more generalized dystonia. In these cases, after surgery, a temporary flare-up of such other features as blepharospasm, oromandibular dyskinesia, or tremor may be observed. Rarely, a flare-up of generalized dystonia may occur. The authors have experienced two such cases: one with temporary and the other with permanent exacerbation of more generalized dystonic symptoms.
5. Pure rotatory torticollis and its combination with mild inclination and/or extension are the forms of spasmodic torticollis that show the best results.
6. Previous surgical procedures, pre-existing fibrosis, or severe arthrosis have been shown to impair the postoperative results.

Functional Distribution of Cervical Nerves Based on Recent Data From Intraoperative Stimulation

Unipolar stimulation is used as the surgeon progressively exposes the posterior rami of the upper cervical nerves. Near-threshold stimulation is performed on nerve branches that have been previously isolated with the help of a hook to avoid current diffusion. This procedure provides important knowledge about the anatomical distribution of the main posterior nerve divisions and their fine branches at each cervical level (see Figure 3), as well as essential data on their specific muscular innervation, as follows.

C1: At this level, the posterior ramus of C1 is found near the vertebral artery. Its peripheral threshold stimulation (0.5 V) elicits selective strong contraction of the ipsilateral suboccipital triangle (rectus and oblique) muscles. As the dissection progresses in a medial direction, over the notch of the posterior arch of the atlas, there is an anterior nerve division. It is located below and beneath the vertebral artery and its threshold stimulation (0.5 V) produces strong contraction of the ipsilateral anterior throat muscles only: the omohyoid, sternohyoid, and sternothyroid muscles. This anterior branch should be spared, because it innervates throat muscles that are important in the process of deglutition, thus avoiding postoperative dysphagia, particularly when a bilateral ramisectomy is performed. The section should be done peripherally, where stimulation of C1 elicits contraction of the posterior muscles only.

C2: This posterior branch is twice as thick as that of C1. Its peripheral threshold stimulation (1.0 V) provokes strong contraction of the ipsilateral obliquus capitis inferior, splenius capitis, and semispinalis capitis muscles. There is also an anterior branch at this level, which, with the same threshold stimulation, will produce strong contraction of the same ipsilateral anterior throat muscles mentioned above. It should also be spared. Data from cadaver dissections performed recently by the authors confirm that these anterior divisions of C1 and C2 branches join the hypoglossal nerve and form what is called the ansa cervicalis (ansa hypoglossi), which is essential for innervation of the anterior throat muscles.[63] Also at this level, denervation must be restricted to the posterior division.

C3: This is the level where more posterior branches are found: one main branch and usually one or two fine branches. The threshold stimulation of the main branch is lower (1.0-1.5 V) due to the fact that it is more superficial than the fine branches, which may suffer from neurapraxia as the dissection continues. Stimulation of these branches elicits selective contraction of the ipsilateral splenius capitis and semispinalis capitis muscles. During cadaver dissections, it was found that at the level of C3, there is the greatest ramification of the posterior division. During surgery, it is usually possible to identify an average of three branches, four in rare cases, possibly because they are within the paravertebral muscles. It seems that the remaining branches are responsible for the recuperation of normal movements postoperatively or for residual abnormal movements when that is the case.

When denervation of the ipsilateral levator scapulae is attempted, in the case of laterocollis, dissection is carried out anteriorly at this level. After visualizing the fascicles of the levator scapulae and cutting them, one may observe one or two branches at this level that run in the same oblique direction as the fascicle previously sectioned. Threshold stimulation of these branches produces contraction of both the levator scapulae and the trapezius muscles. Usually, at least one branch elicits stronger or exclusive contraction of the levator scapulae, and sometimes both branches do; this branch or both branches should be sectioned. If one of these branches promotes strong contraction of the trapezius muscle, it is spared, even knowing that the trapezius muscle will also receive important supplementary innervation from the ipsilateral ventral ramus of C4 and from branches of the spinal accessory nerve.

C4: There are usually one or two thinner posterior branches that, with higher threshold stimulation (around 3.0 V), produce weak contraction of the splenius capitis and semispinalis capitis muscles and stronger contraction of the splenius cervicis and semispinalis cervicis muscles. In cases of denervation of the levator scapulae, when dissecting more anteriorly at this level, one or two oblique branches may be found. The same principle described above applies here to preserve the trapezius muscle. Often, electrical stimulation of this ventral ramus elicits contraction of the diaphragm. This is observed as small depressions in the CO_2 monitoring curve simultaneous with the electrical stimulation. In this situation, the branch must be spared.

C5: At this level, there is a posterior branch that at high threshold stimulation (4.0 V) produces weak contraction of the splenius cervicis and semispinalis cervicis muscles. However, in the early cases of retrocollis treated in this manner, one of the two posterior roots of C5 was spared for fear of impairing extension of the neck. The results were incomplete, demonstrating the importance of C5 in the innervation of the posterior cervical group. The results are very good when both posterior cervical branches are sectioned, and the stability of the neck is not compromised. The fact that even a much higher threshold stimulation elicits weak muscular contraction may be due to neurapraxia caused by longer contact with the retractor during surgery.

C6: At this level, there is a tiny posterior branch that even with high threshold stimulation (4.0-5.0 V) provokes an extremely weak contraction of the splenius cervicis and semispinalis cervicis muscles. Due to its size and response to stimulation, this posterior branch does not seem to be as important as the former ones for the innervation of the cervical muscles.

Surgical Technique

The aim of selective denervation remains that of abolishing abnormal movements while preserving normal or near-normal movements of the neck. This requires denervation of all of the nerve branches that innervate the muscles responsible for the abnormal movements, as evidenced from intraoperative stimulation. Any involved residual branch will maintain part or all of the abnormal movements. On the other hand, excessive sectioning, which may result in limitation of movements of the neck, must be avoided. Accurate knowledge of the distribution of the branches of C1 and C2 will no doubt contribute to simplifying the exposure, because it has been established that the anterior divisions of C1 and C2 innervate exclusively the anterior muscles of the throat (omohyoid, sternohyoid, and sternothyroid), without any contribution to the innervation of the posterior cervical musculature. That is why these anterior divisions must not be sectioned; on the contrary, they should be carefully spared. Only the posterior divisions of C1 and C2 need to be exposed and sectioned peripherally.

In the first few years of the author's (CMB) use of this procedure, the intervention was carried out through a posterolateral incision starting inside the mastoid and coasting along the articular facets. This was replaced by an inverted L-shaped incision (Figure 2). The vertical portion of the incision extends from the occipital protuberance to the spinal process of C7, along the linea alba; the horizontal branch starts at the external occipital protuberance, continuing laterally for 5 cm on the side chosen to be denervated. The posterior primary divisions are found in the plane of cleavage between the undersurface of the semispinalis and the paravertebral muscles. Because only the posterior divisions of C1 and C2 need to be exposed and the posterior divisions of C3, C4, and C5 can be readily identified as they exit from the intervertebral foramen, it may be that a more conservative lateral approach will suffice.

The operation is performed with the patient

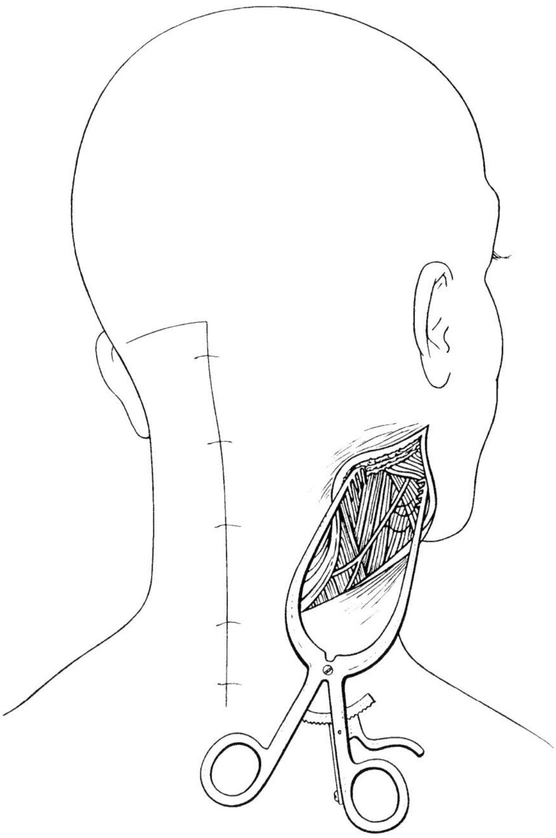

Figure 2: Schematic drawing of the dissection of the spinal accessory nerve to denervate the right sternocleidomastoid muscle. The left side of the retractor is placed on the trapezius muscle and the right side on the sternocleidomastoid muscle. With this exposure, the spinal accessory nerve is seen. When stimulated (0.5 or 1.0 V), the main trunk elicits strong contraction of the trapezius and sternocleidomastoid. At the lower portion of the trapezius, there usually are found one or two main branches that, at the same stimulation level, produce selective contraction of the trapezius; these branches should be spared. As the dissection of the spinal accessory nerve is carried out to the level of the styloid process, there are about three to six branches at different levels that with threshold stimulation (approximately 1 V) will elicit selective contraction of the sternocleidomastoid muscle. These branches should be sectioned. Rarely, one of these branches may be near the styloid process. At the end of the dissection, the main trunk remains free from any connection to the sternocleidomastoid and giving off only the spared one or two branches to the trapezius. Stimulation of the main trunk should now provoke only contraction of the trapezius muscle. After this denervation, the sternocleidomastoid muscle is sectioned transversely to prevent its reinnervation by the ventral rami of C2 and C3.

in the sitting position with the head fixed and inclined slightly forward. This avoids excessive bleeding from the large paravertebral venous plexuses, which in the sitting position can be coagulated as they present themselves. Also, because there is no bone dissection, the risk of air emboli is minimal when using careful invasive and noninvasive monitoring. The latter includes electrocardiography, measurement of arterial blood pressure and temperature, pulse oximetry, capnography, measurement of the fraction of inspired oxygen, precordial Doppler monitoring, measurement of urine output, and use of an esophageal stethoscope. Invasive monitoring includes determination of intra-arterial blood pressure, pulmonary artery pressure with a Swan-Ganz catheter, and central venous pressure. Possible air emboli were detected in 3 of 200 patients. The procedure was suspended temporarily in two of them. In one case the patient was brought back to the horizontal position, but the procedure could be resumed afterward. There were no major complications. If the signs of emboli persist, surgery should be interrupted.

Surgery is performed with the patient under light anesthesia. Curare paralysis is reversed during operative electric stimulation.

Unipolar stimulation (2 or 3 V) is used to identify the nerve divisions and their rootlets before denervation. It is also used to confirm that certain branches, such as those to the trapezius muscle, should be spared when denervating the sternocleidomastoid. Near-threshold stimulation is used on isolated branches. The dissection is done carefully to avoid neurapraxia, which may lead the surgeon to believe that the muscle has been completely denervated. At the end of the procedure, strong stimulation is used to ensure that denervation is adequate.

In order to review the technical aspects, the denervation of the right sternocleidomastoid muscle and contralateral left posterior ramisectomy is described as perfomed in a typical case of rotatory spasmodic torticollis.

Denervation of the Sternocleidomastoid Muscle

For denervation of the sternocleidomastoid muscle, the incision starts, as described previously, at the mastoid process and curves backward as it continues downward along the posterior limit of the sternocleidomastoid muscle, to finish near the point of penetration of the spinal accessory nerve into the trapezius at the junction of the vertical and horizontal portions of the trapezius (see Figure 2). Whenever possible, the greater auricular nerve is spared to avoid temporary numbness along the base of the ear. Stimulation is used to identify the spinal accessory nerve and its branches to the sternocleidomastoid and the trapezius muscles. Dissection is carried out to the level of the styloid process. One must be careful about a kink along the course of the main nerve trunk, as it gives off branches that go to the sternocleidomastoid muscle. Because it is exposed along its entire length, any traction or compression of the main trunk must be carefully avoided to prevent paresis of the trapezius. All the isolated branches that, when stimulated (1 V), produce selective contraction of the sternocleidomastoid are sectioned peripheral to the clip previously placed and then avulsed. There are usually three to six branches to the sternocleidomastoid. Rarely, one may find a branch near the styloid process. At the end of this procedure, only the main trunk remains, giving off the spared one or two main branches to the trapezius. After its denervation is finished, the sternocleidomastoid muscle itself is sectioned transversely, but the aponeurosis is sutured to preserve the contour of the neck. Myectomy of the sternocleidomastoid is necessary because, besides innervation from the spinal accessory nerve, this muscle also receives innervation from the ipsilateral ventral rami of C2 and C3. This explains an occasional recurrence of movements, but not enough to require further denervation.

Posterior Ramisectomy

At present, there have been few changes in the approach for posterior ramisectomy (Figure 3). Because only the posterior primary divisions of C1 and C2 need to be exposed, this procedure could be even more conservative. The vertical portion of the incision extends from the external occipital protuberance to the spinous process of C7. The muscles are separated along the linea alba. Extending from the occipital protuberance, a 5-cm horizontal incision is made on the side to be denervated. This provides a better exposure and avoids unnecessary retraction, which may cause neurapraxia and thus inability to stimulate accurately. The occipital aponeurosis and the trapezius, splenius capitis, and semispinalis capitis muscles are sectioned below their insertion on the occipital bone, so that they can be resutured properly to restore normal movements postoperatively. The posterior arch of the atlas and the articular facets of C2, C3, C4, C5, and C6 are exposed along the natural plane of cleavage on the undersurface of the semispinalis capitis. From this point on, magnifying glasses and frontal light are used, because they are adequate and more convenient than the microscope. The posterior division of C1 is identified as it emerges under the vertebral artery in the notch of the posterior arch of the C1 vertebra. It is then isolated carefully from the vertebral artery and dissected peripherally where its stimulation elicits a response only from the ipsilateral rectus and oblique muscles, sparing the above-mentioned anterior branch, which innervates the anterior throat muscles only. After the proximal stump is clipped, the distal portion is sectioned peripheral to the clip and then avulsed.

On the posterior arch of C2, the inferior oblique muscle is usually sectioned transversely, so that the large posterior division of C2 can be readily seen as it emerges between the posterior arch of the axis and the atlas. Again, the proximal stump is clipped and sectioned peripherally at a level where threshold stimulation elicits contraction of the splenius capitis and semispinalis capitis muscles only, once again sparing the anterior branch responsible for innervation of the anterior throat muscles. The distal part of C2 is avulsed along a few centimeters.

The posterior primary divisions of C3, C4, C5, and C6 are identified individually or by stimulation in the plane of cleavage underneath the semispinalis capitis muscle, or they can be found as they emerge between the articular facets. Either way, they must be followed as closely as possible to their point of emergence from the intervertebral foramen. Near-threshold

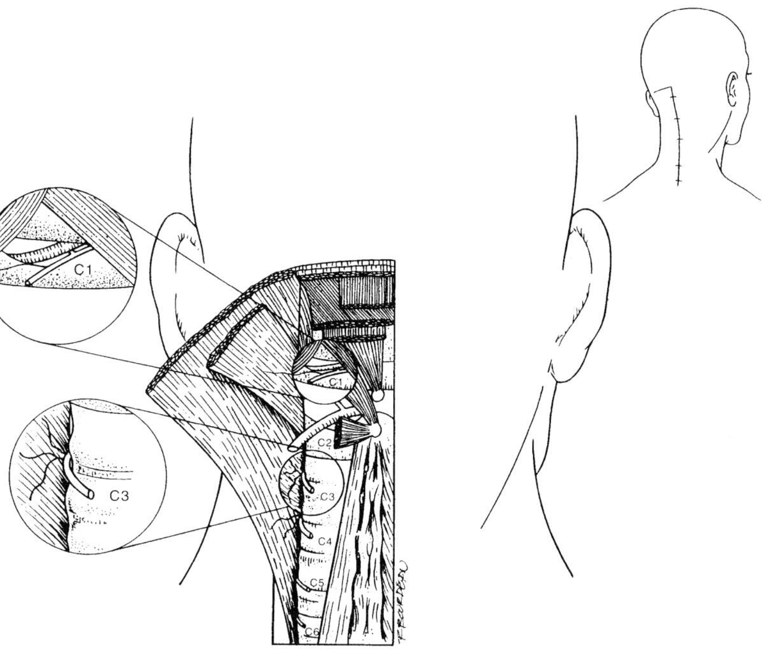

Figure 3: Left) Drawing of the surgical exposure for a left posterior cervical ramisectomy. The emergence of the C1 nerve is underneath the vertebral artery on the left. In the *upper circle,* the drawing shows the nerve root of C1 as it divides into its anterior and posterior branches. The anterior branch should be spared because, together with the anterior division of C2, it innervates only the anterior throat muscles responsible for deglutition. Between the posterior arches of C1 and C2, the nerve root of C2 is visualized as it divides into its anterior and posterior branch. The posterior primary divisions (rami) of C3, C4, C5, and C6 are visualized as they emerge from the intervertebral foramina and come around to innervate the posterior cervical muscles. In the *lower circle,* the nerve root of C3 is shown with its fine collateral branches coming out near the foramen and penetrating into the muscles. **Upper right)** The skin incisions for a typical case of rotatory torticollis to the left: the incision under the right ear for exposure of the right spinal accessory nerve, and the inverted L-shaped incision for the left posterior ramisectomy.

stimulation is very important to reveal the presence of fine early rising branches, particularly at C3 (two or three small branches) and sometimes at C4. Mainly at the level of C3, and also at C4, all these fine branches must be identified and sectioned, with avulsion of the distal portion, because they are important for denervation of the hyperactive medial cervical muscles.

At C5, there is a thinner posterior branch that, with high stimulation, elicits weak contraction of the splenius cervicis and semispinalis cervicis muscles, maybe because of neurapraxia caused by the use of the retractor. This branch should also be sectioned and avulsed distally. In retrocollis, when bilateral posterior divisions from C1 to C5 are sectioned, C6 is not exposed. The importance of the posterior division of C6 is questionable, but in cases of unilateral ramisectomy it has been sectioned as well. Afterward, strong stimulation (5 V) at the foramina levels from C1 to C6 should not elicit any response in the posterior cervical group of muscles.

Although in Table 1 there are listed some muscles also innervated by C7 and C8, such as the splenius cervicis and semispinalis cervicis, in the authors' experience, proper denervation to C6 is enough to provide good postoperative results and avoid residual abnormal movements.

When there is an indication for denervation of the levator scapulae muscle, in cases in which there is a component of lateral tilting of the head or pure laterocollis, dissection is carried out more anteriorly at the level of C3 and C4 until the surgeon visualizes the four fascicles of the levator scapulae, each one attached respectively to the spinous processes of C1, C2, C3 and C4

TABLE 2

RESULTS AFTER SELECTIVE DENERVATION IN PATIENTS SURGICALLY TREATED BETWEEN 1982 AND 1993*

	No. of Cases					
Results	35	91	111	131	260	Last 50
Excellent	34%	31%	31%	37%	41%	54%
Very good	54%	57%	57%	51%	48%	34%
Combined	88%	88%	88%	88%	89%	88%
Fair	9%	10%	10%	10%	10%	10%
Poor	3%	2%	2%	2%	1%	2%

* Excellent = no detectable abnormal movement; very good = slight deviation or slight residual abnormal movements, not bothersome for the patient; combined = sum of the above excellent and very good percentages; fair = appreciable amount of residual abnormal movements; poor = no improvement or worse.

(see Figure 1). After sectioning the fascicles at the C3 and C4 levels, it is possible to see and isolate ventral branches, usually one or two at each level, which, when stimulated, elicit contraction of either the trapezius or the levator scapulae muscle or both. The branches that produce selective or stronger contraction of the levator scapulae should be sectioned. The ones that innervate exclusively or mostly the trapezius should be spared. Care must be taken at the level of C4, where stimulation of an anterior branch can cause contraction of the diaphragm. In this case it should be spared. After its proper denervation, myectomy of the levator scapulae is performed, sectioning, if possible, its four fascicles. Sometimes the first one, attached to C1, is difficult to reach.

At the end of the ramisectomy, the head is brought back to facilitate closure. After careful hemostasis, all of the large muscles and the aponeurosis are sutured before skin closure. As much as possible, the integrity of the muscles should be preserved. The authors have seen a few patients with continuing postoperative stiffness and limitation of neck movements, probably due to excessive sectioning of some neck muscles.

After surgery, the patient should be kept in a semi-sitting position. Patients are given dexamethasone postoperatively, in tapered doses during the following 3 days. This helps to prevent excessive swelling and stiffness of the neck, mainly in cases of bilateral ramisectomy. Opiates may be given for pain for a period of 24-48 hours. The patient is usually up on the first or second day after operation. Specific active physiotherapy starts on the third postoperative day. Patients are discharged 4-5 days after surgery, but physiotherapy should be pursued at least three times a week for the next 6-12 weeks in order to retrain the antagonists, which may be inhibited, and to restore normal or near normal movements of the neck.

RESULTS

On reviewing the analysis of the results in the author's (CMB) last five publications[7,9,11,13,15] between 1982 and 1993, concerning 35, 91, 111, 131, and 260 patients who underwent selective denervation, there is a consistent figure. The results were considered excellent (no residual abnormal movements) or very good (very slight residual movements, not bothersome for the patient) in 88% of the cases (Table 2). The main change over time has been the percentage of patients without any residual movements: it has increased from 34% to 54%. This is probably due to better knowledge of the extent of nerve ramification, mainly at C3 and possibly at C4, so that the search for and dissection of deeper remaining branches at these levels is carried out more rigorously nowadays. Including the authors' patients and patients reported by Arce and Russo,[3] Davis et al,[27] and Braun and Richter,[19] more than 800 patients have undergone selective peripheral denervation with satisfactory results.

Within 2-4 days after surgery, one may have a fair idea of the end result. At that time, the patient is up and moves the head voluntarily, even if the movements are still limited by swelling and pain. Other dystonic features already existent before surgery, such as head tremor or orofacial dyskinesias, could become temporarily more severe during the first week or 10 days after surgery.

Pure rotatory torticollis and its combination with mild inclination and/or extension are the types of spasmodic torticollis that show the best results postoperatively. Sometimes there is residual abnormal head tilting, which now is successfully relieved with the denervation and myectomy of the levator scapulae muscle. A preview of a series of the first 20 patients presenting with either pure laterocollis or, more frequently, combined with rotatory torticollis, who had the levator scapulae denervated to improve the abnormal lateral inclination of the head, has been presented recently.[49] The results were similar to those described above. Patients did not show limitation of movement of the ipsilateral shoulder, probably due to the integrity of the ipsilateral trapezius muscle.

What then are the main causes of failure in 12% of the cases? In the majority of these cases it is probably due to a failure in identifying one or more fine branches at C3 or C4. In a few patients with long-standing torticollis, it may be due to severe osteoarthrosis or fibrosis that developed over the years, which limits the movements of the head even after proper denervation. Whenever passive movements are restricted, it is worthwhile to repeat such movements with the patient under light anesthesia so that the patient may have an idea of what to expect postoperatively. Sometimes, it is difficult or impossible to straighten the patient's head, even under anesthesia. In two of the authors' patients, the movements were maintained by the contralateral semispinalis muscle, which acted as a rotator of the head. Remaining rotation of the head combined with slight contralateral inclination and extension is a very characteristic abnormal posture due to the contralateral obliquus capitis superior muscle (see Table 1).

In one patient with laterocollis for 10 years, the contralateral musculature was so weak and elongated that it was no longer possible to bring the head back to the vertical position. One patient went home 2 or 3 days after operation and did not perform enough physiotherapy to restore normal movement of the head. Finally, one patient with generalized dystonia had a flare-up of his symptoms postoperatively. It seems that in cases of generalized dystonia, surgery should not be performed during the active, progressive stage of the disease. The minimum period of 1 year of stabilization of symptoms should be taken into account to avoid postoperative flare-ups. In the other eight patients with generalized dystonia, there was a marked improvement in posture.

Retrocollis involving only the upper cervical muscles usually improves a great deal with bilateral posterior ramisectomy from C1 to C5. On the other hand, when retrocollis is due to significant involvement of lower cervical and dorsal muscles, also causing spinal deformities, such denervation does not suffice for relief of symptoms.

The importance of a limited muscle section and restoration of normal muscle attachments, as well as early physiotherapy, must be emphasized. Usually, with proper technique, sequelae are not significant. Sensory loss is limited to the distribution of the greater occipital nerve. A few patients have complained of paresthesias or a sensation of tightness or fullness. Three patients had an occasional, sudden tic-like pain, which subsided in a few weeks. Muscular atrophy is usually not apparent.

The results appear to be well maintained over the years. There may be an occasional reinnervation of the sternocleidomastoid muscle, but not enough to cause appreciable abnormal movements. In a previous review[11] of 167 patients operated on more than 5 years ago and 64 patients more than 10 years ago, the benefit of the operation has persisted. In rare instances the initial benefit may be due partly to neurapraxia, and some movements may recur after a few months.

Comments

As mentioned above, the fact that the functional distribution of the anterior and posterior divisions has been confirmed is a great help in selective denervation. It has also been demonstrated that bilateral rhizotomy should not be considered now that it has been established that the anterior branches of C1and C2 contribute only to the innervation of the infrahyoid muscles of the throat, responsible for swallowing. They have no role in the innervation of the posterior cervical musculature. In selective peripheral denervation, only the posterior divisions need and should be denervated.

It has also been established that the posterior divisions from C1 to C5 must be interrupted bilaterally to eliminate the abnormal movements in cases of retrocollis. This procedure does not interfere materially with extension of the neck. As for C6, it has such a small local distribution that its posterior division is left intact in cases of bilateral selective ramisectomy.

The collateral branches of the posterior divisions of C4, and particularly C3, still require further study. At present, at these levels, all collateral branches that respond to stimulation are sectioned and avulsed in order to avoid residual abnormal movements. It is known from cadaver dissections that, mainly at C3, there exist more fine nerve branches than it is possible to isolate during surgical denervation, even when performing careful and meticulous dissection at the C3 and C4 levels. This may be due to the fact that these fine branches burrow within the muscles. Probably the remaining branches suffice to preserve normal movements of rotation on the operated side, contrary to the authors' initial expectation. It was a pleasant surprise to find that normal or near-normal range of movements had been preserved. However, this requires a limited dissection of the neck, and restoration of as much as possible of the anatomy of the muscles at the end of the procedure. Equally important is that early and intensive physiotherapy be instituted.

As for laterocollis, it has been shown that the great contributor is the levator scapulae muscle, not the trapezius muscle. Furthermore, the intact trapezius is sufficient to maintain normal movements of the shoulder and to provide lateral inclination of the head once the ipsilateral levator scapulae is denervated. This complementary surgical procedure has greatly improved the results in cases of laterocollis. Possibly, this could be performed through a lateral incision, thus avoiding increasing section of neck muscles, particularly in cases in which the contralateral levator scapulae is denervated.

There has been neither mortality nor major complications in this group of patients. However, when using the sitting position, careful and constant monitoring is essential to prevent possible air emboli, which may require bringing the patient back to a horizontal position temporarily. The performance of this technique involves very few possibilities for air emboli if the paravertebral venous plexuses are coagulated during exposure. Even with these required precautions, the sitting position is highly preferable to operating with the patients lying on their side, as was done in the beginning. The approach through the paravertebral venous plexuses was unsatisfactory and the search for collateral branches of C3 and C4 was quite difficult.

The increasing knowledge of the functional distribution of the different cervical branches opens up the possibility of a simplified and more conservative technique in the near future. As it is, a well-trained neurosurgeon contemplating the performance of selective peripheral denervation should be familiar with the anatomy of the neck through cadaver dissections, and also spend some time in a center where selective denervation is performed regularly, remembering that any residual nerve will maintain the abnormal movement.

References

1. Adams CBT: Spasmodic torticollis resulting from neurovascular compression. **J Neurosurg 66:**635, 1987 (Letter)
2. Adams CBT: Vascular catastrophy following the Dandy McKenzie operation for spasmodic torticollis. **J Neurol Neurosurg Psychiatry 47:**990-994, 1984
3. Arce C, Russo L: Selective peripheral denervation: a surgical alternative in the treatment of spasmodic torticollis. Review of fifty-five patients. **Mov Disord 7:**128, 1992 (Abstract)
4. Batten FE: On the diagnostic value of the position of the head in cases of cerebellar disease. **Brain 26:** 71-80, 1903
5. Benabou R, Marino R Jr, Benabou S, et al: Therapeutic effects of Flunitrazepam in patients with dystonia. **Mov Disord 9:**41, 1994 (Abstract)
6. Benabou R, Molina-Negro P, Bouvier G: Selection criteria for selective peripheral denervation (SPD) for spasmodic torticollis (ST). **Can J Neurol Sci 22:**S26, 1995 (Abstract)
7. Bertrand C, Molina-Negro P, Bouvier G, et al: Obser-

vations and analysis of results in 131 cases of spasmodic torticollis after selective denervation. **Appl Neurophysiol 50:**319-323, 1987

8. Bertrand C, Molina-Negro P, Martinez SN: Combined stereotactic and peripheral surgical approach for spasmodic torticollis. **Appl Neurophysiol 41:** 122-133, 1978
9. Bertrand C, Molina Negro P, Martinez SN: Technical aspects of selective peripheral denervation for spasmodic torticollis. **Appl Neurophysiol 45:**326-330, 1982
10. Bertrand CM: Peripheral versus central surgical approach for the treatment of spasmodic torticollis, in Marsden C, Fahn S (eds): **Movement Disorders.** London: Butterworth, 1982, pp 315-318
11. Bertrand CM: Selective peripheral denervation for spasmodic torticollis: surgical technique, results and observations in 260 cases. **Surg Neurol 40:**96-103, 1993
12. Bertrand CM: Stereotactic and peripheral surgery for the control of movement disorders, in Barbeau A (ed): **Disorders of Movements. Current Status of Modern Therapy.** Lancaster, England: MTP Press, 1981, pp 191-208
13. Bertrand CM: Surgical management of spasmodic torticollis and adult-onset dystonia with emphasis on selective denervation, in Schmidek H, Sweet W (eds): **Operative Neurosurgical Techniques.** Orlando, Fla: Grune & Stratton, 1988, pp 1261-1269
14. Bertrand CM: The treatment of spasmodic torticollis with particular reference to thalamotomy, in Mortley T (ed): **Current Controversies in Neurosurgery.** Philadelphia, Pa: WB Saunders, 1976, pp 455-459
15. Bertrand CM, Molina-Negro P: Selective peripheral denervation in 111 cases of spasmodic torticollis: rationale and results, in Fahn S, Marsden C, Calne D (eds): **Dystonia 2. Advances in Neurology.** New York, NY: Raven Press, 1988, pp 637-643
16. Bertrand CM, Molina-Negro P, Bouvier G, et al: Surgical treatment of spasmodic torticollis, in Youmans RJ (ed): **Neurological Surgery.** Philadelphia, Pa: WB Saunders, 1995, pp 3701-3712
17. Bertrand CM, Molina-Negro P, Martinez SN: Stereotactic targets for dystonias and dyskinesias: relationship to corticobulbar fibers and other adjoining structures. **Adv Neurol 24:**395-399, 1979
18. Brain WR: On the rotated or "cerebellar" posture of the head. **Brain 49:**61-76, 1926
19. Braun V, Richter HP: Selective peripheral denervation in patients with spasmodic torticollis. **Stereotact Funct Neurosurg 57:**113-122, 1991
20. Brissaud E: **Leçons sur les Maladies Nerveuses. Recueillies et publieés par H. Meige.** Paris: Masson & Cie; 1895
21. Bronstein AM, Rudge P: Vestibular involvement in spasmodic torticollis. **J Neurol Neurosurg Psychiatry 49:**290-295, 1986
22. Bronstein AM, Rudge P: The vestibular system in abnormal head postures and in spasmodic torticollis. **Adv Neurol 50:**493-500, 1988
23. Cooper IS: Effect of thalamic lesions on torticollis. **N Engl J Med 270:**967-972, 1964
24. Couch JR: Dystonia and tremor in spasmodic torticollis. **Adv Neurol 50:**245-258, 1976
25. Cushing H: **Tumors of the Nervus Acusticus and the Syndrome of the Cerebellopontile Angle.** Philadelphia, Pa: WB Saunders, 1917
26. Dandy WE: An operation for the treatment of spasmodic torticollis. **Arch Surg 20:**1021-1032, 1930
27. Davis DH, Ahlskog JE, Litchy WJ, et al: Selective peripheral denervation for torticollis: preliminary results. **Mayo Clin Proc 66:**365-371, 1991
28. Déjerine JJ: **Semiologie des Affections du Systeme Nerveux.** Paris: Masson & Cie, 1914, pp 500-501
29. Fahn S: High dosage anticholinergic therapy in dystonia. **Neurology 33:**1255-1261, 1983
30. Freckmann N, Hagenah R, Herrmann HD, et al: Bilateral microsurgical lysis of the spinal accessory nerve roots for treatment of spasmodic torticollis. Follow up of 33 cases. **Acta Neurochir 83:**47-53, 1986
31. Freckmann N, Hagenah R, Herrmann HD, et al: Treatment of neurogenic torticollis by microvascular lysis of the accessory nerve root—indication, technique, and first results. **Acta Neurochir 59:**167-175, 1981
32. Friedman AH, Nashold BS Jr, Sharp R, et al: Treatment of spasmodic torticollis with intradural selective rhizotomies. **J Neurosurg 78:**46-53, 1993
33. Gilbert GJ: Familial spasmodic torticollis. **Neurology 27:**11-13, 1977
34. Greene P, Shale H, Fahn S, et al: Treatment of torticollis with injections of botulinum toxin. **Neurology 37 (Suppl 1):**123, 1987 (Abstract)
35. Hamby WB, Schiffer S: Spasmodic torticollis: results after cervical rhizotomy in 50 cases. **J Neurosurg 31:** 323-326, 1969
36. Hassler R, Dieckmann G: Stereotactic treatment of different kinds of spasmodic torticollis. **Confin Neurol 32:**135-143, 1970
37. Hedreen JC, Zweig RN, Delong MR, et al: Primary dystonias: a review of the pathology and suggestions for new directions of study. **Adv Neurol 50:**123-132, 1988
38. Isaac K, Cohen JA: Post-traumatic torticollis. **Neurology 39:**1642-1643, 1989 (Letter)
39. Jankovic J, Schwartz K: Botulinum toxin injections for cervical dystonia. **Neurology 40:**277-280, 1990
40. Jho HD, Jannetta PJ: Microvascular decompression for spasmodic torticollis. **Acta Neurochir 134:**21-26, 1995
41. Korein J, Brudny J: Integrated EMG feedback in the management of spasmodic torticollis and focal dystonia: a prospective study of 80 patients, in Yard MD (ed): **Basal Ganglia.** New York, NY: Raven Press, 1976, pp 385-424
42. Lee MC: Spasmodic torticollis and other idiopathic torsion dystonias. Medical management. **Postgrad Med 75 (15):**139-146, 1984
43. Magnus R: **Koperstellung.** Berlin: Springer-Verlag, 1924
44. Marino R Jr, Benabou R, Benabou S: Therapeutic effects of Flunitrazepam in dystonias and torticollis: preliminary communication. **Arq Neuropsiquiatr 51:** 285-286, 1993
45. Marsden C, Fahn S (eds): **Movement Disorders.** London: Butterworth, 1981
46. Marsden CD: The problem of adult-onset idiopathic torsion dystonia and other isolated dyskinesias in adult life (including blepharospasm, oromandibular dystonia, dystonic writer's cramp and torticollis, or axial dystonia). **Adv Neurol 14:**259-276, 1976
47. Marsden CD, Marion MH, Quinn N: The treatment of severe dystonia in children and adults. **J Neurol Neurosurg Psychiatry 47:**1166-1173, 1984

48. McKenzie KG: Intrameningeal division of the spinal accessory and roots of the upper cervical nerves for the treatment of spasmodic torticollis. **Surg Gynecol Obstet 39:**5-10, 1924
49. Molina-Negro P, Bouvier G, Benabou R: Treatment of laterocollis by selective peripheral denervation. **Can J Neurol Sci 22:**S26, 1995 (Abstract)
50. Ozelius L, Kramer PL, Moskowitz CB, et al: Human gene for torsion dystonia located on chromosome 9q32-q34. **Neuron 2:**1427-1434, 1989
51. Pagni CA, Naddeo M, Faccani G: Spasmodic torticollis due to neurovascular compression of the 11th nerve. Case report. **J Neurosurg 63:**789-791, 1985
52. Perot PL Jr: Upper cervical ventral rhizotomy and selective section of spinal accessory rootlets for spasmodic torticollis, in Wilson CB (ed): **Neurosurgical Procedures: Personal Approaches to Classic Operations.** Baltimore, Md: Williams & Wilkins, 1992, pp 163-168
53. Peterson EW, Magoun HW, McCulloch WS, et al: Production of postural tremor. **J Neurophysiol 12:** 371-384, 1949
54. Plant GT, Kermode AG, du Boulay EP, et al: Spasmodic torticollis due to a midbrain lesion in a case of multiple sclerosis. **Mov Disord 4:**359-362, 1989
55. Podivinský F: Torticollis, in Vinken P, Bruyn G (eds): **Handbook of Clinical Neurology. Vol 6: Diseases of the Basal Ganglia.** Amsterdam: North Holland, 1968, pp 567-603
56. Poirier LJ, Péchadre JC, Larochelle L, et al: Stereotaxic lesions and movement disorders in monkeys. **Adv Neurol 10:**5-22, 1975
57. Rossitch E Jr, Khoshbin S, Black PM, et al: Kenneth McKenzie, Harvey Cushing, and the early neurosurgical treatment of spasmodic torticollis. **Neurosurgery 28:**278-282, 1991
58. Shima F, Fukui M, Kitamura K, et al: Diagnosis and surgical treatment of spasmodic torticollis of 11th nerve origin. **Neurosurgery 22:**358-363, 1988
59. Svien HJ, Cody DTR: Treatment of spasmodic torticollis by suppression of labyrinthine activity: report of a case. **Mayo Clin Proc 44:**825-827, 1969
60. Taira T, Hitchcock E: [Torticollis as an initial symptom of adult-onset dystonia musculorum deformans.] **No To Shinkei 42:**867-871, 1991 (Jpn)
61. Tarlov E: On the problem of the pathology of spasmodic torticollis in man. **J Neurol Neurosurg Psychiatry 33:**457-463, 1970
62. Walker FO, Walker JM, Matsumoto RR, et al: Torticollis, midbrain and sigma receptors. **Mov Disord 5:** 265, 1990 (Letter)
63. Williams PL, Bannister LH (eds): **Gray's Anatomy. Anatomical Basis of Medicine and Surgery.** New York, NY: Churchill Livingstone, 1995, p 1258
64. Yahr MD (ed): **The Basal Ganglia.** New York, NY: Raven Press, 1976

CHAPTER 19

Ablative Procedures for Dystonia

Ronald R. Tasker, MD, FRCS(C)

The term "dystonia" was first used in 1911 by Oppenheim[81] to describe what today is known as primary dystonia or dystonia musculorum deformans, although the condition had apparently been previously described in 1908 by Schwalbe,[88] who thought it was a psychogenic disorder. In current usage, dystonia refers to two groups of conditions: primary dystonia and secondary dystonia, both of which are most likely to appear in childhood rather than adult life. Primary dystonia can be further divided into various clinical types, but is essentially of uncertain etiology, with conventional imaging and autopsy studies of the brain being normal. Secondary dystonia results from a disparate variety of insults to the nervous sytem,[66] amongst which it is difficult to discern a common feature. Prominent causes include perinatal or childhood trauma, although the dystonias that may accompany stroke (Dejerine-Roussy syndrome[17]) and levodopa (L-DOPA)-induced dyskinesia are adult-onset diseases. Levodopa-induced dyskinesia, which responds dramatically to pallidotomy,[20,65] will not be further discussed in this chapter. In a personal series of 30 cases of secondary dystonia treated by thalamotomy,[100] 30% followed birth injury and 30% childhood head injury. The curious thing about secondary dystonia is that, despite the fact that it may be caused by a finite event of brain injury, such as trauma, its onset may be delayed and its course progressive over years,[100] much like central pain syndrome.[98] Interestingly, Dejerine-Roussy syndrome as originally described consisted of central pain and dystonia on the side of the body contralateral to the stroke. In a study by the author, in the 6 patients with dystonia of 73 with stroke-induced pain, all had thalamic lesions.[98]

Primary dystonia, on the other hand, can develop with or without a hereditary pattern, and the latter may be autosomal dominant, autosomal recessive, or X-linked recessive.[66] It is often classified into childhood- (0-12 years), adolescent- (13-20 years), or, rarely, adult-onset primary dystonia.[21]

Both primary dystonia and secondary dystonia can also be classified by distribution: focal, segmental, multifocal (rare), generalized, and hemidystonia.[21] The term "focal dystonia" is usually used to refer to such variants of primary dystonia as blepharospasm, hemifacial spasm, spasmodic torticollis, and writer's cramp, which will not be considered further in this chapter because their management rarely involves intracranial stereotactic destructive procedures, with injections of botulinum toxin being particularly useful in some cases.

Indications for Surgical Treatment of Dystonia

Patients being considered for surgery should have failed to improve under exhaustive medical management, keeping in mind the subsets of primary dystonia that respond dramatically to trihexyphenidyl (Artane) or L-DOPA.[22,75,89] The disease must be inflicting sufficient disability to warrant the surgery, keeping in mind the outcome statistics described below. There should be no contraindications, such as bleeding diatheses or significant psychiatric or cognitive impairment. The disabling features of the disease should be amenable to surgical control, and it must be pointed out to the patients and their families that surgery will not alter the progress of the dystonia and has no chance of benefiting the fixed neurological deficits, such as hemiparesis, that are so common in secondary dystonia. In fact, underlying hemiparesis may be masked by dystonic movements and the patient must be warned that such weakness may be much more apparent if the movements stop. In the author's experience, surgery is much more useful for the relief of peripheral limb than of proximal limb and axial dystonia, whether tonic or phasic in nature. It must also be remembered that dystonia is often bilateral and bilateral thalamotomy carries a significant risk of dysarthria,[99] while bilateral pallidotomy may result in cognitive disorders (in the author's experience) or interfere with speech (Burchiel KJ, Favre J, Taha JM: Risk of speech deterioration after pallidotomy. Presented at the Congress of Neurological Surgeons Annual Meeting, Montreal, 1996). The results of thalamotomy in dystonia may be erratic, with some patients showing striking improvement and others with apparently similar disease enjoying little benefit, while even striking improvement may fade rather abruptly over time. Patients with rapidly progressive primary or secondary dystonia are probably poor candidates for surgery, because postoperative progression of the disease may soon swallow up any modest improvement achieved by surgery. Patients with secondary dystonia manifesting bulbar or pseudobulbar deficits are prone to develop dysphagia and/or respiratory complications, while those who are borderline ambulatory may become wheelchair-bound postoperatively if they experience what appear to be minor changes in muscle tone or gait control.

Surgical Procedures Available for Dystonia

Meyers[69] introduced the concept of treating movement disorders with ablative lesions in the basal ganglia rather than in the corticospinal tract, thus offering the possibility of ameliorating the movements without inducing paresis. Since that time, pallidotomy has been used in many centers in the treatment of hyperkinetic disorders, including dystonia. Because dystonia was relatively uncommon, no one center generated large numbers of cases. For example, Cooper,[14] with probably the largest reported series, treated 155 cases of dystonia and over 5000 patients with Parkinson's disease in the same time frame, while in the Toronto Hospital experience, the author's dystonia caseload was one tenth that seen for Parkinson's disease.[100] Thalamotomy superseded pallidotomy as the usual operation for the relief of Parkinson's disease, and subsequently for primary and secondary dystonia; most of the published experience with ablative surgery for dystonia is with thalamotomy. The earlier series describing pallidotomy in dystonia contained few cases, often intermingled with a variety of other types of movement disorder, so that it is difficult, to evaluate pallidotomy as it was performed in those early years to treat dystonia. Similarly, it was not always clear in earlier reports on thalamotomy just what structures were lesioned in "ventrolateral thalamotomy." The more recent rekindling of interest in pallidotomy for Parkinson's disease[53,54] includes an increased understanding of the pathophysiology of that condition, as it affects the basal ganglia.[7,18] Given this, together with the serendipitous discovery that pallidotomy dramatically controls levodopa-induced dystonia,[20,54,65] much more effectively than does thalamotomy,[74,97,99,112] it is anticipated that the effect of pallidal lesions on both primary and secondary dystonia will be carefully re-examined in the near future. Furthermore, with the availability of reliable equipment for chronic deep brain stimulation, including its application in the thalamus,[6] subthalamic nucleus of Luys,[82] and globus pallidus[32,93] to treat Parkinson's disease, it was inevitable that deep brain stimulation applied in various sites is also being explored in the treatment of dystonia (see Chapter 11, "Chronic Deep Brain Stimulation: Indications and Techniques").

It is essential to discover more effective means of treating dystonia surgically. Despite the striking benefit of thalamic stimulation and lesion-making on tremor and of globus pallidus stimulation and lesion-making on levodopa-induced dyskinesia, surgical amelioration of dystonia is modest.

Of the long list of surgical options proposed over the years for the treatment of dystonia, many do not appear to be in common use today, including stimulation of the caudate nucleus,[95] stimulation and lesioning of the dentate nucleus or cerebellum,[16,24,26,33,45,70,86,87,91,110,111,117,120,121] pulvinarotomy,[48] dorsomedian thalamotomy,[96] lesioning of the substantia nigra[48] putamenotomy,[48] and capsulotomy[19,41] (Poblete M, Mancini R, Aranda L: Stereotaxic posterior capsulotomy in hemiballismus. Presented at the World Society for Stereotactic and Functional Neurosurgery Meeting, Sao Paulo, 1977). Other techniques, such as dorsal column stimulation,[23,29,30,35,40,55,92,113,114] thalamic stimulation[6,67,68,90,106,107] (Benabid AL, Pollak P, Limousin P, et al: Chronic stimulation of the ventrolateral thalamic nucleus in dystonia. Presented at Focus on Dystonia Meeting, Rome, 1994), and baclofen infusion,[3] are beyond the scope of this chapter.

Technique of Thalamotomy

In most centers, the technique of thalamotomy for dystonia is similar to that used for Parkinson's disease, which has been abundantly described.[23,27,34,49,56,62,77,78,100,102,103,105] In the author's practice, a Leksell G frame (Elekta Instruments, Tucker, Georgia) is attached to the head as closely as possible, in a midsagittal position, after local anesthetic blockade of the occipital and supraorbital nerves. Stereotactic magnetic resonance imaging (MRI) is then performed exactly as it would be for a stereotactic biopsy. However, because it is difficult to visualize the surgical target in the thalamus from an MRI, its location is determined indirectly. The three-dimensional stereotactic coordinates of the anterior commissure (AC) and posterior commissure (PC) are measured using the software available in the scanner. Although some surgeons believe ventriculography is essential for accurate work, MRI has proven very adequate in the author's experience and superior to computed tomography, with which it is difficult to precisely identify the location of the AC.[50] Using the patient's AC and PC coordinates, the sagittal plates from the Schaltenbrand and Bailey[84] and Schaltenbrand and Wahren[85] atlases are stretched or shrunk in the anterior-posterior direction as needed until they match the patient's AC-PC distance; the resulting diagrams are ruled in stereotactic coordinates for the particular application of the Leksell frame to the patient's head, a manipulation accomplished with a software program based on a personal computer.[101]

In order to maintain MRI accuracy, careful calibration is important, the frame must be free of magnetic materials, a suitable filler for the fiducial tubes is necessary, and the image of interest should be as close as possible to the center of the field. Because accuracy is greater in axial images, the AC and PC are usually identified on sagittal scout films bracketing the midsagittal plane, following which axial cuts are made to bracket, in turn, the positions of the AC and PC. From the redrawn sagittal brain diagrams, the stereotactic coordinates of the manual tactile relay nucleus—the inferior third of Hassler's ventral caudal nucleus[41] in the 15-mm sagittal plane—are read off preparatory to advancing an electrode to the center of this nucleus. This is done through a 1/8-inch twist drill hole made through a puncture wound in the scalp in the same sagittal plane as the expected lesion (15 mm from the midline). No attempt is made to coagulate dura or cortex, both of which are breached with a pointed probe prior to introducing the electrode for physiological localization. The author has not observed any greater incidence of significant surface hemorrhage compared to that seen with an incision and burr hole

(1%-2%) in the course of about 100 functional stereotactic procedures performed in 1 year.

Physiological localization is the next step.[56,57,100,102-105] Both microstimulation and microelectrode recording are performed with the same electrode as the electrode is advanced from about 10 mm above to as far as 10 mm below the expected target. Threshold stimulation is carried out every 1.0 mm and recording is done continually along the entire trajectory. The manual tactile relay nucleus is identified by inducing sharply localized, low-threshold areas of paresthesia in the fingers (projected fields) and/or with the recording of neuronal discharges evoked by light tactile stimulation at similar sites (receptive fields).[1,2,8,9,25,28,34,38,46,49,79] As soon as projected and receptive fields related to digits 1, 2, and 3 are defined, the electrode is moved 2 mm rostrally and the process repeated. In this second trajectory, stimulation should induce paresthesias at higher thresholds in the hand or upper limb and may drive or suppress the dystonia, while recording identifies neurons with receptive fields in the upper limb responding to deep pressure, muscle squeezing, or joint bending (kinesthetic cells).[36,37,46,58,76,80,116] In Parkinson's disease, "tremor cells" are found here,[59,63] although only occasionally are "dystonia cells" identified.[60] These are cells whose firing pattern is evoked by the tremor or dystonia, respectively. Because dystonic movements are unpredictable, dystonia cells are more difficult to identify. If the sought-after responses are not found, additional trajectories must be similarly explored, usually at 2-mm intervals. In some patients, "voluntary cells" that fire in advance of a particular contralateral voluntary movement will be found, usually rostral to the kinesthetic cells.[15,39,43,46,62,83,109] For the relief of tremor, the lesion should be placed at a thalamic site where kinesthetic and/or voluntary and tremor cells are located and where stimulation most completely abolishes tremor at the lowest threshold. However, in the author's experience, meeting these criteria alone is not sufficient. The optimal site for lesion-making is about 2 mm above the AC-PC line and 2 mm rostral to the rostral border of the digital manual tactile relay nucleus[61,62] (Albe-Fessard D: Physiopathologie du Parkinson. Presented at Le Point sur la Maladie de Parkinson Symposium, organized by Merck Sharp & Dohme, Brussels, 1973). This is an area that is difficult to define physiologically; tremor cell activity here is most tightly linked to tremor as demonstrated on electromyography. It may be the site that Wester and Hauglie-Hanssen[115] were referring to when they stated that the best predictor of a thalamotomy target site was the abolition of tremor by the mere introduction of a probe into the area, together with tremor arrest from stimulation. Lesions made in the appropriate cell zone where tremor arrest occurs but outside this crucial area may result in tremor recurrence, and making lesions large enough to increase the likelihood of encompassing the critical site may cause the complications of hand ataxia, dysarthria, and gait disturbance.[47,118,119] In thalamotomy for dystonia, this same optimal site probably applies, but it is generally agreed that the lesion for dystonia must be larger and extend more rostrally than for the control of tremor.[14,72,73]

At the author's institution, a radiofrequency (RF) lesion is made with the OWL Universal RF System (Diros Technology, Toronto, Ontario, Canada) using a 1.1-mm diameter electrode with a 3-mm bare tip, which is heated to 80°-90°C for 60 seconds, usually requiring a current of 50-70 μA. The lesion is made with sequential temperature increases, starting at 50°C, and serial neurological testing and evaluation of the dystonia are performed continually. Usually multiple overlapping lesions are required, guided by their effect on the dystonia. In Cooper's experience,[12] the lesion encroached on the ventral caudal nucleus and included Hassler's ventral oral nuclei,[41] as well as the centromedian nucleus. It must be emphasized that in patients with primary dystonia and brains of normal dimensions and narrow third ventricles, the internal capsule may lie much closer to the midline than expected, so that a lesion typical for secondary dystonia or Parkinson's disease (14-15 mm from the midline) may induce paresis.[42]

Pallidotomy

At the author's institution, pallidotomy is performed in the same way as thalamotomy, except that the target coordinates are chosen from the redrawn 20-mm lateral sagittal atlas diagram in the internal portion of the globus pallidus (GPi). With microelectrode recording[64] in a parasagittal trajectory, neurons whose firing patterns are typical of the external portion of the globus pallidus (GPe) are sought superiorly. These are replaced with typical GPi cells deeper along the trajectory, some of which may fire synchronously with tremor and/or in response to passive movements of contralateral and often ipsilateral limb joints. Microstimulation usually has little observable effect in the GPi and GPe. Inferiorly, cellular activity fades and sites are sought where flash-evoked potentials can be recorded from the axons of the optic tract or stimulation-induced phosphenes can be produced in the contralateral visual fields, precisely marking the site in the optic tract. Caudal tracts are also sought in which stimulation induces tetanization of the contralateral face or upper limb, in order to define the position of the internal capsule. Occasionally more medial or lateral sagittal planes must be explored before suitable responses are found, whereupon a graded RF lesion is made for 90 seconds with temperatures up to 90°C. Serial assessments of the contralateral power and visual fields are made and the effects on dyskinesia noted.

Outcome of Stereotactic Ablative Surgery in Dystonia

In the author's opinion, published information concerning only two destructive procedures warrants review: thalamotomy and pallidotomy. A historical overview of the field of stereotactic surgery for movement disorders is presented in the literature[41,48,94] and in Chapter 2, "History of Surgery for Movement Disorders."

Pallidotomy

Most published data concerning pallidotomy for dystonia emanate from the earlier years of stereotactic surgery, when limitations of technique compromised the precision of lesion localization and outcome measurement. When interest in thalamotomy superseded that in pallidotomy, thalamotomy became the treatment of choice for dystonia.[48]

Burzaco[10] compared pallidotomy in 37 patients and thalamotomy in 45 patients with various movement disorders, including primary and secondary dystonia. After pallidotomy, improvement was reported in 50% of the patients with bilateral dystonic hyperkinetic disorders, 75% of those with focal dystonia, 80% with bilateral primary dystonia, and 57% with spasmodic torticollis. After thalamotomy, improvement occurred in 46%, 81%, 69%, and 57%, respectively, of these patient groups. Thus, there appeared to be little choice between the two procedures.

Although it is known that most centers that currently use pallidotomy to treat Parkinson's disease also use the procedure on patients with dystonia, there are few published reports. Iacono et al[44] described dramatic improvement in a 17-year-old man with a 9-year history of primary dystonia after simultaneous bilateral pallidoansotomy. Kwon and Whang[51] treated a patient with secondary dystonia using the Gamma Knife to make a posteroventral pallidal lesion. The dystonia improved, but the patient developed homonymous hemianopsia. The author's colleague Andres Lozano performed bilateral pallidotomy exactly as for Parkinson's disease in a bedridden child with generalized primary dystonia, under general anesthesia, with striking improvement in both axial and appendicular movements (personal communication, 1997). In the first week after surgery, the patient was able to walk with a walker, and has progressed to normal ambulation at 16 months postoperatively.

Thalamotomy

Kandel[48] reported his experience with 102 destructive lesions in the globus pallidus, ventral lateral (VL) nucleus of the thalamus, and the subthalamic area (not to be confused with the subthalamic nucleus of Luys) in 86 patients with a mixed group of hyperkinetic disorders, 31% of whom suffered from hemidystonia. He reported "good" results in 35% of the overall group of patients and marked improvement in 30%, the results being best in patients who had had lesions made in the VL nucleus or the VL nucleus plus the subthalamic area.

There is a large experience with thalamotomy in cerebral palsy, a disorder that often manifests dystonic movements. According to Kandel,[48] Balasubramanian et al reduced spasticity by ≥50%

in 71% of patients with cerebral palsy and reduced hyperkinesia in 43% after making lesions in the VL, centromedian, and ventral intermediate (VIM) nuclei. Kandel made pallidal lesions 8 times, VL nucleus lesions 126 times, and VL nucleus plus subthalamic area lesions 68 times in 174 patients with cerebral palsy. Some patients had lesions made in the dentate nucleus and pulvinar. Twelve percent of these patients enjoyed a "good" result and 22% showed significant improvement; 15% of the procedures were followed by complications, including a 1.7% mortality rate. Results were best in patients with bilateral lesions in the VL nucleus and subthalamic area. Narabayashi[71] treated 165 cerebral palsy patients mainly with thalamotomy. Their disabilities varied widely in severity and seemed to determine surgical outcome. Excellent results occurred in 38% of the least affected patients who were followed, with significant improvement in 24%. Marked improvement occurred in only 6% of the most severely affected survivors (18.8% died) who could be followed, while 31% showed useful improvement.

Kandel[48] performed 272 procedures in 188 cases of primary dystonia, with some patients operated on bilaterally. Lesions were usually made in the VL nucleus or the VL nucleus plus subthalamic area, and sometimes also in the globus pallidus and dentate nucleus. Postoperatively, 22% of patients enjoyed "good" results and 54% showed significant improvement, at the expense of 1.8% mortality and a 10% rate of other complications.

Cooper[12-14] made large thalamic lesions, usually in the VIM, ventral caudal, and centromedian nuclei but sometimes in the pulvinar, to treat 104 primary dystonia patients with unilateral surgery and 122 with bilateral surgery. In the short term, 67% showed mild to moderate improvement, which tended to fade over time. The mortality rate was 2%. Cooper believed that Jewish patients with familial disease who were operated on between the ages of 11 and 15 years had the best outcome (85% improved), although surgery had to be repeated frequently because of movement recurrence. Cooper found axial and appendicular movements to be relieved equally well.

Gros et al[31] noted deterioration over time but no age preference in the outcomes for surgery to treat primary dystonia. In their experience, phasic movements responded best.

Tsukamoto et al[108] reported good results in a 10-year-old girl with what they termed "Hallervorden-Spatz" disease. The patient was able to sit for several hours a day and to write a little with support after bilateral VL thalamotomy repeated on each side. She suffered a left hemiparesis as a complication.

Cardoso et al[11] reported that 47% of their 17 patients with dystonia who underwent thalamotomy of the ventral oral anterior and posterior nuclei between 1980 and 1994 showed early moderate improvement, which was sustained in 35% while 12% improved further over time. Patients with secondary dystonia fared better than those with primary dystonia (50% vs. 43% moderately or markedly improved at longest follow-up). Complications affected 35% of patients, but persistent paresis, dysarthria, and pseudobulbar palsy affected only one patient.

The author's experience[100] with 57 cases of dystonia (30 secondary, 20 primary, 7 atypical), 28% of whom where operated on bilaterally, is shown in Table 1. Reduction of distal limb movements, whether phasic or tonic, was the only significant gain in these patients: 50%-57% in the upper limbs and 39%-69% in the lower limbs, depending upon whether movements were phasic or tonic and caused by primary or secondary dystonia. The 38% improvement in dexterity in the primary dystonia group compared with 17% in the secondary dystonia group probably reflects underlying hemiparesis in the latter patients. Otherwise, any improvement in speech, facial movement, neck and trunk movement, and gait are modest and similar in the two groups of patients. Postoperative regression occurred in 31% of the secondary dystonia and 40% of primary dystonia cases, occurring as late as 6 years after the operation. This deterioration tended to cancel out the benefits achieved by surgery. One secondary dystonia patient died of respiratory complications and one required a permanent tracheotomy for the same reason (Table 2); both suffered from bilateral disease with pseudobulbar symptoms. Two primary dystonia patients developed moderate hemiparesis (the syndrome of the narrow third ventricle referred to above[42]). Significant worsening of dysarthria was seen chiefly after bilateral surgery.

TABLE 1

THALAMOTOMY IN DYSTONIA

Feature	% Significantly Improved	
	Primary Dystonia (20 pts)	Secondary Dystonia* (29 pts)
Speech	2	12
Facial movement	22	35
Neck movement	29	19
Trunk movement	28	31
Gait	13	12
Dexterity	38	17
Upper limb movements		
Phasic	53	52
Tonic	57	50
Lower limb movements		
Phasic	39	53
Tonic	69	41

*Procedure abandoned in one patient.

TABLE 2

COMPLICATIONS OF THALAMOTOMY FOR DYSTONIA

Complication	% of Cases	
	Primary Dystonia (20 pts)	Secondary Dystonia* (29 pts)
Death	0	3.4
Permanent tracheotomy	0	3.4
Hemiparesis	10	0
Transient dysphagia	5	6.9
Significant persistent dysarthria	20	6.9
Mild persistent dysarthria	30	6.9
Transient dysarthria	20	6.9
Persistent gait disturbance	20	6.9
Transient gait disturbance	0	20.7
Transient hand ataxia	15	3.4
Transient dysphagia	0	3.4
Transient numbness	20	17.2
Superficial wound infection	5	6.9
Epileptic seizure	5	3.4

*Procedure abandoned in one patient.

TABLE 3

PUBLISHED OUTCOMES IN THALAMOTOMY FOR DYSTONIA

Author(s) & Year	No. of Cases	Diagnosis	% Patients With Long-Term Improvement		% Patients With Worsened Symptoms	Complications
			Marked	Moderate		
Laitinen,[53] 1965	10	Cerebral palsy, dystonia		50	17	
Cooper,[13-15] 1969, 1976	208	Various dystonia	24.5	45.2	12	2% deaths
Gross et al,[32] 1976	25	Various dystonia	50	50		4% deaths 16% significant
Andrew et al,[4,5] 1974, 1983	16	Various dystonia	25			7% permanent cognitive deficits 15% hemiparesis 11% dysarthria 28% hand ataxia 2% seizure
Tasker et al,[102] 1988	29	Secondary dystonia	34	21		See Table 2
	20	Primary dystonia	32	30	10	
Kandel,[49] 1989	188	Primary dystonia	22	54	5	10% complications 2.7% mortality 1.6% paresis 1.0% dysphagia

Table 3 presents in tabular form the overall results of thalamotomy in the larger published series, showing a fairly consistent marked improvement in 22%-50% of cases and moderate improvement in 21%-54%, usually with a significant complication rate.

CONCLUSIONS

Thalamotomy results in modest amelioration of dystonic symptoms. Outcome after pallidotomy is probably similar, but only small series of cases have been reported, with few using modern techniques, and often the results are clouded because the small number of dystonia patients is included with patients with other hyperkinetic conditions. In view of the dramatic effects of GPi pallidotomy and deep brain stimulation on levodopa-induced dyskinesia, which is as striking as the relief of parkinsonian tremor by lesions or deep brain stimulation in the VIM nucleus, a modern, careful evaluation of unilateral and bilateral pallidal surgery for dystonia is warranted and may yield surprising results. Because of the small number of cases seen, such a study would best be a multicenter one. Moreover, the widening experience with deep brain stimulation in the subthalamic nucleus of Luys to treat patients with Parkinson's disease will surely lead to its investigation for treatment of dystonia. It is likely that, based on experience with parkinsonian and other types of tremor, the effect on dystonia of deep brain stimulation in the thalamus will be only modest, similar to that of thalamotomy. Indeed, Benabid et al applied deep brain stimulation to the VL nucleus in seven patients with primary dystonia, with moderate contralateral improvement in 57%, although speech, gait, and axial dystonia did not improve. However, deep brain stimulation in the GPi may be more promising.

The author's colleague Andres Lozano carried out bilateral deep brain stimulation of the GPi in a patient with generalized primary dystonia, with dramatic amelioration of axial and appendicular movements (see Chapter 11).

References

1. Albe-Fessard D, Arfel G, Guiot G, et al: Dérivations d'activités spontanées et évoquées dans les structures cérébrales profondes de l'homme. **Rev Neurol 106:** 80-105, 1962
2. Albe-Fessard D, Guiot G, Hardy J: Electrophysiological localization and identification of subcortical structures in man by recording spontaneous and evoked activities. **EEG Clin Neurophysiol 15:** 1052-1053, 1963 (Abstract)
3. Albright AL, Barry MJ: Intrathecal baclofen for dystonic cerebral palsy. **J Neurosurg 84:**349A-350A, 1996 (Abstract)
4. Andrew J, Edwards JM, Rudolf N de M: The placement of stereotaxic lesions for involuntary movements other than in Parkinson's disease. **Acta Neurochir Suppl 21:**39-47, 1974
5. Andrew J, Fowler CJ, Harrison MJG: Stereotaxic thalamotomy in 55 cases of dystonia. **Brain 106:** 981-1000, 1983
6. Benabid AL, Pollak P, Gao D, et al: Chronic electrical stimulation of the ventralis intermedius nucleus of the thalamus as a treatment of movement disorders. **J Neurosurg 84:**203-214, 1996
7. Bergman H, Wichmann T, De Long MR: Reversal of experimental parkinsonism by lesions of the subthalamic nucleus. **Science 249:**1436-1438, 1990
8. Bertrand G, Jasper H, Wong A: Microelectrode study of the human thalamus: functional organization in the ventro-basal complex. **Confin Neurol 29:** 81-86, 1967
9. Bertrand G, Martinez SN, Hardy J, et al: Stereotactic surgery for Parkinsonism. Microelectrode recording, stimulation, and oriented sections with a leucotome. **Prog Neurol Surg 5:**79-112, 1973
10. Burzaco J: Stereotactic pallidotomy in extrapyramidal disorders. **Appl Neurophysiol 48:**283-287, 1985
11. Cardoso F, Jankovic J, Grossman RG, et al: Outcome after stereotactic thalamotomy for dystonia and hemiballismus. **Neurosurgery 36:**501-508, 1995
12. Cooper IS: 20-year followup study of the neurosurgical treatment of dystonia musculorum deformans. **Adv Neurol 14:**423-452, 1976
13. Cooper IS: Dystonia: surgical approaches to treatment and physiologic implications, in Yahr MD (ed): **The Basal Ganglia.** New York, NY: Raven Press, 1976, pp 369-383
14. Cooper IS: **Involuntary Movement Disorders.** New York, NY: Harper & Row, 1969, pp 160-292
15. Crowell RM, Perret E, Siegfried J: "Movement units" and "tremor phasic units" in the human thalamus. **Brain Res 11:**481-488, 1968
16. Davis R, Engle H, Kudzma J, et al: Update of chronic cerebellar stimulation for spasticity and epilepsy. **Appl Neurophysiol 45:**44-50, 1982
17. Dejerine J, Roussy G: Le syndrome thalamique. **Rev Neurol 14:**521-532, 1906
18. DeLong MR: Primate models of movement disorders of basal ganglia origin. **Trends Neurosci 13:** 281-285, 1990
19. Dierssen G: Treatment of dystonic and athetoid symptoms by lesions in the sensory portion of the internal capsule. **Confin Neurol 26:**404-406, 1965
20. Dogali M, Fazzini E, Kolodny E, et al: Stereotactic ventral pallidotomy for Parkinson's disease. **Neurology 45:**753-761, 1995
21. Fahn S: Concept and classification of dystonia. **Adv Neurol 50:**1-8, 1988
22. Fahn S: High dosage anticholinergic therapy in dystonia. **Neurology 33:**1255-1261, 1983
23. Fahn S: Lack of benefit from cervical cord stimulation for dystonia. **N Engl J Med 313:**1229, 1985 (Letter)
24. Fasano VA, Urciuoli R, Broggi G, et al: New aspects in the surgical treatment of cerebral palsy. **Acta Neurochir Suppl 24:**53-57, 1977
25. Fukamachi A, Ohye C, Narabayashi H: Delineation of the thalamic nuclei with a microelectrode in stereotaxic surgery for Parkinsonism and cerebral palsy. **J Neurosurg 39:**214-225, 1973
26. Galanda M, Nádvorník P, Šramka M: Combined transtentorial dentatotomy with pulvinarotomy in cerebral palsy. **Acta Neurochir Suppl 24:**21-26, 1977
27. Gildenberg PL: Functional neurosurgery, in Schmidek HH, Sweet WH (eds): **Operative Neurosurgical Techniques: Indications, Methods, and Results.** 2nd ed. New York, NY: Grune & Stratton, 1982, pp 993-1043
28. Gillingham FJ: Depth recording and stimulation. **J Neurosurg 24 (Suppl):**382-387, 1966
29. Goetz CG, Penn RD, Tanner CM: Efficacy of cervical cord stimulation in dystonia. **Adv Neurol 50:** 645-649, 1988
30. Groen RJ, Lambooy N, Tavy DLJ: Myoclonic dystonia: effective treatment by cervical cord stimulation. A case report. **Surg Neurol 32:**72-74, 1989
31. Gros C, Frerebeau PH, Perez-Dominguez E, et al: Long term results of stereotaxic surgery for infantile dystonia and dyskinesia. **Neurochirurgica 19:** 171-178, 1976
32. Gross C, Rougier A, Boraud T, et al: Alleviation of motor signs of Parkinson's disease after stimulation of the internal segment of the globus pallidus. Experimental evidence in human. **Soc Neurosci 20:** 1779, 1994 (Abstract)
33. Guidetti B, Fraioli B: Neurosurgical treatment of spasticity and dyskinesias. **Acta Neurochir Suppl 24:** 27-39, 1977
34. Guiot G, Hardy J, Albe-Fessard D: [Precise delimitation of the subcortical structures and identification of thalamic nuclei in man by stereotactic electrophysiology.] **Neurochirurgica 5:**1-18, 1962 (Fr)
35. Gutstein HS, Waltz JM: Spinal cord stimulation in the treatment of dystonia. **Neurology 35 (Suppl 1):** 273-274, 1985
36. Hardy TL, Bertrand G, Thompson CJ: Position and organization of thalamic cellular activity during diencephalic recording. I. Pressure-evoked activity. **Appl Neurophysiol 43:**18-27, 1980
37. Hardy TL, Bertrand G, Thompson CJ: Position and organization of thalamic cellular activity during

diencephalic recording. II. Joint- and muscle-evoked activity. **Appl Neurophysiol 43:**28-36, 1980
38. Hardy TL, Bertrand G, Thompson CJ: Thalamic recordings during stereotactic surgery. II. Location of quick-adapting touch-evoked (novelty) cellular responses. **Appl Neurophysiol 42:**198-202, 1979
39. Hardy TL, Bertrand G, Thompson CJ: Topography of "bilateral-movement-evoked" thalamic cellular activity found during diencephalic recording. **Appl Neurophysiol 43:**67-74, 1980
40. Harris GF, Millar EA, Hemmy DC, et al: Neuroelectric stimulation in cerebral palsy: long-term quantitative assessment. **Stereotact Funct Neurosurg 61:** 49-59, 1993
41. Hassler R: Stereotactic brain surgery for extrapyramidal motor disturbances, in Schaltenbrand G, Bailey P (eds): **Introduction to Stereotaxis with an Atlas of the Human Brain.** Stuttgart: Georg Thieme Verlag, 1959, Vol 1, pp 472-488
42. Hawrylyshyn PA, Tasker RR, Organ LW: Third ventricular width and the thalamocapsular border. **Appl Neurophysiol 39:**34-42, 1976/1977
43. Hongell A, Wallin G, Hagbarth KE: Unit activity connected with movement initiation and arousal situations recorded from the ventrolateral nucleus of the human thalamus. **Acta Neurol Scand 49:** 681-698, 1973
44. Iacono RP, Kuniyoshi SM, Lonser RR, et al: Simultaneous bilateral pallidoansotomy for idiopathic dystonia musculorum deformans. **Pediatr Neurol 14:** 145-148, 1996
45. Ivan LP, Ventureyra ECG: Chronic cerebellar stimulation in cerebral palsy. **Appl Neurophysiol 45:** 51-54, 1982
46. Jasper HH, Bertrand G: Thalamic units involved in somatic sensation and voluntary and involuntary movements in man, in Purpura DP, Yahr MD (eds): **The Thalamus.** New York, NY: Columbia University Press, 1966, pp 365-390
47. Jones MW, Tasker RR: The relationship of documented destruction of specific cell types to complications and effectiveness in thalamotomy for tremor in Parkinson's disease. **Stereotact Funct Neurosurg 54/55:**207-211, 1990
48. Kandel EI: **Functional and Stereotactic Neurosurgery.** Translated by Watts G, translation edited by Walker AE. New York, NY: Plenum Press, 1989
49. Kelly PJ, Ahlskog JE, Goerss SJ, et al: Computer-assisted stereotactic ventralis lateralis thalamotomy with microelectrode recording control in patients with Parkinson's disease. **Mayo Clin Proc 62:** 655-664, 1987
50. Kondziolka D, Dempsey PK, Lunsford LD, et al: A comparison between magnetic resonance imaging and computed tomography for stereotactic coordinate determination. **Neurosurgery 30:**402-407, 1992
51. Kwon Y, Whang CJ: Stereotactic Gamma Knife radiosurgery for the treatment of dystonia. **Stereotact Funct Neurosurg 64 (Suppl 1):**222-227, 1995
52. Laitinen LV: Short-term results of stereotaxic treatment for infantile cerebral palsy. **Confin Neurol 26:** 258-263, 1965
53. Laitinen LV, Bergenheim AT, Hariz MI: Leksell's posteroventral pallidotomy in the treatment of Parkinson's disease. **J Neurosurg 76:**53-61, 1992
54. Laitinen LV, Bergenheim AT, Hariz MI: Ventroposterolateral pallidotomy can abolish all parkinsonian symptoms. **Stereotact Funct Neurosurg 58:**14-21, 1992
55. Leis AA, Dimitrijevic MR, Delapasse JS, et al: Modification of cervical dystonia by selective sensory stimulation. **J Neurol Sci 110:**79-89, 1992
56. Lenz FA, Dostrovsky JO, Kwan HC, et al: Methods for microstimulation and recording of single neurons and evoked potentials in the human central nervous system. **J Neurosurg 68:**630-634, 1988
57. Lenz FA, Dostrovsky JO, Tasker RR, et al: Single-unit analysis in the human ventral thalamic nuclear group: somatosensory responses. **J Neurophysiol 59:** 299-316, 1988
58. Lenz FA, Kwan HC, Dostrovsky JO, et al: Single unit analysis of the human ventral thalamic nuclear group. Activity correlated with movement. **Brain 113:**1795-1821, 1990
59. Lenz FA, Kwan HC, Martin RL, et al: Single unit analysis of the human ventral thalamic nuclear group. Tremor-related activity in functionally identified cells. **Brain 117:**531-543, 1994
60. Lenz FA, Martin R, Kwan HC, et al: Thalamic single-unit activity occurring in patients with hemidystonia. **Stereotact Funct Neurosurg 54/55:**159-162, 1990
61. Lenz FA, Normand SL, Kwan HC, et al: Statistical prediction of the optimal site for thalamotomy in Parkinsonian tremor. **Mov Disord 10:**318-328, 1995
62. Lenz FA, Tasker RR, Kwan HC, et al: Selection of the optimal lesion site for the relief of Parkinsonian tremor on the basis of spectral analysis of neuronal firing patterns. **Appl Neurophysiol 50:**338-343, 1987
63. Lenz FA, Tasker RR, Kwan HC, et al: Single unit analysis of the human ventral thalamic nuclear group: correlation of thalamic "tremor cells" with the 3-6 Hz component of Parkinsonian tremor. **J Neurosci 8:**754-764, 1988
64. Lozano A, Hutchison W, Kiss Z, et al: Methods for microelectrode-guided posteroventral pallidotomy. **J Neurosurg 84:**194-202, 1996
65. Lozano AM, Lang AE, Galvez-Jimenez N, et al: Effect of GPi pallidotomy on motor function in Parkinson's disease. **Lancet 346:**1383-1387, 1995
66. Marsden CD: The investigation of dystonia. **Adv Neurol 50:**35-44, 1988
67. Mazars G, Merienne L, Cioloca C: Control of dyskinesias due to sensory deafferentation by means of thalamic stimulation. **Acta Neurochir Suppl 30:** 239-244, 1980
68. Mazars G, Mérienne L, Cioloca C, et al: Intermittent thalamic stimulation in the management of intractable pain. **Adv Neurosurg 3:**243-248, 1975
69. Meyers HR: Surgical procedure for postencephalitic tremor, with notes on the physiology of premotor fibers. **Arch Neurol Psychiatry 44:**455-459, 1940
70. Nádvorník P, Šramka M, Lisý L, et al: Experience with dentatotomy. **Confin Neurol 34:**320-324, 1972
71. Narabayashi H: Choreoathetosis and spasticity, in Schaltenbrand G, Walker AE (eds): **Stereotaxy of the Human Brain. Anatomical Physiological and Clinical Applications.** Stuttgart: Thieme, 1982, pp 532-543
72. Narabayashi H: Experiences of stereotaxic surgery on cerebral palsy patients. **Acta Neurochir Suppl 24:** 3-10, 1977
73. Narabayashi H: Stereotaxic surgery for athetosis or

the spastic state of cerebral palsy. **Confin Neurol 22:** 364-367, 1962
74. Narabayashi H, Yokochi F, Nakajima Y: Levodopa-induced dyskinesia and thalamotomy. **J Neurol Neurosurg Psychiatry 47:**831-839, 1984
75. Nygaard TG, Marsden CD, Duvoisin RC: Dopa-responsive dystonia. **Adv Neurol 50:**377-384, 1988
76. Ohye C: Neurons of the thalamic ventralis intermedius nucleus—their special reference to tremor. **Adv Neurol Sci 29:**224-231, 1985
77. Ohye C: Selective thalamotomy for movement disorders: microrecording stimulation techniques and results, in Lunsford LD (ed): **Modern Stereotactic Surgery.** Boston, Mass: Nijhoff, 1988, pp 315-331
78. Ohye C, Fukamachi A, Miyazaki M, et al: Physiologically controlled selective thalamotomy for the treatment of abnormal movement by Leksell's open system. **Acta Neurochir 37:**93-104, 1977
79. Ohye CH, Fukumachi A, Narabayashi H: Spontaneous and evoked activity of sensory neurons and their organization in the human thalamus. **Z Neurol 203:**219-234, 1972
80. Ohye CH, Narabayashi H: Physiological study of presumed ventralis intermedius neurons in the human thalamus. **J Neurosurg 50:**290-297, 1979
81. Oppenheim H: Ueber eine eigenartige Krampfkrankheit des kindlichen und jugendlichen Alters (Dysbasia lordotica progressiva, Dystonia musculorum deformans). **Neurol Centralbl 30:** 1090-1107, 1911
82. Pollak P, Benabid AL, Gross C, et al: Effets de la stimulation du noyau sous-thalamique dans la maladie de Parkinson. **Rev Neurol 149:**175-176, 1993
83. Raeva S: Localization in human thalamus of units triggered during "verbal commands," voluntary movements and tremor. **EEG Clin Neurophysiol 63:** 160-173, 1986
84. Schaltenbrand G, Bailey P: **Introduction to Stereotaxis with an Atlas of the Human Brain.** Stuttgart: Thieme, 1959
85. Schaltenbrand G, Wahren W: **Atlas for Stereotaxy of the Human Brain.** Stuttgart: Thieme, 1977
86. Schvarcz JR, Sica RE, Morita E: Chronic self-stimulation of the dentate nucleus for the relief of spasticity. **Acta Neurochir Suppl 30:**351-359, 1980
87. Schvarcz JR, Sica RE, Morita E, et al: Electrophysiological changes induced by chronic stimulation of the dentate nucleus for cerebral palsy. **Appl Neurophysiol 45:**55-61, 1982
88. Schwalbe W: Eine eigentumliche tonische Krampfform mit hysterischen Symptomen. Inaug Diss. Berlin: G Schade, 1908
89. Segawa M, Nomura Y, Tanaka S, et al: Hereditary progressive dystonia with marked diurnal fluctuation—consideration on its pathophysiology based on the characteristics of clinical and polysomnographical findings. **Adv Neurol 50:**367-376, 1988
90. Sellal F, Hirsch E, Barth P, et al: A case of symptomatic hemidystonia improved by ventroposterolateral thalamic electrostimulation. **Mov Disord 8:** 515-518, 1993
91. Siegfried J: Stereotaxic cerebellar surgery. **Confin Neurol 33:**350-360, 1971
92. Siegfried J, Lazorthes Y, Broggi G: Electrical spinal cord stimulation for spastic movement disorders. **Appl Neurophysiol 44:**77-92, 1981
93. Siegfried J, Lippitz B: Bilateral chronic electrostimulation of ventroposterolateral pallidum: a new therapeutic approach for alleviating all Parkinsonian symptoms. **Neurosurgery 35:**1126-1130, 1994
94. Spiegel EA: **Guided Brain Operations Methodological and Clinical Developments in Stereotactic Surgery Contribution to the Physiology of Subcortical Structures.** Basel: Karger, 1992
95. Spiegel EA, Szekely EG: Prolonged stimulation of the head of the caudate nucleus. **Arch Neurol 4:** 55-65, 1961
96. Spiegel EA, Wycis HT: **Stereoencephalotomy. Part II. Clinical and Physiological Applications. Monographs in Biology and Medicine II.** New York, NY: Grune & Stratton, 1962
97. Tasker RR: Significance and etiology of induced abnormal movements: physiological implications, in Barbeau A, McDowell FH (eds): **L-Dopa and Parkinsonism.** Philadelphia, Pa: Davis, 1970, pp 159-163
98. Tasker RR, De Carvalho G: Pain in thalamic stroke. **Proc Annu Meet Inter-Urban Stroke Academic Assoc:**1-25, 1990
99. Tasker RR, De Carvalho GC, Li CS, et al: Does thalamotomy alter the course of Parkinson's disease? **Adv Neurol 69:**563-583, 1996
100. Tasker RR, Doorly T, Yamashiro K: Thalamotomy in generalized dystonia. **Adv Neurol 50:**615-633, 1988
101. Tasker RR, Dostrovsky JO: Computers in functional stereotactic surgery, in Kelly PJ, Kall BA (eds): **Computers in Stereotactic Neurosurgery.** Boston, Mass: Blackwell, 1992, pp 155-164
102. Tasker RR, Lenz FA, Dostrovsky JO, et al: The physiological basis of VIM thalamotomy for involuntary movement disorders, in Struppler A, Weindl A (eds): **Clinical Aspects of Sensory Motor Integration.** Berlin: Springer-Verlag, 1987, pp 265-276
103. Tasker RR, Lenz F, Yamashiro K, et al: Microelectrode techniques in localization of stereotactic targets. **Neurol Res 9:**105-112, 1987
104. Tasker RR, Organ LW, Hawrylyshyn P: **The Thalamus and Midbrain of Man: A Physiological Atlas Using Electrical Stimulation.** Springfield, Ill: Charles C Thomas, 1982
105. Tasker RR, Yamashiro K, Lenz FA, et al: Thalamotomy in Parkinson's disease: microelectrode techniques, in Lunsford D (ed): **Modern Stereotactic Surgery.** Boston, Mass: Martinus Nijhoff, 1988, pp 297-313
106. Tsubokawa T, Katayama Y, Yamamoto T: Control of persistent hemiballismus by chronic thalamic stimulation. Report of two cases. **J Neurosurg 82:**501-505, 1995
107. Tsubokawa T, Yamamoto T, Katayama Y: Chronic thalamic stimulation for control of involuntary movements caused by stroke or head injury, in Gildenberg PL, Tasker RR (eds): **Textbook of Stereotactic and Functional Neurosurgery.** New York, NY: McGraw-Hill, 1998, pp 1109-1114
108. Tsukamoto H, Inui K, Taniike M, et al: A case of Hallervorden-Spatz disease: progressive and intractable dystonia controlled by bilateral thalamotomy. **Brain Dev 14:**269-272, 1992
109. Umbach W, Ehrhardt KJ: Micro-electrode recording in the basal ganglia during stereotaxic operations. **Confin Neurol 26:**315-317, 1965
110. Upton ARM, Cooper IS, Amin I: Quantitative

assessment of stereotactic and functional neurosurgery. **Appl Neurophysiol 45:**281-290, 1982

111. Vaernet K: Chronic cerebellar stimulation in spastic choreo-athetosis. **Acta Neurochir Suppl 24:**59-63, 1977
112. van Manen J, Speelman JD, Tans RJJ: Indications for surgical treatment of Parkinson's disease after levodopa therapy. **Clin Neurol Neurosurg 86:**207-212, 1984
113. Waltz JM: Computerized percutaneous multi-level spinal cord stimulation in motor disorders. **Appl Neurophysiol 45:**73-92, 1982
114. Waltz JM: Surgical approach to dystonia, in Marsden CD, Fahn S (eds): **Movement Disorders.** New York, NY: Raven Press, 1981, pp 300-307
115. Wester K, Hauglie-Hanssen E: The prognostic value of intra-operative observations during thalamotomy for parkinsonian tremor. **Clin Neurol Neurosurg 94:** 25-30, 1992
116. Wetzel N, Snider RS: Neurophysiological correlates in human stereotaxis. **Q Bull Northwest Univ Med School 32:**386-392, 1958
117. Whittaker CK: Cerebellar stimulation for cerebral palsy. **J Neurosurg 52:**648-653, 1980
118. Yasui N, Narabayashi H, Kondo T, et al: Slight cerebellar signs in stereotactic thalamotomy and subthalamotomy for Parkinsonism. **Appl Neurophysiol 39:**315-320, 1976/1977
119. Yoshida M, Okada K, Watanabe M, et al: Analysis of tremulous movements after thalamotomy correlated to intrathalamic therapeutic lesions. **Appl Neurophysiol 39:**311-314, 1976/1977
120. Zervas NT: Long-term review of dentatectomy in dystonia musculorum deformans and cerebral palsy. **Acta Neurochir Suppl 24:**49-51, 1977
121. Zervas NT, Horner FA, Pickren KS: The treatment of dyskinesia by stereotaxic dentatectomy. **Confin Neurol 29:**93-100, 1967

INDEX

Page numbers for figures and tables are followed by *f* and *t*, respectively.

D

E

F

G

H

I

J

L

M

R

S

T

U

V

W

Previously Published Books in the *Neurosurgical Topics* Series

Advanced Techniques in Central Nervous System Metastases
Edited by Robert J. Maciunas, MD

Physician's Perspective on Medical Law, Volumes I & II
Edited by Howard H. Kaufman, MD, and Jeff L. Lewin, JD

Pediatric Neurosurgical Intensive Care
Edited by Brian Andrews, MD, and Gregory Hammer, MD

Subarachnoid Hemorrhage: Pathophysiology and Management
Edited by Joshua B. Bederson, MD

Syringomyelia and the Chiari Malformations
Edited by John A. Anson, MD, Edward C. Benzel, MD, and Issam A. Awad, MD

Neurosurgical Aspects of Pregnancy
Edited by Christopher M. Loftus, MD

Endovascular Neurological Intervention
Edited by Robert J. Maciunas, MD

Benign Cerebral Glioma, Volumes I & II
Edited by Michael L.J. Apuzzo, MD

Contemporary Management of Spinal Cord Injury
Edited by Edward C. Benzel, MD, and Charles H. Tator, MD

Philosophy of Neurosurgery
Edited by Issam A. Awad, MD

Neurosurgical Emergencies, Volumes I & II
Edited by Christopher M. Loftus, MD

Interactive Image-Guided Neurosurgery
Edited by Robert J. Maciunas, MD

Spinal Instrumentation
Edited by Edward C. Benzel, MD

Current Management of Cerebral Aneurysms
Edited by Issam A. Awad, MD

Spinal Trauma: Current Evaluation and Management
Edited by Gary L. Rea, MD, and Carole A. Miller, MD

Surgery of the Cranial Nerves of the Posterior Fossa
Edited by Daniel L. Barrow, MD

Degenerative Disease of the Cervical Spine
Edited by Paul R. Cooper, MD

Neurosurgery for the Third Millennium
Edited by Michael L.J. Apuzzo, MD

Cerebrovascular Occlusive Disease and Brain Ischemia
Edited by Issam A. Awad, MD

Practical Approaches to Peripheral Nerve Surgery
Edited by Edward C. Benzel, MD

Complications and Sequelae of Head Injury
Edited by Daniel L. Barrow, MD

Neurosurgical Aspects of Epilepsy
Edited by Michael L.J. Apuzzo, MD

Complications of Spinal Surgery
Edited by Edward C. Tarlov, MD

Neurosurgical Treatment of Disorders of the Thoracic Spine
Edited by Edward C. Tarlov, MD

Intracranial Vascular Malformations
Edited by Daniel L. Barrow, MD

Malignant Cerebral Glioma
Edited by Michael L.J. Apuzzo, MD

Management of Posttraumatic Spinal Instability
Edited by Paul R. Cooper, MD

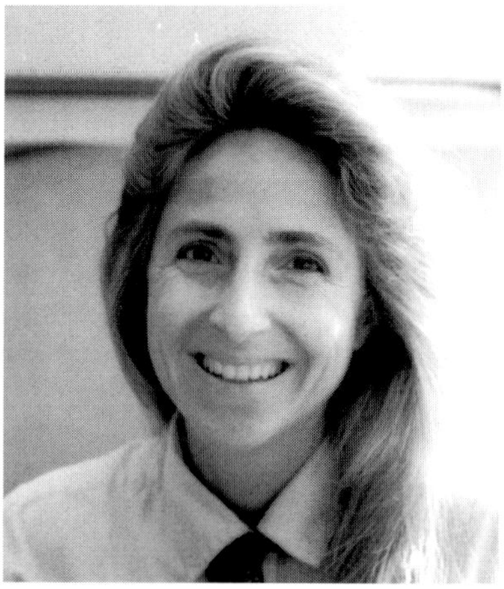

Isabelle M. Germano, MD, is Associate Professor of Neurosurgery and Neurology at the Mount Sinai School of Medicine in New York. Her clinical interest is dedicated to stereotaxy and computer-guided neurosurgery for surgical treatment of movement disorders, brain tumors, and epilepsy. Her laboratory research is focused on molecular mechanisms at the basis of epilepsy and brain tumors. She is the Director of Stereotaxy and Functional Neurosurgery at the Mount Sinai Medical Center.

Neurosurgical Treatment of Movement Disorders is Dr. Germano's first contribution to the Neurosurgical Topics series.

AANS Publications Office
Lebanon, New Hampshire

Editors
Joanne B. Needham
Gay Palazzo

Administrative Assistant
Deirdre Barry

Compositor
Barbara Homeyer

Indexer
Nancy Fontaine

Reference Editor
Kim DeVillers